# Textbook of Histology

# Textbook of Histology

**Upendra Kumar Gupta** MBBS, MS (Anatomy)
Professor and Head
Department of Anatomy
National Institute of Medical Sciences and Research
Jaipur, Rajasthan

**Rashee Mittal** MSc (Medical Anatomy)
Assistant Professor
Department of Anatomy
National Institute of Medical Sciences and Research
Jaipur, Rajasthan

**CBS Publishers & Distributors** Pvt Ltd

New Delhi • Bengaluru • Chennai • Kochi • Kolkata • Mumbai
Hyderabad • Jharkhand • Nagpur • Patna • Pune • Uttarakhand

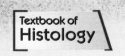

**ISBN:** 978-93-86478-29-0

Copyright © Authors and Publisher

**First Edition: 2017**

Published by Satish Kumar Jain and produced by Varun Jain for

**CBS Publishers & Distributors** Pvt Ltd

4819/XI Prahlad Street, 24 Ansari Road, Daryaganj, New Delhi 110 002, India.
Ph: 23289259, 23266861, 23266867   Website: www.cbspd.com
Fax: 011-23243014                   e-mail: delhi@cbspd.com; cbspubs@airtelmail.in.
*Corporate Office:* 204 FIE, Industrial Area, Patparganj, Delhi 110 092

Ph: 4934 4934          Fax: 4934 4935      e-mail: publishing@cbspd.com; publicity@cbspd.com

*Branches*

- **Bengaluru:** Seema House 2975, 17th Cross, K.R. Road, Banasankari 2nd Stage, Bengaluru 560 070, Karnataka
  Ph: +91-80-26771678/79          Fax: +91-80-26771680          e-mail: bangalore@cbspd.com
- **Chennai:** 7, Subbaraya Street, Shenoy Nagar, Chennai 600 030, Tamil Nadu
  Ph: +91-44-26680620, 26681266          Fax: +91-44-42032115          e-mail: chennai@cbspd.com
- **Kochi:** Ashana House, No. 39/1904, AM Thomas Road, Valanjambalam, Ernakulam 682 016, Kochi, Kerala
  Ph: +91-484-4059061-65          Fax: +91-484-4059065          e-mail: kochi@cbspd.com
- **Kolkata:** 6/B, Ground Floor, Rameswar Shaw Road, Kolkata-700 014, West Bengal
  Ph: +91-33-22891126, 22891127, 22891128          e-mail: kolkata@cbspd.com
- **Mumbai:** 83-C, Dr E Moses Road, Worli, Mumbai-400018, Maharashtra
  Ph: +91-22-24902340/41          Fax: +91-22-24902342          e-mail: mumbai@cbspd.com

*Representatives*

- **Hyderabad**  0-9885175004
- **Jharkhand**  0-9811541605
- **Nagpur**  0-9021734563
- **Patna**  0-9334159340
- **Pune**  0-9623451994
- **Uttarakhand**  0-9716462459

*Printed at* Shree Maitrey Printech Pvt. Ltd., Noida, U.P., India

# Foreword

**Prof (Dr.) Balvir S. Tomar**
M.B.B.S., M.D., M.C.H. (USA), M.I.A.P., M.A.H.T. (England),
F.I.A.P. (USA), F.A.A.P. (USA), F.I.C.A. (USA), F.A.C.U. (London)
Pediatric-Gastroenterology: Kings College Hospital School of Medicine,
University of London, London (England)
Pediatric Nutrition: Harvard University (USA),
W.H.O. Fellow in Child Health in USA,
Commonwealth Medical Fellow in London (England)
**President** - Society of Pediatric Gastroenterology, Hepatology, Transplant & Nutrition
**Director** - Institute of Pediatric Gastroenterology and Hepatology
**Chancellor** - Nims University, Jaipur

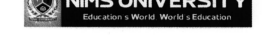

Knowledge and competencies in preclinical, clinical and paraclinical subjects are critical in medical education. Anatomy continues to be one of the fundamental subjects in undergraduate medical education and enables students to excel during postgraduate level and beyond during their professional careers. Being an essential tool of biology and medicine, the origin of histology is traced back to early 17th century. As a science of studying microscopic anatomy of cells and tissues, histology was acknowledged as an academic discipline since 19th century. Credit goes to histologists, Camillo Golgi and Satigo Ramon Y Cajal, who were awarded with Nobel Prize in Physiology or Medicine in 1906.

*Textbook of Histology* in your hands is a matter of pride for academia of the NIMS University. The book is the outcome of devotion and commendable efforts made by Prof (Dr) UK Gupta and Mrs Rashee Mittal. Micrographs with similar looking H&E pencil sketches are the hallmark of the present book. The book embodies comparison tables, quick reviews, and clinical correlates that demonstrate knowledge, authority and wisdom of both the authors.

I am sure that the present book will occupy its unique presence in libraries of medical colleges/universities and will provide sustained support to students across the years. The present effort is just a beginning and I firmly believe that both the authors will come up with more innovative ideas in the future. I congratulate both the authors and wish them to be widely referred and acknowledged in the galaxy of intellectuals.

**Prof (Dr) Balvir S Tomar**

# Preface

"Rare things in medicine are not rare, only observers are rare."
— Prof HR CLOUSTON

Histology is a very vast field of medical science which involves the study of microscopic structures of the human body. This book is an outcome of long-term feedback received from the students as they found difficulty in recognition of slides and drawing diagrams according to what they see in the microscope. We hope that this book will cater to the needs of students perfectly.

World class labeled color micrographs with clarity and the best pencil sketches drawn with H&E pencils looking similar to micrographs for easy identification and reproduction in the manuals are provided in this book. Micrographs of special staining are even provided at suitable places. An old Chinese saying "A good picture is better than a thousand words" is fitting very well for this book.

All important details have been covered sufficiently with labeled micrographs and sketches. The text is provided in an interesting and easy to follow language. The highest number of comparison tables has been provided at the end of the book in Appendix I. For last-minute revision and spotting, three points on every slide as 'quick review' have been provided in Appendix II. Clinical correlates of normal histology are provided separately in colored boxes to exploit the importance of histology in pathology.

For self-assessment and preparation for postgraduate entrance examinations, MCQs are provided at the end of every chapter.

**Upendra Kumar Gupta**
**Rashee Mittal**

# Acknowledgements

The authors, Dr Upendra Kumar Gupta and Mrs Rashee Mittal, wish to acknowledge Prof (Dr) Balvir S Tomar, Chancellor, NIMS University, for providing an appropriate academic atmosphere in the University; and Dr Neelam Bapna, Dr SK Agrawal and other faculty members of Department of Anatomy, NIMS University, for their generous help.

Mrs Rashee Mittal wishes to acknowledge Dr DS Chowdhary for his unconditional guidance and support like a father to her. She also wishes to acknowledge Dr Sushma Kataria, Professor and Head, Department of Anatomy, Dr SN Medical College, Jodhpur, for creating interest in histology. She wishes to acknowledge all her colleagues and friends, Dr Ritu Agrawal, Dr Himanshi Chowdhary, Dr Usha, Dr Pradeep Bokariya, Dr Vijaylaxmi Sharma, Dr Savita Chowdhary, Dr Lovesh Shukla, Dr UL Gajbe, Dr VK Chimurkar, Dr Anjali Wanjari, Dr Prafful Nikam, Dr Harsha Bobade, Dr Lalit Waghmare, Dr Amardeep Bissa, Dr Rekha Parashar, Dr Suresh Sharma and Dr Kamlesh Rundla, for their time to time support. She is indebted to her husband for always being there during the preparation of this book. She thanks her twins, Nitya and Naman, for giving so much love and for their understanding not to disturb her in studies at an age of three and a half years. She also thanks her parents and family for their love.

Last but not the least, the authors wish to acknowledge Mr YN Arjuna (Senior Vice President Publishing, Editorial and Publicity) and his entire team comprising Ms Ritu Chawla (AGM Production), Mr Sanjay Chauhan (graphic artist), Mr Dinesh Chandra Arya (DTP operator) and Mr Prasenjit Paul (copyeditor) for their continuous help in publication of this book.

**Upendra Kumar Gupta**
**Rashee Mittal**

# Contents

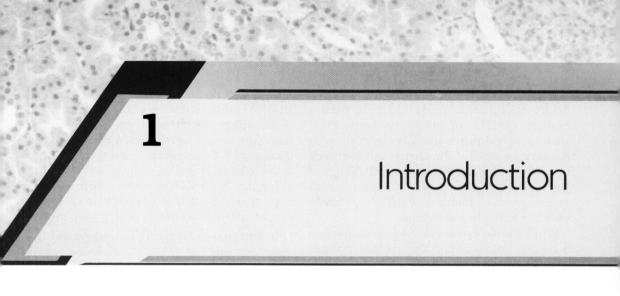

# 1

# Introduction

The name "Histology" is derived from the Greek words *histos* (web or tissue) and *logos* (the study of), which means that histology is the study of structure, composition, and functions of the tissues in organisms. Tissue is a group of similar cells working together to perform a similar function.

**Marie Francois Xavier Bichat is considered as the "father of modern histology and pathology".** He was a French anatomist and physiologist born at Thoirette on November 14, 1771. He was the first person to look beyond the recognizable organ systems and suggest that each part of the body was composed of various kinds of tissues. Using only a hand-lens, he identified 21 different kinds of tissues, such as fibrous, glandular, and mucous tissue in the body.

Tissues maintain body functions through the collaborative efforts of their individual cells. Our body is composed of four basic tissues:

- **Epithelial tissue:** It is derived from all the three germ layers. It covers all the exterior surfaces as well as lines both internal closed cavities and tubes that communicate with the exterior. Epithelial cells rest on a non-cellular basement membrane.
- **Connective tissue:** It is derived from mesoderm and consists of individual cells scattered within an extra cellular matrix. It forms the stroma of the organ, protects against microorganisms, repairs damaged tissues, and also stores fat.

- **Muscular tissue:** It is derived from mesoderm. Each muscle is composed of numerous contractile cells. The cells generate force through contraction to produce movement of the body and in the body.
- **Nervous tissue:** It is derived from ectoderm. It is one of the highly differentiated tissues in the body. It is composed of specialized interconnected cells called neurons. Nervous tissue manifests optimally the two properties of protoplasm—irritability, and conductivity.

The basic tissues of our body can also be classified as:

- **Morphological tissue:** Epithelial and connective tissue
- **Functional tissue:** Muscular and nervous tissue
- **Mixed tissue:** Myoepithelial tissue (functionally muscular, but morphologically epithelial)

Cell is the fundamental, structural and functional unit of the body. Our body contains about $60 \times 10^{12}$ cells of about 200 different types which are having a common structural plan although they vary widely in size and shape. Cells within tissues function in a unified manner and can communicate each other and distinctly placed tissues by receiving signals from signaling molecules involving the intercellular junctions, specific membrane receptors, and neural innervations.

To understand the true histological structure ideally microscopic study of living tissues should be carried out, but study of only a few small living primitive animals can be done in this way as most of the tissues are too thick for study under the microscope. Histological study is mainly done on killed tissues, which are preserved in such a way that they closely resemble to the living tissues.

When tissues are affected by diseases such as cancer, inflammation, etc. certain changes occur in their specific histological structure. The histological study of these changes is known as **histopathology** and to understand it knowledge of normal structure is essential.

Today the concept of histology is not restricted to the study of tissues alone; it also includes understanding of the structure and function of cells, tissues, organs and systems, which can better be described as **"microscopic anatomy"**.

## Section Interpretation

In histology, three-dimensional tissues are viewed in two dimensions; therefore, it is extremely important to interpret the three-dimensional structure from the two-dimensional image. To understand this sections are studied in different planes. Sometimes a single section does not show all the details of the tissue; therefore, serial sectioning is required for accuracy. Serial sectioning is sometime not feasible as in larger specimens so sectioning at regular intervals (e.g. every eighth section) may give a good idea of structure of whole specimen—this is known as step sectioning.

Different planes (Fig. 1.1) to understand the structures are:

a. **Longitudinal plane:** Any plane that is parallel to the longitudinal axis of any part.

b. **Transverse (horizontal or cross) plane:** A plane at right angles to the longitudinal plane or at right angle to the longitudinal axis of any part.

c. **Oblique (tangential) plane:** A plane at any angle between longitudinal and transverse planes results in oblique section.

## Units of Measure

Millimeter (mm) = 1/1000 meter
Micron (μ), micrometer (μm) = 1/1000 mm
Nanometer (nm) = 1/1000 μm
Angstrom (Å) = 1/10 nm

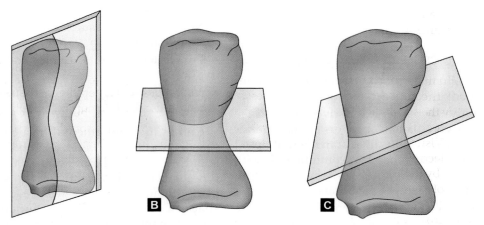

**Fig. 1.1:** Diagram of bone showing different planes. (A) Longitudinal, (B) transverse, and (C) oblique

# 2

# Histological Tools

## MICROSCOPES

The word microscope is derived from the *Greek* words *micros* (small) and *skopeo* (look at), which means by microscope we can look at whole mounts of microorganisms, and structural details of minute objects, which are not visible with naked eyes.

For examination of histological sections, microscope used should complete three tasks:

1. Production of a magnified image of the specimen (magnification),
2. Separation of the details in the image (resolution), and
3. Provide the details to the eye, camera, or other imaging device (contrast).

## LIGHT MICROSCOPE/OPTICAL MICROSCOPE

The light microscope functions on the basis of optical theory of lenses by which it can magnify the image obtained by the movement of an electromagnetic wave through the sample. Visible light occupies a very small part of the electromagnetic spectrum and can be detected by the human eye. The range of wavelengths of visible light is from approximately 400 nm (deep violet) to 800 nm (far red). As light microscope uses visible light as a source of illumination, it is also called bright-field microscope.

Light microscope is a compound microscope, as it has two lens systems: An objective lens and an ocular lens. It is one of the most commonly used microscopes in histology laboratories. Historians credit the **invention of the compound microscope** to the **Dutch spectacle maker, Zacharias Janssen,** around the year 1590.

### Some Common Terms

- **Magnification:** It means enlargement of the image. It is the function of both objective and ocular lenses. The objective lens forms a magnified image of the specimen and the ocular lens again magnifies it to provide details to the eye, camera, or other imaging device. Total magnification is achieved by multiplying the magnifying power of the objective lens and the magnifying power of the ocular lens.

- **Resolution:** It is the ability to see two objects as separate, discrete entities. Two objects can be distinctly seen only if they are far enough apart for light to pass between them. Resolution of human eye is 0.1–0.2 mm and resolution of light microscope is 0.2 µm (a light microscope cannot distinguish between two points closer together than 0.2 µm). For a specific microscope, the actual limit of resolution can be calculated as:

$$D = \frac{\lambda}{NA_{Condenser} + NA_{Objective}}$$

Where D = minimum distance at which two points can be resolved; $\lambda$ = wavelength of light; $NA_{Condenser}$ = numerical aperture of condenser; $NA_{Objective}$ = numerical aperture of objective.

- **Numerical aperture (NA):** It is a measure of ability of lens to "capture" light coming from the specimen and use it to make the image. Use of oil in between the specimen and the objective lens increases numerical aperture and in turn, makes the limit of resolution smaller. Value of NA is engraved on the side of each objective lens and it ranges from 0.5 to 1.4.

- **Refractive index:** It is a measure of the bending or refraction of a beam of light when passing from one medium into another. Refractive index of air is 1 and of oil immersion is 1.51.

## Parts of the Microscope

It can be divided into two groups: Mechanical and Optical.

### A. Mechanical Parts

The mechanical parts in the light microscope are (Fig. 2.1):

a. **Base/foot:** It provides support to the microscope, i.e. the microscope rests on it.

b. **Arm/limb:** It holds the body tube, stage, substage, and mirror or the light source.

c. **Body tube:** Its lower end holds the revolving nose piece. At the upper end body tube contains a sliding draw tube, which carries the eyepiece at its upper end. Generally the body tube length is fixed to 160 mm or 170 mm (only in Leitz). In modern microscopes, these fixed tube lengths have been replaced

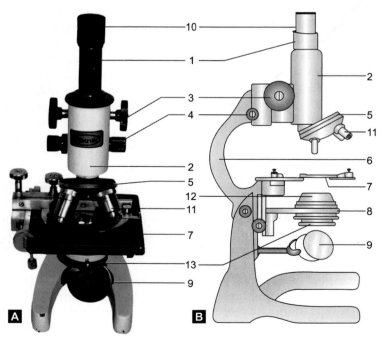

**Fig. 2.1:** Light microscope showing mechanical and optical parts, (A) photograph, (B) schematic diagram. Mechanical parts are: Draw tube (1), body tube (2), coarse focus control knob (3), fine focus control knob (4), revolving nosepiece (5), arm (6), stage (7), substage (8) and mirror (9). Optical parts are: Eyepiece (10), objective lens (11), condenser (12) and iris diaphragm (13)

by infinity corrected objectives which can extend the tube length and even permit the addition of other devices in the light path. Infinity corrected objectives come in a wide range of magnification from 1.5X to 200X.

d. **Revolving nosepiece/turret:** It is 12 mm to 18 mm thick circular plate with holes for the attachment of objective lenses. In modern microscopes, up to six objectives are mounted onto a nosepiece to enable rapid change in magnification from one to another.

e. **Stage:** It is the flat platform where slides are placed and has an opening for passing the light. Stage clips hold the slides in place. Concentric X–Y control knobs are attached to the stage, which move the slides forward/back or left/right. The slide can be placed in any given position by means of Vernier scale attached to the stage.

f. **Substage:** It is placed below the stage and carries the condenser.

g. **Focus controls:** They are located on the lateral side and consist of two knobs. The larger of the two knobs is the coarse focus control (used to locate the specimen at 4X and 10X) and the smaller knob is the fine focus control (used to bring specimen into sharp focus at 40X and 100X, but only after initial focusing at lower magnification).

h. **Light source/mirror:** Some microscope has low-voltage electric lamp and other has mirrors for illumination. The electric lamp work through a transformer and requirements of intensity can be adjusted in them. The mirror possesses two surfaces: A concave and a plane. If low power objective is used or when there is no condenser in the microscope, concave side of the mirror is used to direct the light to the slide. When high-power objectives are used, it is necessary to use the condenser and in this condition, only the plane surface of the mirror is used to direct the light. The larger instruments have their light sources for illumination (in-built light source).

## B. Optical Parts

The optical parts in the light microscope are:

a. **Condenser:** It is made up of a system of convex lenses that gather the light coming from the source and concentrate that light in parallel beams onto the tissue section. In this way, it controls the quality of the image which will be formed by the objective lens. It can be focused up and down with the control located below the stage on the left side of the microscope.

b. **Field (Iris) diaphragm:** It is situated below the condenser and opening and closing of it controls the amount of light reaching the objective lens. It is adjusted with the lever protruding from the front of the condenser. If the field diaphragm is closed too much, the contrast of image will be very high, whereas if the field diaphragm is left wide open, then the image will be brighter and contrast will be less. In both cases the resolution of the image is poor. For the correct setting of the field diaphragm the numerical aperture of the condenser should be matched to the numerical aperture of the objective lens.

c. **Objective lenses:** They gather the light passing through the tissue section and then project an accurate and magnified image of the specimen up into the body of the microscope. A revolving nosepiece holds the objective lenses. The lenses are of 4X, 10X, 40X, and 100X power. The high power objective lenses are retractable. This means that if they hit a slide, the end of the lens will push in (spring loaded), thereby protecting the lens and the slide. The objective lenses can also be coded with colored rings.

　i. *4X Lens:* It is used to get an overview of the structures present in a section and to find areas for more detailed observation. It is denoted by a red ring.

　ii. *10X Lens:* It is the most useful objective lens to identify tissues and it is denoted by a yellow ring.

iii. **40X Lens**: It is used to see the details of cell and tissue organization. It is denoted by a blue ring.

iv. **100X Lens**: It is used primarily to see subcellular details and requires the use of immersion oil. It is denoted by a white ring.

d. **Eyepiece/ocular lens:** It again magnifies the image projected by the objective lens and presents the eye with a virtual image. A microscope with one ocular lens (eyepiece) is monocular microscope and with two ocular lenses is binocular microscope. Its magnification is imprinted on its upper metallic rim (normally 10X).

## Image Formation by Light Microscope

Image formation begins with light coming from an external or internal light source. It passes through the condenser lens which concentrates the light and illuminates the specimen. Light passing through the specimen enters one of the objective lenses, which produce a magnified real image. This image is again magnified by the ocular lens of the eyepiece and this resulting magnified virtual image is then focused on the retina of the eye.

## Setting up the Microscope

a. Adjustment of light is done by using artificial or natural light. Light intensity can be increased by bringing the light source nearer to the mirror, if the light source is not in-built.

b. If the condenser is in use, the plane side (if condenser is not in use, then concave side) of the mirror is used to reflect the light accurately up in the optical axis of the microscope. Raise the condenser to bring near the underside of the stage and open the iris diaphragm.

c. Place a clean, stained slide on the stage and use the concentric X–Y knobs to position the slide over the hole in the stage.

d. Always start with the lowest power objective lens first. Once the image is sharp with the lowest power lens, then you can simply click in the next high power lens and do minor adjustments with the focus control knobs. As the microscopes are par focal, so once they are in focus with one objective lens, they are in focus for all objective lenses. High power objective lenses require more light, thus the iris diaphragm will need to be opened.

e. Use the coarse and fine focus control knob to bring it into focus. Use coarse focus control knob to get minimum working distance. Use only the fine focus control knob to sharpen the focus.

f. The iris diaphragm should now be closed just to the point where glare is eliminated and the microscope is now set up for use.

## SPECIAL TYPES OF MICROSCOPE

### A. Dark-field Microscope

**This microscope is used for demonstration of specific bacteria such as spirochetes, and trypanosomes and to study the large transparent objects (e.g. living protozoa, crystals, and spicules, etc.), which are otherwise invisible with a light microscope.**

Dark-field microscope requires blocking out of the central light rays that normally pass through or around the specimen and allowing only oblique rays to illuminate the specimen. These oblique rays are created by using a modified or special condenser, which is a single lens with plane upper and lower surface and sides are slightly convex. Center of the lower surface is masked by a black disc and a ring of light can enter around the edge. The numerical aperture of the objective lens must be lower than the numerical aperture of the condenser lens (in light microscope the numerical aperture of both is matched). Everything is visible regardless of color, usually bright white against a dark background. The main limitation of this microscope is that only a small portion of light can enter the objective lens. Therefore, specimen must be strongly illuminated to produce a clear final image.

## B. Phase Contrast Microscope

**This microscope is used to view living cells in their natural state (as in tissue culture), and also for quick examination of unstained paraffin-embedded sections and for frozen sections.**

The human eye is only sensitive to the differences in amplitude (brightness) and wavelength (color), but not to the phase change. But for most biological samples light only induces phase change and a small amount of change in amplitude and wavelength. The phase contrast microscope consists of a circular annulus in the condenser which produces a cone of light. This cone is super-imposed on a similar sized ring within the phase-objective lens. Every objective lens has a different size ring, so for every objective lens another condenser setting has to be chosen. The ring in the objective lens reduces the intensity of direct light, but more importantly, it creates an artificial phase difference of about a quarter wavelength. This microscope translates the minute variations in phase into corresponding changes in amplitude, thus resulting in a difference in brightness and making the transparent object shine out in contrast to its surroundings.

Two modifications of the phase contrast microscope are **interference microscope,** which is used for the examination of parts of living cells and the **differential interference microscope** (using Nomarski discs), which is useful for enhanced visualization of immuno-histochemical preparations.

## C. Polarizing Microscope

**This microscope is used especially for samples which show birefringence such as numerous crystals, pigments, proteins, lipids, fibrous structures, and amyloid deposits.**

This microscope uses polarized light (waves of light beam that lack symmetry) to analyze structures that are birefringence (which splits single light ray with different propagation speeds due to the different refractive indices of the substance). A typical polarized light microscope has two polarizing filters that are conventionally called polarizer and the analyzer. Polarizer is placed below the condenser under the stage and an analyzer is placed in the light pathway between the objective lens and the eyepiece. Light first passes through the polarizer, which eliminates all wave of light except those in a single plane. The analyzer then eliminates all waves of light except those in a specific plane of polarization. Thus, these two polarizing filters allow user to define the plane of polarization of light reaching the eyepiece. Because the sample is birefringence, so appears bright against dark background.

## D. Fluorescent Microscope

**This microscope is used to visualize specimens that fluoresce, i.e. emit light of a different color (always higher wavelength) than the light absorbed by the specimen.**

This microscope uses ultraviolet (UV) light generated by a high pressure mercury lamp to excite fluorescence of the specimen. Two filters are required for fluorescent microscope. The first one is an exciter filter, which is placed between the light source and the specimen. This filter cuts out visible light but transmits UV light. The specimen is now illuminated with this UV light and will fluoresce and gives off some visible light. Second filter, barrier or suppression filter, is placed before the eyepiece. It only allows visible light rays to pass through the eyepiece and absorbs UV light to prevent the damage of the retina of the eye. Fluorescence occurs after light is absorbed either because of naturally occurring fluorescent materials (autofluorescence or primary fluorescence) in the cells such as vitamin A, porphyrins, and some neurotransmitters or fluorochromes have been used to stain the cells (secondary or induced fluorescence). Fluorochromes are fluorescent dyes or chemicals that are used to label biological material. The resolution of fluorescent microscope is about 100 nm.

## E. Confocal Microscope

**This microscope is used for production of high resolution 3D images of subsurfaces in specimens such as microbes.**

The light from a laser source travels to the specimen through a beam splitter and then through two movable scanning mirrors (scan in both X- and Y- directions. Finally, the laser beam enters in the fluorescent microscope and illuminates the specimen. The emitted light from the specimen travels back through the fluorescent microscope, mirrors, beam splitter and finally focused onto the detector's pinpoint aperture. Light received by pinpoint aperture is registered by the detector attached to a computer that builds the digital image. Digital images captured at many individual spots allow digital reconstruction of a 3D image. The point light source, the focal point of the lens, and the detector's pinpoint aperture are all optically conjugated or aligned to each other in the focal plane (confocal).

## F. Electron Microscope

This microscope uses a beam of electrons, instead of photons (light) to "illuminate" the specimen. This allows a dramatic increase in magnification and resolution (up to 0.2 nm). However, electrons possess a very poor penetrating power, so very thin sections are required. Electron microscope uses electromagnets rather than the glass lenses used in light microscopy.

There are two kinds of electron microscope: Transmission electron microscope (TEM) and Scanning electron microscope (SEM).

a. **Transmission electron microscope (TEM): This microscope is used to reveal the substructure or ultrastructure of cells and tissues.**
This microscope works much like a light microscope, transmitting a beam of electrons through a thin specimen and then focusing the electrons to form a two-dimensional image on a screen or on film. The source of the electrons is a heated tungsten filament. The electron beam is accelerated down in a vertical column located under vacuum by high voltage (40 to 100 kV) and focused by electromagnets. Electrons cannot be focused by glass lenses. In fact, even very thin glass can stop an electron beam. Electromagnetic condenser lens changes the diameter of the electron beam. After passing through the specimen the beam is then focused and magnified by the electromagnetic diffraction and intermediate lenses. An image of the specimen is viewed on a phosphor-coated fluorescent screen and the final pictures, called electron micrographs, are made on photographic plates or film. The resolution of a modern TEM is about 0.2 nm.

b. **Scanning electron microscope (SEM): This microscope is used to produce the 3D image of external and internal surface of cells.**
This microscope is quite different from a TEM because electrons are not used to directly produce the image of the specimen, instead they are used to excite the specimen in such a way that it gives out secondary electrons. These secondary electrons are collected by detectors and used to form the image. However, the beam not only causes the generation of secondary electrons, but scatters them as well. These backscattered electrons can also be used to form an image. Electrons collected by detectors passed through a scanning amplifier and then reach to a cathode ray tube (CRT), which acts like a television screen. In modern SEM instead of cathode ray tube digital images are captured using sensitive detectors and CCD for display on a computer. The surface contours of the specimen are visualized in a 3D image showing remarkable details with great depth of focus. The resolution of SEM is 10 nm.

For comparison between light and electron micro-scopes, *see* Table 1 given in Appendix I.

## TYPES OF HISTOLOGICAL PREPARATIONS

The specimen in histology can be prepared as:

### A. Whole Mount

These are preparations made by placing a whole microorganism or specimen on a slide. These preparations should not be more than 0.2–0.5 mm in thickness.

### B. Sections

To obtain sections tissue processing is done. The tissue sample is cut in about 2–4 mm thick pieces and then it is processed by a microtome. Finally, 4–6 µm thick sections are stained and mounted permanently.

### C. Smears

Smears are made from blood, bone marrow, or any fluid. A drop is placed on one end of a slide and spread with another slide into a uniform monolayer. This slide is then quickly air dried and finally stained to see under the microscope. Smears are also made by crushing soft tissue between two slides or by pressing a slide against the moist surface of a tissue (impression smears).

## TISSUE PROCESSING

To examine the tissue components under a light microscope, it is necessary to process the tissue. The steps of tissue processing are:

### A. Fixation

It is the process of preservation of tissue samples to prevent autolysis (decomposition of tissue by own enzymes) and putrefaction (decomposition by bacterial enzymes). The substances used for fixation are known as fixatives. The tissue specimen is first cut into small pieces (approximately 2–4 mm thick) and then kept overnight (usually) into the fixative for the purpose of fixation. Roles of fixatives are:

a. Preservation of the tissues in its most natural state.

b. Quick penetration in the tissue, so that it stabilizes sufficiently for subsequent histological procedures.

c. Hardening of all the constituents of the cells for easy manipulation as a result of either cross-linking or denaturing protein molecules.

d. No swelling and shrinking of components of tissues.

e. Allows the use of all kinds of stains.

f. Cheap, non-toxic, and non-irritant.

But there is no ideal fixative. Generally, a mixture of two or more fixative is used, so that deficiencies of one fixative can be compensated by the other. Formaldehyde is a gas but is soluble in water to the extent of 37–40% w/v. This solution of formaldehyde in water is called formalin. Pure formalin is not a suitable fixative as it over hardens the tissue. A 10% dilution in water is normally used as a fixative. It penetrates rapidly, causes a little distortion, does not destroy any of the cellular consti-tuents and can be followed by almost all staining methods.

The major problem with formalin-fixed, paraffin embedded tissue has been the loss of antigen immunorecognition and problems in analysis of mRNA and DNA. It does not protect the tissues from the shrinking agents employed in embedding and sectioning, so it is often used in combination with other fixatives. Other commonly used fixatives are: Alcohol, glutaraldehyde (in electron micro-scopy), picric acid, mercuric chloride, and acetic acid.

**Decalcification** Some tissue components, such as teeth and bones, are extremely firm due to high calcium deposits. Decalcification is done to assure that the specimen is soft enough to allow cutting with the microtome. If the tissue is not completely decalcified, the sections will be torn and ragged, and may damage the cutting edge of microtome knife. The criteria for suitable decalcifying agents are:

a. Complete removal of calcium.

b. Absence of damage to tissue cells or fibers.

c. Subsequent staining not altered.

d. Little time required for decalcification.

Decalcifying agents are nitric acid, hydrochloric acid, formic acid, picric acid, and EDTA (ethylene-diaminetetraacetic acid).

## B. Embedding

The purpose of embedding is to process the tissue into a form in which it can be cut into thin microscopic sections; usually this is done with the paraffin embedding.

Following are the steps in paraffin embedding:

a. **Dehydration:** It means removal of water. Since water and paraffin do not mix, the first step in embedding with paraffin is to replace the water in the tissues with a solvent (dehydrant) that is miscible with paraffin. This is usually done with a series of alcohols: 30%, 50%, 70% and 90%. Time required for dehydration depends upon the thickness of the tissue sample. At the end of this procedure, water will be completely replaced by alcohol.

Dehydration should be accomplished slowly. Excessive dehydration will make the tissue hard, brittle, and shrunken; while incomplete dehydration will impair the penetration of clearing reagents.

b. **Clearing:** The purpose of this procedure is to remove the dehydrant (alcohol) with a substance, which is miscible with the embedding medium (paraffin). The tissue is immersed in the clearing agent until it becomes translucent. Prolonged exposure to most clearing agents causes the tissue to become brittle and therefore, more difficult to section. The commonest clearing agent is xylene (prolonged use over hardens the tissue). Others are dioxan (extremely toxic to nasal mucosa and conjunctiva), chloroform (slow penetration and not gives adequate transparency) and cedar wood oil (traces remains in the tissue).

c. **Infiltration and embedding:** Paraffin wax is the most popular infiltration and embedding medium as it is compatible with most routine and special stains. For complete impregnation with wax, it is necessary to form a solid block containing the tissue. This is done by filling a mold with molten paraffin wax, which is heated at a temperature 2–3°C above the melting point. The amount of wax should be 25–50 times the volume of tissue. The tissue is transferred from clearing agent to molten wax. The most commonly used mold is Leuckhart's L pieces (two L of metal resting on a metal or glass plate). Molds are lightly smeared with glycerin to prevent the wax sticking. As soon as a film of solid wax is formed on the surface, the whole block with mold are submerged in cold water. When blocks are set hard, they are removed from the mold.

Other embedding medium are: Synthetic resin (used in electron microscopy and also for calcified bone), gelatin (used in frozen sections), celloidin (used especially in the examination of eye and brain), and ester wax (used for cutting thin sections).

## C. Sectioning

To cut the specimen into sections; block is then mounted on an instrument called microtome (Fig. 2.2). Microtome is a slicing machine, which serves for cutting uniform sections of appropriate thickness with the help of steel or razor blade knife. Mostly, the rotary microtome is used for paraffin wax-embedded tissues. When we move the block forward it, almost touches the knife. The section thickness is set between 10 and 30 μ to trim away any surplus wax. On exposing a suitable area of tissue the section thickness is set at 4–6 μ. The microtome is now moved in an easy rhythm with right hand operating the microtome and

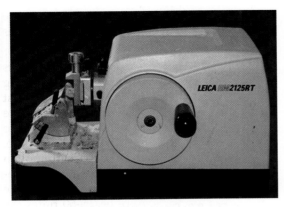

**Fig. 2.2:** Photograph of rotary microtome

left hand holding the sections away from the knife. The ribbon is formed due to the slight heat generated during cutting, which causes the edges of the sections to adhere.

Once sections are cut, they are floated on a warm water bath that helps in removing wrinkles. Then they are picked up on a glass slide. The glass slides are then placed in a warm oven for about 15 minutes to help the section adhere to the slide. Even Meyer's egg albumin is used as an adhesive in some laboratories.

### D. Staining

It is an auxiliary technique used to enhance contrast in microscopic image. Staining procedure consists of three steps:

a. **Deparaffinization:** Paraffin sections mounted on glass slides require the removal of paraffin wax before staining. Two changes (baths) of xylene are used for deparaffinization.

b. **Hydration:** Xylene is not miscible with water and the most dye solutions are aqueous based, so xylene must be replaced. This is usually done with a series of alcohols: Absolute, 90%, 70%, 50% and 30%. After that washing for 5 min in running tap water is done.

c. **Staining:** Regression method is used for staining. In this method, tissue is firstly overstained with hematoxylin and then washed in running tap water. The differentiation of cells is checked under low power of the microscope. If overstained, then the slide is dipped in 1% acid alcohol and then again it is washed in running tap water. After this it is stained with 1% eosin. If the tissue gets overstained with eosin, the slide should be washed with running water to remove the excess stain.

In routine histology, the combination of hematoxylin and eosin stain is used which is commonly referred to as H and E stain. Hematoxylin is extracted from the *Hematoxylin campechianum* tree. Hematein, the oxidation product of hematoxylin, is used as a stain. Hematoxylin is a basic stain with deep purple or blue color. Structures (ribosomes and chromatin) that are stained by basic stains are described as basophilic ("base-loving"). Cell nuclei look purple because of presence of chromatin. Hematoxylin may be used after almost any fixative and it is a permanent stain.

Eosin being an acid aniline dye binds to and stains acidophilic or oxyphilic or eosinophilic ("acid-loving") structures pink. Most of the cytoplasm of cells is stained by eosin. Bone matrix is also stained by eosin. Eosin combines with hemoglobin to give an orange color. It may be used after any fixative and is used as a counter-stain in many combinations in addition to hematoxylin.

### E. Mounting

Once any staining technique has been completed; the cover slip must be mounted on the section to protect the tissue from being scratched, to provide better optical quality and to preserve the tissue section for years to come. Mounting media, which are non-miscible with water, are mostly used. Sections are firstly processed through alcohol series: Absolute, 90%, 70%, 50% and 30%. Then two baths of xylene are done and finally mounting is done with Canada balsam or Dpx or synthetic resin.

**Frozen sections:** When rapid production of sections for urgent intra-operative diagnosis is required, tissue is frozen. Freezing can be done by using liquefied nitrogen, carbon dioxide gas, dry ice, aerosol sprays, and isopentane cooled by liquid nitrogen. After freezing the tissue becomes firm, as ice works as an embedding medium. The consistency of frozen block can be altered by variations in temperature. If the temperature is less, then the block will be hard and if the temperature is more, then the block will be soft. For the good quality of frozen sections the tissue should be fresh and should be frozen as rapidly as possible. Cryostat (Fig. 2.3) is a refrigerated cabinet in which a special microtome is housed to section the frozen tissue block. The frozen sections are then placed on slides for rapid staining and microscopic examination. Freezing is also effective in histochemical study of enzymes and small molecules.

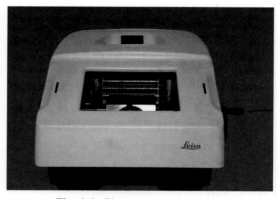

**Fig. 2.3:** Photograph of cryostat

### F. Examination

The slides thus prepared can be examined under the light microscope by the proper adjustment of light path.

### SPECIAL STAIN

In histology, the term "routine staining" refers to the H and E stain as they are used "routinely" with all tissue specimens to reveal the underlying tissue structures. The term "special stains" refer to a large number of alternative staining techniques that are used when the H and E does not provide all the information. It covers a wide variety of methods that may be used to visualize particular tissue structures, elements, or even microorganisms not identified by H and E staining. The images below will illustrate some of the special stains and the appearance of stained structures.

### A. Giemsa Stain (Fig. 2.4)

It is a classic blood film stain for blood smears and bone marrow specimens. It is

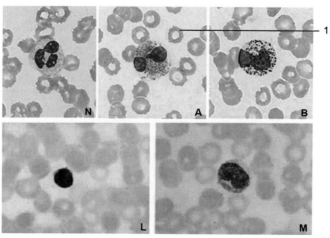

**Fig. 2.4:** Peripheral blood smear preparation stained by Giemsa [RBC (1)]

also used to display transverse bands in mitotic (metaphase) chromosomes and to identify protozoan parasites.

**RBCs:** Pinkish grey

**Leukocytes:**

Neutrophils (upper row left)

- *Nucleus:* Deep blue to violet
- *Cytoplasm:* Pale pink
- *Granules:* Purple to liliac

Eosinophils (upper row center)

- *Nucleus:* Deep blue to violet
- *Granules:* Orange to pink

Basophils (upper row right)

- *Nucleus:* Deep blue to violet
- *Granules:* Deep blue to violet

Lymphocytes (lower row left)

- *Nucleus:* Deep blue to violet
- *Cytoplasm:* Light blue

Monocytes (lower row right)

- *Nucleus:* Deep blue to violet
- *Cytoplasm:* Light blue

**Platelets:** Red purple granules in the center.

**B. Acid Phosphatase Stain** (Fig. 2.5)

It is used in histochemical techniques to recognize lysosomes due to their acid phosphatase content. Sites of acid phosphatase activity will stain dark brown to black.

**C. Thionin Stain** (Fig. 2.6)

It is specific for DNA and Nissl substance, which is primarily ribosomal RNA. It imparts a deep blue color to Nissl substance of neurons and a pale blue color to the nuclear chromatin of both neuronal and non-neuronal cells.

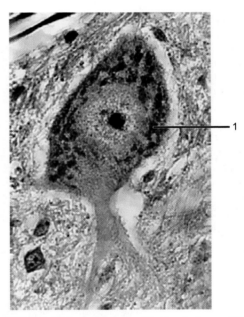

**Fig. 2.6:** Thionin stain for Nissl substance (1)

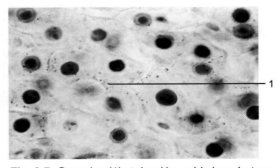

**Fig. 2.5:** Granules (1) stained by acid phosphatase

## D. Luxol Fast Blue Stain (Fig. 2.7A, B)

It has affinity for phospholipid of myelin. Under the stain, myelin fibers appear blue, neuropil appears pink, and nerve cells appear purple.

## E. Osmium Stain (Fig. 2.8)

It has an affinity to combine lipids in membranes. Lipid droplets will appear black. Myelin sheaths of nerves will appear as black annular structures because of the presence of lipids.

## F. PAS (Periodic Acid Schiff) + Hematoxylin Stain (Fig. 2.9A, B and C)

This is used for detection of glycogen in tissues such as liver, cardiac and skeletal muscle on formalin-fixed, paraffin-embedded tissue sections, and may be used for frozen sections as well. The glycogen will be stained deep red or magenta. Goblet cells will be stained magenta. Basement membranes and brush borders will be stained pink.

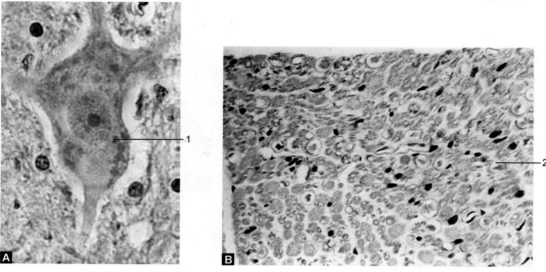

**Fig. 2.7:** Luxol fast blue stain. (A) Nissl substance (1), (B) myelin sheath (2)

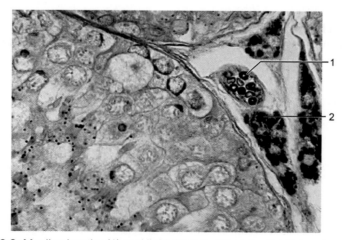

**Fig. 2.8:** Myelin sheaths (1) and lipid droplets (2) stained with osmium stain

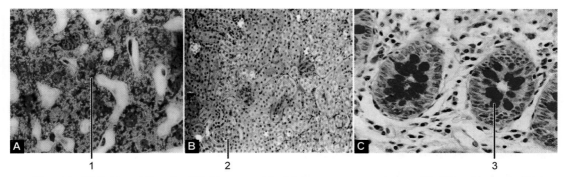

**Fig. 2.9:** PAS+H and E stain. (A) Glycogen (1), (B) basement membrane (2), (C) goblet cells (3)

### G. Silver Stain (Fig. 2.10)

This is an impregnation method. The fresh tissue is treated with silver nitrate and exposed to strong light, which reduces the silver. The intercellular borders of epithelium will appear black.

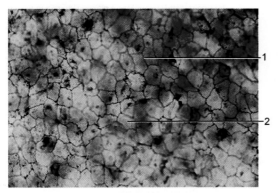

**Fig. 2.10:** Simple squamous epithelium stained by silver stain. Intercellular borders (1), epithelial cell (2)

### H. PAM + H and E Stain (Fig. 2.11)

PAM (periodic acid methenamine silver) mainly stains polysaccharides. By this method the basement membranes will appear black as they are impregnated with methenamine silver.

### I. Toluidine Blue Stain (Fig. 2.12)

The property of this stain is metachromasia. This means that tissue component stains a

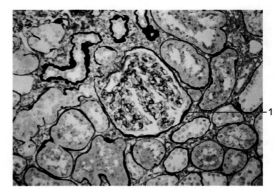

**Fig. 2.11:** Basement membrane (1) stained by PAM+H and E stain

different color than the dye itself. Mast cell granules and polysaccharides will appear purple instead of blue color.

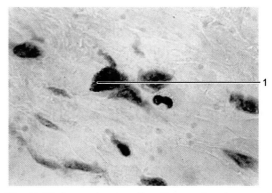

**Fig. 2.12:** Loose connective tissue showing mast cell granules (1) by toluidine blue stain

### J. Grimelius Silver Stain (Fig. 2.13)

It is used for demonstration of granules containing cells such as enteroendocrine cells. The cell granules will appear black by this method.

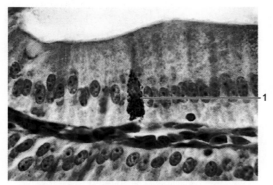

**Fig. 2.13:** Enteroendocrine cells stained by Grimelius silver stain. Granules within the enteroendocrine cell (1)

## Summary

1. A microscope is used to see structures which are not visible with naked eyes.

2. Magnification of compound light microscope = magnification of objective lens × magnification of ocular lens.

3. Condenser gathers the light coming from the light source and concentrates that light in parallel beams onto the specimen.

4. 10X is a most useful objective lens to identify tissues.

5. Dark field microscopes are used for demonstration of specific structures, as it required strongly illuminated specimen.

6. Phase contrast microscope is used to view living structures in their natural state.

7. Electron microscope is of 2 types: TEM and SEM.

8. Steps of tissue preparation: Fixation → dehydration → clearing → infiltration and embedding → sectioning → deparaffinization → hydration → staining → mounting → examination.

9. H and E stain is most commonly used in routine histology.

10. Hematoxylin stains basophilic structures purple, while eosin stains eosinophilic structures pink.

| Self Assessment |
| --- |

1. What is the another name for bright field microscope?
   a. Light microscope
   b. Phase contrast microscope
   c. Polarizing microscope
   d. Transmission electron microscope

2. How the total magnification is achieved with a compound microscope?
   a. By magnification of objective lens
   b. By magnification of ocular lens
   c. By magnification of ocular lens added to the magnification of the objective lens
   d. By multiplying the magnifying power of the objective lens and the magnifying power of the ocular lens

3. Which microscope is used to view living cells in their natural state?
   a. Light microscope
   b. Phase contrast microscope
   c. Transmission electron microscope
   d. Scanning electron microscope

4. Which microscope does not rely on visible light?
   a. Simple microscope
   b. Compound microscope
   c. Phase contrast microscope
   d. Transmission electron microscope

5. Which of the following is an acid dye?
   a. Azure II
   b. Toluidine blue
   c. Methylene blue
   d. Eosin

6. What color does hematoxylin stain structures?
   a. Orange          b. Purple
   c. Pink            d. Red

7. Which of the following stains is used for routine histological examination?
   a. Giemsa stain
   b. Hematoxylin and eosin stain
   c. Luxol fast blue stain
   d. Masson's trichrome stain

8. Which of the following would be best suited to visualize basement membrane?
   a. Wright's stain
   b. Hematoxylin and eosin stain
   c. PAM stain
   d. Silver impregnation

9. What does osmium stain used primarily for?
   a. Blood
   b. Fat
   c. Myelin sheath
   d. Elastic fibers

10. Which of the following stains gives tissue component a different color than the dye itself?
   a. Toluidine blue
   b. Osmium stain
   c. Silver stain
   d. H and E stain

## Answers

1. a,    2. d,    3. b,    4. d,    5. d,    6. b,    7. b,    8. c,    9. c,
10. a

# 3

# The Cell

The cell is the fundamental structural and functional unit of life. Each cell houses the genetic material-genes, in the nucleus. The cell takes nutrients in, converts these nutrients into energy, and carries out specialized functions. The term "cell" is derived from the Latin word *cellule*, which means a small room. It was given by Robert Hooke in 1663 when he found that a cork if seen under a micrographia (designed by him) consists of small compartments.

There are two general categories of cells: **Prokaryote** and **eukaryote**.

Prokaryotic cells are the simplest and the first type of cells to evolve, which lack a nuclear membrane. These cells also lack many organelles, such as mitochondria, chloroplasts and the Golgi apparatus, whose functions are taken over by the prokaryotic plasma membrane.

Eukaryotic cells (Fig. 3.1) are generally larger than the prokaryotic cells. The major

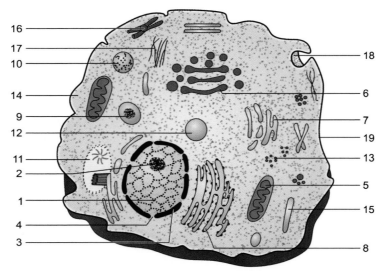

**Fig. 3.1:** Eukaryotic (animal) cell: Schematic diagram showing nucleus (1), nucleolus (2), nuclear envelope (3), nuclear pore (4), mitochondria (5), Golgi apparatus (6), smooth endoplasmic reticulum (7), rough endoplasmic reticulum (8), lysosome (9), peroxisome (10), centrioles (11), vacuole (12), ribosomes (13), cytoplasm (14), microtubules (15), intermediate filaments (16), actin filaments (17), pinocytic vesicle (18) and plasma membrane (19)

and extremely significant difference between prokaryotes and eukaryotes is that eukaryotic cells contain membrane-bound organelles in which specific metabolic activities take place. Most important among these is the presence of a nucleus, which is a double membrane bound organelle that houses the eukaryotic cell's DNA. It is this nucleus, which gives the eukaryotes, its name (in Greek *Eue*, true, + *Karyon*, Nucleus).

The nucleus is lodged in a jelly-like semi-solid substance known as cytoplasm. Cytoplasm is enclosed by a selectively permeable membrane known as plasma membrane.

For comparison between prokaryotic and eukaryotic cells *see* Table 2 given in Appendix I.

## PLASMA MEMBRANE (PLASMALEMMA)

It is about 8–10 nm thick lipid-bilayer membrane, which is visible with transmission electron microscope. It forms a thin boundary of the cytoplasm and is selectively permeable in nature. It consists of a phospholipid bilayer along with cholesterol and associated proteins (Fig. 3.2).

**The plasma membrane and the membrane surrounding the cytoplasmic organelles** differ slightly in their thickness and protein contents, but they all have the same basic trilaminar structure. Because of the universality of this appearance, this trilaminar structure has been designated as unit membrane.

A phospholipid molecule has a polar head, which is attracted to water (hydrophilic) and a non-polar tail end, which repels water (hydrophobic). Heads of lipid molecules face towards outer and inner surface of the membrane, while the tails face towards each other. When the plasma membrane is fixed with osmium tetroxide, osmium binds to the heads and produces two parallel black lines enclosing the light line of osmium-free fatty acid tails. The lipid bilayer provides permeability to the lipid soluble molecules.

**Phospholipids** are of four major types: Sphingomyelin, phosphatidylserine, phosphatidylcholine, and phosphatidylethanolamine. Composition of phospholipids varies in different membranes and even phospholipids present in outer and inner layer are also different. In membranes of RBCs phosphatidylcholine and sphingomyelin are more abundant in the outer layer, whereas phosphatidylserine and phosphatidylethanolamine are more abundant in the inner layer (adjacent to the cytoplasm).

Cholesterol is incorporated within the gaps between phospholipids equally on both sides of the membrane and stabilizes the plasma membrane. In most plasma membranes, protein molecules contain approximately half of the total membrane mass. Proteins either span the entire phospholipid bilayer as integral (trans) membrane proteins or are attached on the external surface as peripheral membrane proteins. Peripheral membrane proteins may also be coated with a polysaccharide material that forms the glycocalyx or cell coat. The cell coat has important roles in the formation of intracellular adhesions, in cell recognition, and in the adsorption of the molecules to the cell surface. The cell coat even

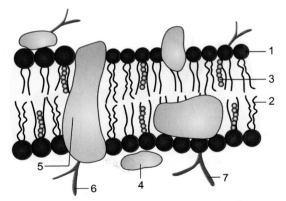

**Fig. 3.2:** Plasma membrane: Schematic diagram showing polar head (1), non-polar tail (2), cholesterol (3), peripheral membrane protein (4), integral membrane protein (5), glycoprotein (6) and glycolipid (7)

provides mechanical and chemical protection to the cell membrane and also serves as receptor sites for some hormones.

In 1972, Singer and Nicolson suggested the "fluid mosaic model" of the plasma membrane. According to them the lipid bilayer is in fluid state within which the globular proteins are embedded or floating at variable depth and even these proteins are free to move laterally unless they are not attached to filaments in the underlying cytoplasm.

For many years the structure of the plasma membrane was explained on the basis of "fluid mosaic model". However, according to recent studies the distribution and movements of proteins within the lipid bilayer is not so random. In the plasma membrane there are localized regions (10–200 nm) containing high concentration of cholesterol and glycosphingolipids. These regions are thicker than surrounding areas and called "lipid rafts" (Fig. 3.3). Because of the thickness of rafts the fluidity is less in these areas. Rafts contain a large number of integral and peripheral membrane proteins, which are involved in receiving and conveying cell-specific signals.

The loosely bound peripheral proteins can be easily separated from the cell membrane, whereas integral proteins are tightly bound and can be separated only by using detergents or organic solvents. When cells are frozen and fractured (cryofracture or freeze fracture technique), splitting of plasma membranes occurs usually along the hydrophobic center, i.e. between the two lipid layers. This technique depicts two faces of the membrane, an E- or extracellular face and P- or protoplasmic face. Most of the proteins are attached to the P-face and only fewer proteins are attached to the E-face (Fig. 3.4).

Integral membrane proteins frequently form ion channels and carrier proteins that facilitate the passage of specific ions and molecules across the cell membrane. Many of these proteins are relatively long and are thus folded so that they make several passes through the membrane and are known as multipass proteins. Membrane proteins are important in cell-cell adhesion, intercellular signaling and for the formation of channels for transport of materials into and out of the cell.

### Functions of the Plasma Membrane

a. It protects the cell and also maintains its shape.

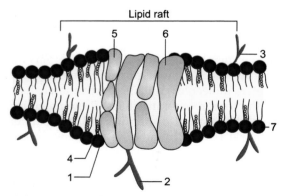

**Fig. 3.3:** Schematic diagram showing the structure of lipid raft. Glycosphingolipid (1), glycoprotein (2), glycolipid (3), cholesterol (4), peripheral membrane protein (5), integral membrane protein (6) and phospholipid (7)

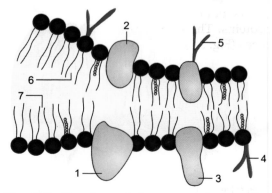

**Fig. 3.4:** Structure of plasma membrane after cryofracture. Protein on E-face (2), protein on P-face (1), peripheral protein (3), glycolipid (4), glycoprotein (5), E-face (6) and P-face (7)

b. It controls the movement of substances in and out of the cell (selectively permeable membrane).

c. It regulates the cell-cell interactions.

d. It acts as an interface between the cytoplasm and the external milieu (tissue fluid). If the cell membrane breaks, cytoplasm may extrude, but it repairs itself to some extent. If the injury is in greater extent, then it leads to cell death.

e. It is capable of recognizing the foreign bodies.

f. It forms a sensory surface and carries various receptors.

### Transport Across Membranes

The main processes by which materials and information transport across cell membranes are:

### A. Passive Diffusion

This process occurs mainly due to concentration gradient across the membrane and it also depends on the size and polarity of the molecules. This process does not require energy. Gases, water, lipids, and lipid soluble molecules can pass freely through the membrane (Fig. 3.5).

### B. Facilitated Diffusion

This process transfers small water soluble molecules. In this process passive diffusion occurs, but requires the presence of transport proteins. The transport proteins are of two types (Fig. 3.5):

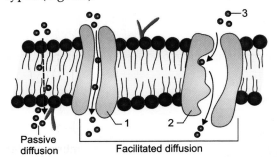

Passive diffusion

Facilitated diffusion

**Fig. 3.5:** Schematic diagram showing transport across the cell membrane. Channel protein (1), carrier protein (2) and molecules (3)

a. **Channel proteins:** These proteins form a water-filled channel across the membrane through which selected molecules or ions can pass depending on concentration, size, and electrical charge.

b. **Carrier proteins:** These proteins bind to a particular molecule or ion and then undergo a change in conformation and release the substrate to the other side of the membrane.

### C. Active Transport

The transport through this process occurs against the electrochemical gradient and thus requires energy, e.g. $Na^+$–$K^+$ pump by which the $Na^+$ ions move out of the cell and $K^+$ ions move into the cell. The required energy for this movement is generated by the conversion of ATP to ADP by $Na^+$–$K^+$ ATPase.

### D. Vesicular Transport (Exocytosis and Endocytosis)

The process by which large molecules or particulate matter (RBCs, bacteria) can go in and out of the cell is called endocytosis and exocytosis, respectively. Plasma membrane takes active participation in both of these processes.

a. **Exocytosis:** In this process, membrane-bound secretory granule of vesicles comes in contact with the inner surface of plasma membrane and fuses with it. This is followed by rupture of fused portion and contents of vesicle are released into the extracellular space (Fig. 3.6). The membrane which is added to the plasma membrane by exocytosis is recovered through an endocytotic process. Exocytosis is of two types:

 i. *Regulated exocytosis:* This process depends on the stimulus and it takes place in cells specialized for release of a large volume of secretory material, e.g. acinar cells of pancreas.

 ii. *Constitutive exocytosis:* This process takes place continuously and secretory products

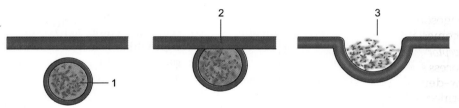

**Fig. 3.6:** Schematic diagram showing the process of exocytosis. Membrane-bound vesicles (1), plasma membrane (2) and extracellular space (3)

are released in small vesicles, e.g. secretion of immunoglobulins by plasma cells.

b. **Endocytosis:** These are of three types:

i. *Fluid-phase pinocytosis:* The process by which a cell 'drinks'. Ingestion of liquid and small protein molecules is done by this process. When liquid molecules come in contact with the plasma membrane, it becomes indented. It forms a pinocytotic vesicle (less than about 150 nm in diameter) by pinching off from its plasma membrane and takes the liquid molecules into the cytoplasm (Fig. 3.7). In most of the cells, these vesicles become endosomes and are finally degraded by the lysosome. However, in many thin cells, pinocytotic vesicles may move to the opposite cell surface where they fuse with the plasma membrane and thus releases their contents outside the cell. This process is called transcytosis and through this mainly bulk transfer of molecules occurs.

ii. *Phagocytosis:* The process by which a cell 'eats'. Ingestion of solid particles such as cell debris, bacteria, and other foreign material is done by this process. When solid particles come in contact with the plasma membrane, the membrane sends processes to enclose the particles. When enveloping processes meet they fuse with each other and particles are drawn inside the cell. The invaginated membrane is then pinched off from the rest of the plasma membrane and forms an intracellular vacuole (more than about 250 nm in diameter), called phagosome (Fig. 3.8).

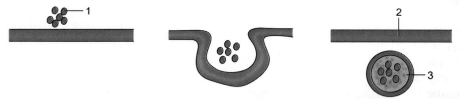

**Fig. 3.7:** Schematic diagram showing the process of pinocytosis. Liquid molecules (1), plasma membrane (2) and pinocytic vesicle (3)

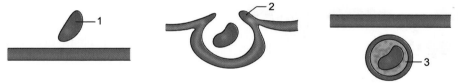

**Fig. 3.8:** Schematic diagram showing the process of phagocytosis. Solid particles (1), enveloping processes (2) and phagosome (3)

Phagosome then receives hydrolases and becomes a late endosome.

iii. *Receptor-mediated endocytosis:* Through this process specific molecule (ligand) such as low-density lipoproteins and protein hormones enter into the cell. Receptors for these ligands are present on the surface of the cell and are called cargo receptors. Binding of ligands to cargo receptors results in aggregation of these ligands in specific regions of the cell membrane (lipid rafts), which then invaginate as coated pits (Fig. 3.9). They are named coated pits because they have aggregations of clathrin molecules on their cytoplasmic surface. These pits then pinched off into the cytoplasm as coated vesicle containing ligands and their cargo receptors.

## CYTOPLASM

It is a jelly-like substance and forms the true internal milieu of the cells. It is part of the cell that lies between the nucleus and the plasma membrane. It contains three different components: Cytoplasmic organelles, cytoplasmic inclusions, and cytoplasmic fluid (cytosol).

## Cytoplasmic Organelles

The human body contains many different organs and each organ performs a different function. Similar to the human body, cells also have a set of "little organs", called organelles. These organelles are adapted and/or specialized for carrying out one or more vital functions. These organelles are of two types: Membrane-bound and non-membranous organelles.

## A. Membrane-bound Organelles

These are found only in eukaryotes. These are:

a. **Mitochondria:** These are known as the powerhouse of the cell, as it converts energy to form ATP, which can be used by the cell.

Mitochondria are dynamic structures, as they can grow in length, they can divide and even they can coalesce. The name "Mitochondria" is derived from the Greek words *mitos* (thread) and *chondros* (granule), as they mainly appear thread like in the light microscope. Mitochondria vary in size, (0.5–2 μm in length) and shape (spherical, filamentous, rod-shaped, or coiled). The number of these organelles correlates with the metabolic activity of different cells. As mitochondria are able to generate ATP, they are present in large numbers in cells, which use large amounts of energy such as cardiac muscle cells. They are also numerous in specific areas where energy is required, such as apical region of ciliated cells, the middle piece of sperm, infoldings of plasma membrane of PCT of kidney, and subsarcolemmal areas of skeletal and cardiac muscle cells. Mitochondria are present in all cells except **red blood cells** and **terminal keratinocytes**.

Mitochondria are normally not seen by light microscope. When stained with H and E stain, they are responsible for eosinophilia of the cytoplasm, as they are acidophilic. They may be stained specifically by histochemical techniques, which reveal some of their component enzymes.

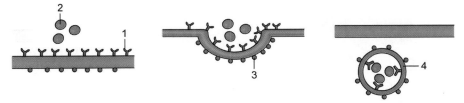

**Fig. 3.9:** Schematic diagram showing the process of receptor-mediated endocytosis. Cargo receptors (1), ligand (2), clathrin molecules (3) and coated vesicle (4)

Mitochondria consist of two membranes (Fig. 3.10). The outer mitochondrial membrane (6–7 nm thick) is smooth and lies in close contact with the cytoplasm. The inner mitochondrial membrane encloses a space, called a matrix. The matrix contains the soluble enzymes of the Krebs cycle and the enzymes involved in β-oxidation of fatty acid. The matrix contains RNA (similar in structure and function of cytoplasmic ribosomes), mitochondrial DNA (less molecular weight than nuclear DNA), suspended granules, and filaments. Mitochondrial DNA consists of the double helix in the form of a circle that contains 37 genes. It is believed that mitochondrial genes are inherited only from mother as head of sperm lacks mitochondria.

The space between two mitochondrial membranes is called inter membranous space. The inner mitochondrial membrane is thinner than the outer mitochondrial membrane and it is convoluted into elongated folds called cristae. In protein-secreting cells cristae are arranged as shelves, while in steroid secreting cells they are arranged in tubules. Cristae tremendously increase the surface area for ATP synthesis and reactions related to the electron transport, i.e. Krebs citric acid cycle, and oxidative phosphorylation. Cristae have numerous knob-like projections; elementary particles, which extend into the matrix of the mitochondria and are rich in enzyme ATP synthase (generate most of the cell's ATP).

Protein densities are higher in both mitochondrial membranes in comparison to other membranes in the cell, therefore, fluidity of mitochondrial membranes is less. The outer membrane is freely permeable for most metabolites, since it contains pores (3 nm in diameter), which form an aqueous channel through which proteins up to 5,000 Daltons can pass and go into inter membranous space. But all proteins cannot get into the matrix as the inner mitochondrial membrane contains phospholipid cardiolipin, which renders it virtually impermeable.

*Functions of the mitochondria:*

• Mitochondria produce most of the cell's ATP, which is used in many chemical reactions.

• Granules present in the matrix store calcium and other cations, so mitochondria also help the cells to maintain the proper concentration of certain ions.

• The mitochondria also help in making some parts of hormones like testosterone and estrogen.

• The mitochondria present in hepatocytes have enzymes which detoxify ammonia.

• The mitochondria also play an important role in the process of apoptosis or programmed cell death. At times of cellular stress, cytochrome C (enzyme present in inter membranous space of mitochondria) is released into the cytoplasm, which activates sets of proteases that degrade all cellular components that result in rapid cell death.

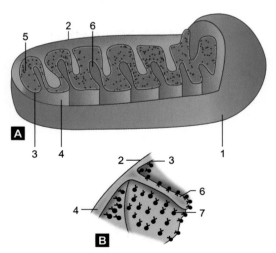

**Fig. 3.10:** Mitochondria (1) (A) schematic diagram, (B) enlarged view showing outer membrane (2), inner membrane (3), inter membranous space (4), matrix (5), cristae (6) and elementary particles (7)

b. **Endoplasmic reticulum (ER):** These are flattened sheets, sacs, and tubes of membrane which extend throughout the cytoplasm and enclose a large intracellular space. The membrane of the endoplasmic reticulum is in structural continuity with the outer membrane of the nuclear envelope. It comprises about half of the total membrane of a cell. The endoplasmic reticulum is of two different types: Rough endoplasmic reticulum (rER) and smooth endoplasmic reticulum (sER). **The rER generally occurs as flattened sheets and studded on its outer surface with the ribosome. The sER is more tubular and lacks attached ribosome.**

Endoplasmic reticulum has two forms, but in most of the cells, only one form usually predominates. Protein secreting cells, such as acinar cells of the pancreas and cells that have the large amounts of the plasma membrane, such as neurons are characterized by an abundance of rough endoplasmic reticulum. Whereas in cells that secrete lipids, lipoproteins or steroid hormones the smooth endoplasmic reticulum predominates, such as lining cells of the small intestine. However, in liver cells, both types of endoplasmic reticulum are present in equal amounts.

*Functions of endoplasmic reticulum:*
- It plays a vital role in the formation of the skeletal framework.
- It provides the increased surface area for cellular reactions.
- Proteins formed by the ribosomes enter in the cavity of rER for processing and sorting.
- The enzymes present in the endoplasmic reticulum are responsible for the synthesis of phospholipids including the phospholipids which are major constituents of cell membranes.
- sER is involved in the metabolism of fat and steroids.
- sER is involved in detoxification of certain lipid soluble drugs and other toxic compounds.

- sER in skeletal muscle is called sarcoplasmic reticulum, which participates in the control of muscle contraction by sequestering calcium ions from the cytosol.

c. **Golgi apparatus:** This organelle is present in all cells except the red blood cells. It is well developed in secretory cells. **It is a system of stacked, membrane bound, flattened sacs, which is involved in modifying, sorting and packaging secretory macromolecules that are delivered to other organelles.** The Golgi apparatus is generally localized above the nucleus, but it may be scattered or dispersed widely in the cytoplasm (e.g. nerve cells).

Golgi apparatus with H and E stain presents a clear area in comparison to surrounding basophilic cytoplasm as it lacks ribosomes; hence called a negative Golgi image. It looks as a network of blackened canals by osmic acid stain or silver impregnation.

Each stack has a *cis-* or forming-face, which is commonly convex in shape (Fig. 3.11) and a *trans-* or maturing-face, which is generally concave. The intermediate part is formed by stacks of flattened saccules called medial Golgi.

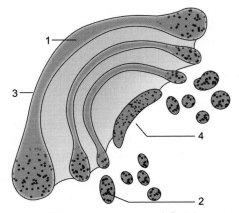

**Fig. 3.11:** Schematic diagram of Golgi apparatus (1) showing *cis*-face (3), *trans*-face (4) and newly formed membrane bound vesicles (2)

The *cis*-face is associated with small transfer vesicles, whereas *trans*-face is associated with larger secretory vesicles.

Vesicles budding off from the sER coalesce with the bottom of the stack of *cis*-face. Some proteins are phosphorylated over here and then this material is transferred to the medial Golgi. Carbohydrate moieties are added over here to form glycoproteins. Finally, all material is transferred to *trans*-face for modification, sorting, packaging, and secretion of proteins in the form of larger secretory vesicles.

*Functions of Golgi apparatus*:
- It does modification, sorting, and packaging of macromolecules that are synthesized by the cells for secretive purposes or for use within the cell.
- It renews integral membrane proteins with integral membrane protein synthesized by the rER.
- It produces glycosaminoglycans, which forms part of connective tissue.

d. **Endosomes:** These are membrane-bound compartments present inside the cells. The compartments, which are located near the cell membrane where vesicles originating from the plasma membrane fuse, are called early endosomes. These endosomes sort out the proteins received through endocytotic vesicles. From here, many vesicles containing receptor proteins return to the plasma membrane. The large numbers of vesicles containing remaining proteins will be transported deeper in the cytoplasm called late endosomes, which later form the lysosomes.

e. **Lysosomes: These electron-dense membrane-bound vesicles measuring 0.2–0.8 μm contain hydrolytic enzymes, mainly acid hydrolases.** These are involved in intracellular digestion. Among the organelles of the cytoplasm, the lysosomes have the thickest covering membrane to prevent the enclosed hydrolytic enzymes from coming in contact with other substances in the cell.

Lysosomes are formed by a complex series of pathways, which transform late endosomes into lysosomes (Fig. 3.12). The synthesis of the hydrolases occurs in the rER; then they are transferred to the Golgi apparatus, where they are modified and packaged and finally transferred through endosomes to the lysosomes. Material taken from outside the cell by endocytosis receives hydrolases to become an endosome, which finally degraded in lysosomes.

Lysosomes also remove excess or nonfunctional organelles and other cytoplasmic structures through a process, called autophagy. A membrane from sER forms around the excess organelle or cytoplasmic structures to be removed, producing an autophagosome which then fuses with lysosome. Autophagy is greater in secretory cells that have accumulated excess secretory granules and at the times of nutritional stress, such as starvation. Digested products from autophagosomes are reused in the cytoplasm. Indigestible materials after the hydrolytic breakdown of the contents of lysosomes are retained within a small vacuolar remnant called residual body.

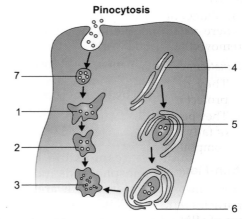

**Fig. 3.12:** Schematic diagram showing the pathway of delivery of materials to lysosome. Early endosome (1), late endosome (2), lysosome (3), sER (4), worn out organelles (5), autophagosome (6) and pinocytotic vesicle (7)

In some cells, these residual bodies may remain for the entire life as granules such as in neurons as lipofuscin granules.

*Functions of the lysosomes:*

- Lysosomes are the cells' garbage disposal system, which degrades endosomes as well as autophagosome.
- Lysosomes are called suicidal bags of the cell as before a cell dies due to lack of oxygen or any other reasons; they destroy all organelles in the cytoplasm.

f. **Peroxisomes (microbodies): These are small spherical organelles (0.2–1 μm in diameter) that are enclosed by a single membrane.** It contains more than 40 oxidative enzymes, particularly catalase and other peroxidases. Almost all oxidative enzymes produce a toxic substance, hydrogen peroxide ($H_2O_2$) as a product of the oxidative reaction. Catalase (major peroxisomal protein) degrades hydrogen peroxide to water and oxygen; thus protects the cell. These organelles resemble the lysosomes in their appearance, but they differ both in function and in biogenesis. They either arise from the growth and division of pre-existing peroxisomes or through budding of precursor vesicles from the sER. Peroxisomes are abundant in the cells of liver and kidney, where many of the toxic substances are removed from the body.

*Functions of the peroxisomes:*

- They degrade hydrogen peroxide to protect the cell.
- They perform detoxification, β-oxidation of fatty acids and metabolism of various compounds.

## B. Non-Membranous Organelles

a. **Ribosomes:** These are small electron-dense particles of 15–20 nm in size and are made up of rRNA and protein. These are found in all cells except the red blood cells. The ribosomes are composed of two subunits: Large (60S) and small (40S). 'S' stands for Svedberg unit of sedimentation rate. The large subunits are synthesized in the nucleolus, whereas the small subunits are synthesized in the nucleus. Then they are transported to the cytoplasm through the nuclear pores. Each subunit contains rRNA of different lengths as well as several different proteins. Groups of ribosomes are often attached to a single strand of mRNA in small circular aggregations, called polyribosomes or polysomes. Ribosomes may be attached to the rER or may be found scattered in the cytoplasm (free ribosomes). Free ribosomes are the site of synthesis for proteins destined for the nucleus, peroxisomes, and mitochondria. Polysomes are the site of synthesis of secretory proteins, membrane proteins, and lysosomal enzymes.

b. **Centrioles:** In a non-dividing, diploid cell usually two centrioles are present. Each rod-shaped centriole is about 0.2 μm long. The centrosome is a specialized region of the cytoplasm located near the nucleus and includes a pair of centrioles and the amorphous dense pericentriolar matrix. The two centrioles are oriented perpendicular to each other and lies in the center of the cell (cytocentrum). Each centriole is made up of a ring of nine triplets of microtubules that are oriented parallel to the long axis of the centriole. Each microtubule triplet consists of one complete (A) and two incomplete (B and C) microtubules fused to each other (Fig. 3.13). The complete microtubule is positioned closest to the center of the cylinder, whereas incomplete microtubule (C) is the farthest away. This arrangement of microtubules appears as a pinwheel in cross section. Multinucleated cells contain several centrioles. The centrioles are self-replicating organelles that duplicate, just before cell division.

*Functions of the centrioles:*

- They provide basal bodies for cilia, and flagella.
- During mitosis, they are responsible for the formation of the spindle.

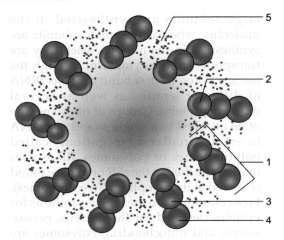

**Fig. 3.13:** Schematic diagram of a cross section of centriole showing nine groups of microtubules triplets (1) formed by one complete microtubule A (2) and two incomplete microtubules B (3) and C (4). These are connected by a pericentriolar matrix (5)

c. **Filaments:** In the cytoplasm, a network of protein filaments is present that interact extensively with each other and with the component of the plasma membrane. This network of filaments forms the shape of the cell and also forms a basis for movement of cell, so known as cytoskeleton. It fixes the organelles in place, helps during endocytosis, and also moves parts of the cell in the process of growth and motility. Three main kinds of cytoskeletal filaments are:

i. *Microtubules:* These are long hollow, thin, tubular structures, and about 20–25 nm in diameter. Each microtubule consists of 13 circularly arranged globular dimeric tubulin molecules. Each tubulin dimer is formed by α- and β-tubulin

subunits (Fig. 3.14). During cell division, microtubules form the mitotic spindle, which distributes chromosomes equally between two daughter cells. These are major components of axons and dendrites. These tubules even participate in the axoplasmic flow of material along these processes. These tubules provide the capability of ciliary and flagellar motion and are also involved in intracellular vesicular transport (e.g. movement of secretory vesicles and melanin transport in pigment cells). Microtubules are also present in other cellular structures like sensory hair, and tail of sperm.

ii. *Intermediate filaments:* These filaments are long, straight or slightly bent (Fig. 3.15) and are intermediate in thickness (8–10 nm) between microtubules and microfilaments. These filaments are

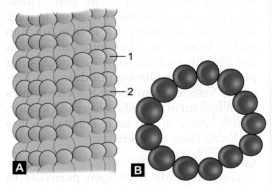

**Fig. 3.14:** (A) Schematic diagram showing microtubules formed by two subunits α-tubulin (1) and β-tubulin (2), (B) cross section showing arrangements of tubulin subunits

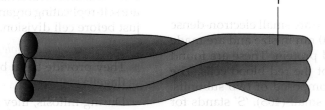

**Fig. 3.15:** Schematic diagram showing intermediate filaments (1)

much more stable than microtubules and microfilaments, so provide the mechanical strength and support. They contain several types of tissue-specific proteins; such as keratins (epithelium, hairs, and nails), desmin (muscles), vimentin (cells of mesodermal origin—endothelial cells, fibroblasts, and chondroblasts), laminin (nuclear lamina), glial fibrillary acidic protein (astrocytes), and neurofilaments (neurons).

iii. *Microfilaments:* These rod-like structures are of about 6–8 nm in diameter and composed mainly of the protein actin (Fig. 3.16). These rods form part of the contractile machinery in both muscle and non-muscle cells. Microfilaments associated with non-muscle cell helps in their motility in the form of ameboid movements. Actin is an important component of the cytoskeleton and occurs in two forms: G (globular)-actin, which is free actin molecules present in the cytoplasm, and F (filamentous)-actin, which is the polymerized form that consists of two protofilaments twisted together to form a helix.

These protofilaments are made up of multiple globular actin monomers (G-actin). The actin filament is then assembled into larger filaments, networks and 3-dimensional structures. Actin filaments form a meshwork beneath the plasma membrane, called cell cortex, which helps to maintain the shape of the cell. These filaments also form the structural core of microvilli.

For comparison among microtubules, intermediate filaments and microfilaments *see* Table 3 given in Appendix I.

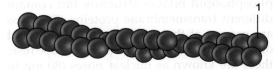

**Fig. 3.16:** Schematic diagram showing microfilaments formed by actin protein (1)

## Cytoplasmic Inclusions

Accumulations of potentially useful or even useless products of metabolism within the cytoplasm are known as cytoplasmic inclusions, such as pigments, glycogen granules, and fat droplets.

### A. Pigments

Some tissues are intrinsically tinted with natural colored compounds, called pigments. The most common pigment in our body (besides hemoglobin) is melanin, which provides protection to the skin. Additionally, in non-dividing cells (e.g. cardiac muscle cells, neurons) and in hepatocytes a yellow-brown pigment lipofuscin is present. This pigment represents a residue of undigested material present in residual bodies. Because the amount of this material increases with age, it is also called aging pigment. Many cells, especially macrophages of the liver and spleen, contain pigmented deposits of hemosiderin granules. Hemosiderin is an iron-storage complex formed by the indigestible residues of hemoglobin. Its presence is related to the phagocytosis of red blood cells.

### B. Glycogen Granules

Glycogen is a D-glucose polymer and it is the most common storage form of glucose, which appears as small clusters. Glycogen granules are not bound by a membrane, but frequently lie in the vicinity of the sER. Hepatocytes and skeletal muscle cells contain the largest glycogen stores, but they differ in function. In hepatocytes glycogen is present in large aggregates (rosettes) and maintains blood glucose levels. In skeletal muscle, glycogen forms ATP through glycolysis.

### C. Fat Droplets

These are the storage form of triglycerides and cholesterol, so often closely associated with sER, where synthesis of lipid, cholesterol, and lipoproteins occurs. Cholesterol is a precursor to steroid hormones, so steroid-secreting cells, such as cells of the adrenal cortex, testis, and ovary also contain many small lipid droplets. Cells of adrenal cortex typically look spongy because of lipid content, so called spongiocytes. Fat droplets are usually nutritive inclusions that provide energy for cellular metabolism. These are mainly present in adipocytes, but they are also present as individual droplets, e.g. hepatocytes. During routine histology (H and E staining), fat gets washed off and looks like empty spaces. However, by the use of osmium, fat can be fixed and seen as grey-black droplets (*see* Fig. 2.8 in Chapter 2).

## Cytoplasmic Fluid (Cytosol)

Cytoplasmic organelles and inclusions are suspended in a fluid, known as cytosol. It occupies nearly half of the total volume of the cell. It also consists of granular bodies such as free ribosome, endoplasmic reticulum with ribosome attached to it, glycogen granules and fat droplets. The cytosol also contains soluble proteins, enzymes, ions and metabolites. It is commonly acidophilic, so stain with acid stains, like eosin.

## NUCLEUS

It is about 3–4 µm in diameter and it is the largest organelle of the cell. The mature red blood cells and blood platelets (cytoplasmic fragments of megakaryocytes) contain no nucleus. **The nucleus is the site of DNA replication and transcription of DNA into precursor RNA molecules**. Enzymes which are required for these processes are contained within the nucleus. The nucleus includes the nuclear envelope, nucleolus, nucleoplasm, and chromatin (Fig. 3.17).

## A. Nuclear Envelope

**The nucleus is surrounded by two parallel membranes separated by a narrow space (40–70 nm) called the perinuclear cistern**. Together, the paired membranes and the perinuclear cistern make up the nuclear envelope, which separates nucleus from the cytoplasm. The

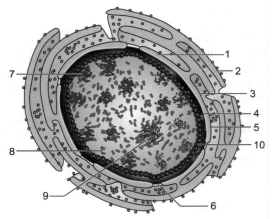

**Fig. 3.17:** Schematic diagram showing the formation of nuclear envelope (1) from rough endoplasmic reticulum (2).Outer nuclear envelope (3), inner nuclear envelope (4), perinuclear cistern (5), nuclear pore (6), heterochromatin (7), euchromatin (8), nucleolus (9) and nuclear lamina (10)

nuclear envelope is made by differentiation of the rER. The inner nuclear membrane is about 6 nm thick and it faces the nuclear contents. It is in close contact with the nuclear lamina, which is a lattice-like network of intermediate filaments (lamins). Lamins attach heterochromatin to the inner membrane and participate in the breakdown (phosphorylation) and reorganization (dephosphorylation) of the nuclear envelope during cell division. The outer nuclear membrane is also 6 nm thick, approximately, and it faces the cytoplasm. It is in continuity with the rER and its cytoplasmic surface, usually possesses ribosomes, which actively synthesize transmembrane proteins that are destined for the outer or inner nuclear membranes. The inner and outer nuclear membranes have the typical phospholipid bilayer structure but contain different transmembrane proteins. The gaps are present at the sites where the inner and outer membranes of the nuclear envelope fuse, these are known as nuclear pores (80 nm in diameter). The number of pores is from dozens to thousands and it depends upon the metabolic activity. These pores contain about 30 different types of proteins, called nucleo-porins that regulate the passage of ions and macromolecules, ribosomal subunits, etc. in and out of the nucleus. The nucleus communicates with the cytoplasmic fluid by these pores. Ions and small molecules diffuse freely through the nuclear pore, while larger molecules, such as mRNA, moving from nucleus to cytoplasm and histones from cytoplasm to nucleus move through the pore by an energy-dependent process.

## B. Nucleolus

**It is a dense, oval and distinct (up to 1 mm in diameter) factory in the nucleus where the rRNA is transcript and ribosomes are produced.** It is not surrounded by a membrane and its size, number, and location may depend on a cell's functional activity. Nucleoli become exceptionally large and prominent in cells that are actively synthesizing proteins. It disappears during prophase of mitosis and reappears during telophase. It contains three morphologically distinct compartments:

a. **Granular compartment (GC) or Pars granulosa:** It is found at the periphery in which maturing ribosomal subunits are assembled.

b. **Dense fibrillar component (DFC) or Pars fibrosa:** It is located in the center and contains ribonuclear protein fibrils.

c. **Fibrillar center (FC):** It is an innermost pale staining compartment and contains DNA that is not being transcripted.

The synthesis of nucleolar RNA is regulated by genes which are located in the secondary constrictions of chromosomes, which are having satellite bodies in their short arms, i.e. chromosomes 13, 14, 15, 21 and 22.

## C. Nucleoplasm

It fills the space between the chromatin and the nucleolus. It is composed mainly of proteins (some of which have enzymatic activity), metabolites, and ions.

## D. Chromatin

It was so named because it is easily stained with dyes; "chroma" means color. Its acidic nature gives it an affinity for basic dyes, such as hematoxylin. It is a complex of DNA and protein, which represents the relaxed, uncoiled chromosomes of interphase nucleus. The genetic material is encoded in the deoxyribo-nucleic acid (DNA) of chromosomes. The DNA stored within the nucleus is essential to the cell because its genes encode the amino acid sequences of the various proteins that the cell must produce to stay alive. The major proteins involved in chromatin are histone proteins, although many other chromosomal proteins have prominent roles too. Chromatin resides within the nucleus as heterochromatin and euchromatin. Heterochromatin appears as coarse granules in the electron microscope and as basophilic clumps in the light microscope. It is a condensed form of chromatin, which is located mostly in the periphery of the nucleus. **Heterochromatin is transcriptionally inactive (e.g. chromatin in the head of sperm) and contains highly repeated DNA sequences.** Euchromatin is visible as a finely dispersed granular material in the electron microscope and as lightly stained basophilic areas in the light microscope. **Euchromatin is an active form of chromatin (e.g. chromatin of neurons and hepatocytes), which is scattered throughout the nucleus.** In euchromatin the genetic material of the DNA is being transcribed into RNA. Nuclei which are large and predominantly made up of euchromatin are called open-face nuclei, while nuclei that are made up mainly of heterochromatin are called closed-face nuclei.

## E. Barr Body

**It is composed of one of the X chromosome (inactive) that remains condensed in interphase, and appears as a dark staining body attached to the nuclear membrane (Fig. 3.18).** The phenomenon was first described by Dr Murray L Barr. Barr bodies can be seen on the nucleus of neutrophils as a drumstick-like

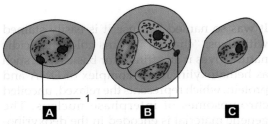

**Fig. 3.18:** Schematic diagram showing features of Barr body (1) (A) in human female oral (buccal) epithelial cell, (B) in polymorphonuclear leukocyte and (C) human male oral (buccal) epithelial cell (no Barr body)

appendage and in the epithelial cells obtained from the lining of the cheek. A normal human female (XX) has only one Barr body per somatic cell; while a normal human male (XY) has none. In females with Turner syndrome (XO) no Barr body is present, while in male with Klinefelter syndrome (XXY) one Barr body is present.

## CELL DIVISION

### A. Mitosis

In the early 1950s, the idea that chromosomes are made up of DNA was generally agreed on. DNA occurs in well-marked unit characteristic of the strain or species. There is a duplication of this number in mitosis and a reduction in meiosis. Centrosomes are the main microtubule organizing centers of the cell. The centrosomes duplicate once per cell cycle, separate and then nucleate the two end points of the mitotic spindle. The function of the microtubule spindle during mitosis is to distribute replicated DNA equally between daughter cells. During mitosis, sister chromatids separate and are reeled into centrosomes at opposite poles of the spindle. The 'bait' that captures the chromatids is the kinetochore, which is a proteinaceous structure that binds both microtubules and centromeric DNA. The kinetochore moves linked sister chromatids back and forth along the spindle during metaphase and separate sister chromatids to the centrosomes during anaphase.

The cell is thought to use two types of regulators to ensure that this crucial duplication takes place: First, cell-cycle factors, which regulate when centrosome duplication occurs; and second, intrinsic factors, which ensure that only one round of duplication occurs per cell cycle. During the cell cycle, a cell goes through a series of sequential events in which one step has to be completed before the next is initiated. In general, cell status can be in preparatory or in dividing phase. Interphase (preparatory phase) is considerably longer than the dividing phase. The interphase is divided into gap1 (G1), synthesis phase (S), and gap2 (G2). During interphase, the cell grows, performs its metabolic function, and replicates its chromosomes in preparation for another division. The division phase is called as M (mitotic) phase and includes mitosis (nuclear division) and cytokinesis (cell division).

The cell immediately enters in G1 phase at the end of M phase. G1 phase is generally the longest and most varied phases of the cell cycle (Fig. 3.19). In G1 phase no DNA synthesis occurs, it is usually a period of cell growth. The S phase follows G1 and in this phase DNA replication takes place, so DNA of the cell is doubled. Once a cell enters into the S phase, it is committed to complete the mitosis. The S phase is followed by G2 phase, in which

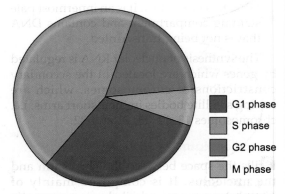

**Fig. 3.19:** Schematic diagram showing subdivisions of mitosis

proteins required for mitosis accumulate and chromosome begins to condense in preparation for cell division.

Nuclear division occurs in four phases: Prophase, metaphase, anaphase, and telophase.

a. **Prophase:** The chromosomes begin to condense; revealing sister chromatids attached at the centromere. Outside the nucleus, the two centriole pairs begin to separate, and move towards opposite poles of the cell. Each chromosome splits longitudinally into two chromatids except at the centromere. As prophase proceeds, nucleoli disappear, and the nuclear membrane disintegrates to release the chromosomes, this marks the end of the prophase (Fig. 3.20).

b. **Prometaphase:** Nuclear membrane completely disappears. The spindle microtubules extend up to chromosomes and bind to the centromere in a junction called the kinetochore. The centrioles are now at the opposite poles.

c. **Metaphase:** Three types of microtubules (MTs) exist in the mitotic spindle-kinetochores MTs, interpolar MTs, and aster MTs. These three align the chromosomes across the metaphase or equatorial plate, perpendicular to the spindle, tugging them equally to each pole.

d. **Anaphase:** The two sister chromatids separate and are pulled by the kinetochore MTs toward the poles. At the end of anaphase the sister chromatids are grouped at either end of the cell and both clusters are diploid in number.

e. **Telophase:** The spindle dissociates; the nuclear membrane and nucleolus reform, the chromosomes begin to uncoil.

f. **Cytokinesis:** A cleavage furrow (puckering of the plasma membrane) forms perpendicular to the orientation of the mitotic spindles. A belt of actin and myosin microfilaments contracts (similar to muscle contraction) to cleave the cytoplasm in half (usually in half, sometimes the two daughter cells are of

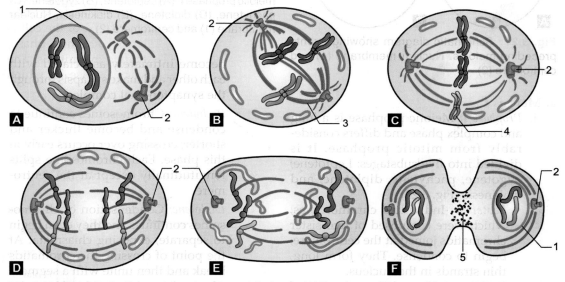

**Fig. 3.20:** Schematic diagram showing stages of mitosis: (A) Prophase, (B) prometaphase, (C) metaphase, (D) anaphase, (E) telophase and (F) cytokinesis. Nuclear membrane (1), centriole (2), mitotic spindle (3), metaphase plate (4) and actin-myosin belt (5)

different sizes). The spindle remnants now disintegrate.

## B. Meiosis

It is the process of cell division that results in the formation of daughter cells whose chromosome number is reduced from diploid (2n) to haploid (n). It occurs only in sex cells during the formation of germ cells (ovum or spermatozoa). When the germ cells are in the S phase of the cell cycle prior to meiosis (Fig. 3.21), the amount of DNA doubled to 4n but the number of chromosomes remains 2n (46 chromosomes). Meiosis begins at the end of interphase in the cell cycle and is completed in two steps: Meiosis I (reduction division) and meiosis II (equatorial division).

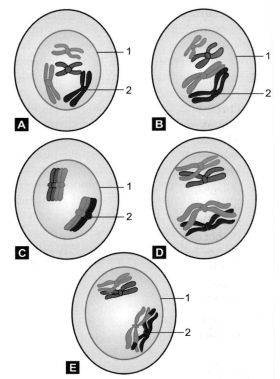

**Fig. 3.22:** Schematic diagram showing events in meiotic prophase I: (A) Leptotene, (B) zygotene, (C) pachytene, (D) diplotene, (E) diakinesis. Nuclear membrane (1) and centromere (2).

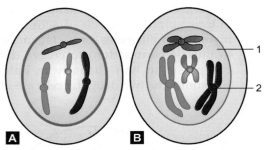

**Fig. 3.21:** Schematic diagram showing events preceding meiosis. Nuclear membrane (1) and centromere (2)

### a. Meiosis I

i. *Prophase I:* Meiotic prophase is a long and complex phase and differs considerably from mitotic prophase. It is divided into five substages: Leptotene, zygotene, pachytene, diplotene, and diakinesis (Fig. 3.22).

- *Leptotene:* Individual chromosomes, which were composed of two sister chromatids joined at the centromere, begin to condense. They form long, thin strands in the nucleus.
- *Zygotene:* Homologous pairs of chromosomes (maternal and paternal copies of the same chromosome)

become intimately associated with each other and make synapsis through the synaptonemal complex.

- *Pachytene:* Chromosomes continue to condense and become thicker and shorter; crossing over occurs early in this phase. Each chromosome splits longitudinally except at the centromere.
- *Diplotene:* Condensation of chromosomes continues and they even begin to separate, exposing chiasmata. At the point of crossing the chromatids break and then unite with a segment of non-sister chromatids of homologous chromosomes. This process is called crossing over.

- *Diakinesis:* The homologous chromosomes condense maximally and the nucleolus disappears, and the nuclear envelope disintegrates.

ii. *Metaphase I:* The homologous pairs of chromosomes, each composed of two chromatids, line up on the metaphase (equatorial) plate of the meiotic spindle. They are attached to the spindle microtubules at the kinetochores of the chromosomes (Fig. 3.23).

iii. *Anaphase I:* The chromosomes separate and are pulled to the poles by the spindle microtubules. The centromeres do not divide. Here homologous chromosomes are separated from one another. Each chromosome with two sister chromatids goes to one of the poles of the spindle.

iv. *Telophase I and cytokinesis:* The nuclear envelope reforms and cytokinesis occurs, essentially as in mitosis except that the daughter cells are now haploid. However, the DNA content is still diploid. Each of the two newly formed daughter cells enters in meiosis II.

b. **Meiosis II:** Each daughter cell formed by the first meiotic division enters straight in metaphase I. In between meiosis I and meiosis II, no DNA replication takes place.

i. *Metaphase II:* The chromosomes align at the metaphase plate and spindle microtubules attach to the kinetochores of each sister chromatid, facing opposite poles (Fig. 3.24).

ii. *Anaphase II:* The centromeres divide and the sister chromatids are separated to form new chromosomes, which are pulled to the opposite poles of the spindle.

iii. *Telophase II and cytokinesis:* The nuclear envelope reforms and the cells divide. Each cell has a daughter chromosome from one of the chromosomes in each pair (the cells are haploid). Unlike the cells produced by mitosis, which are genetically identical to the parent cell, the cells produced by meiosis are genetically unique.

For comparison between mitosis and meiosis, *see* Table 4 given in Appendix I.

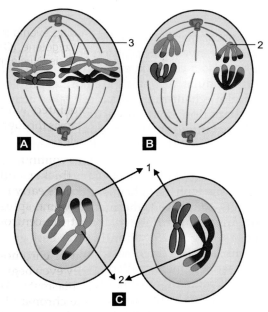

**Fig. 3.23:** Schematic diagram showing events in meiosis I: (A) Metaphase I, (B) anaphase I, (C) telophase I and cytokinesis. Nuclear membrane (1), centromere (2) and chiasmata (3)

## DIFFERENTIATION OF CELLS

Our body contains 200 different types of cells, which are formed from an undifferentiated cell; zygote (totipotent). In adults, undifferentiated cells found among differentiated cells in a tissue or organ that can renew themselves and can differentiate to yield some or all of the major specialized cell types of the tissue or organ. They are not totipotent but they are pluripotent. The primary roles of adult stem cells in a living organism are to maintain and repair the tissue in which they are found. They

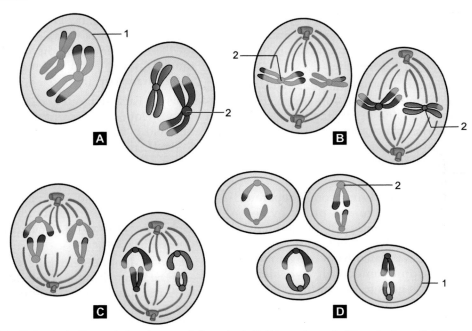

**Fig. 3.24:** Schematic diagram showing events in meiosis II. (A) prophase II, (B) metaphase II, (C) anaphase II, (D) telophase II and cytokinesis. Nuclear membrane (1) and centromere (2)

are also known as somatic stem cells instead of adult stem cell. Unlike embryonic stem cells, which are defined by their origin (the inner cell mass of the blastocyst), the origin of the adult stem cells in mature tissues is unknown.

## CELL DEATH

Cells may die as a result of either tissue injury (necrosis) or programmed cell death.

### A. Necrosis

It is a pathological response which occurs due to exposure of cells to unfavorable conditions such as hypoxia, low pH and radiations. Necrotic cells swell and subsequently rupture. The resulting debris can even induce an inflammatory response.

### B. Apoptosis (Programmed Cell Death)

It was first discovered in developing embryos, where programmed cell death is an essential process for shaping the embryo (morphogenesis). Later investigators observed that apoptosis are also a common event in the tissues of normal adults. Apoptosis is a normal physiological mechanism in which cell takes active participation in its own death (intrinsic cellular suicide). It is regulated by both internal and external stimuli. In apoptosis, the cell and its nucleus become small and condensed (pyknotic nucleus), which can be seen easily with the light microscope. Chromatin gets condensed, the nucleus breaks up, and blebbing of the plasma membrane occurs (Fig. 3.25). Finally, the cell gets shrunk, and it is fragmented into membrane-enclosed fragments called apoptotic bodies. All cell remnants are readily engulfed, or phagocytosed by the macrophages. However, the apoptotic fragments do not trigger the inflammatory process. It is a mechanism for cell deletion in the regulation of cell population.

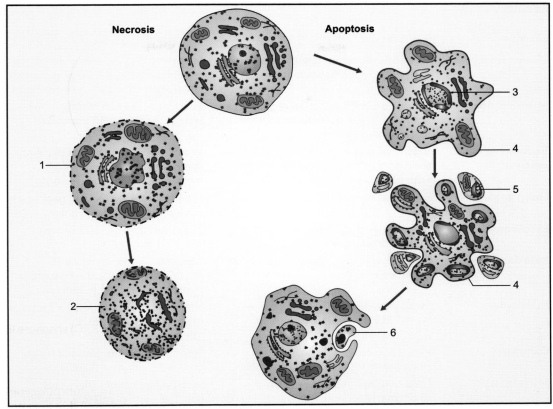

**Fig. 3.25:** Schematic diagram showing comparison in cell death by apoptosis and necrosis. Swelling of cell (1), rupture of cell (2), condensed nucleus and chromatin (3), blebbing of plasma membrane (4), apoptotic bodies (5) and phagocytic clearance (6)

**Mitochondrial Myopathies:** These are a group of neuromuscular diseases caused by damage to the mitochondria. Mitochondria are the powerhouse of the cell. Nerve cells and muscles require a great amount of energy, so they are particularly damaged when mitochondrial dysfunction occurs. Mitochondrial myopathies can be caused by defects in nuclear and mitochondrial DNA.

**Lysosomal Storage Diseases:** These are autosomal recessive disorders. In these diseases, there is an inherited lack of a lysosomal enzyme, catabolism of its substrate remains incomplete, leading to accumulation of the partially degraded insoluble metabolites within the lysosomes. Approximately 40 lysosomal storage diseases have been identified; each result from the functional absence of a specific lysosomal enzyme.

**Stem Cells in Dental Pulp:** Stem cells are generally defined as clonogenic cells capable of both self-renewal and multi-lineage differentiation. Mesenchymal cells are present in dental pulp, which acts as stem cells. These cells are capable of responding to specific environmental signals either to generate new stem cells or to select a particular differentiation program.

## Summary

| Organelle | Structure | Functions |
| --- | --- | --- |
| Plasma membrane | Lipid bilayer containing cholesterol, peripheral and integral membrane proteins | Selectively impermeable membrane which maintains the shape of the cell and regulates the cell–cell interactions |
| Mitochondria | Double membrane-bound organelle with highly folded inner membrane in the form of cristae | Energy production mainly in the form of ATP for activities of cell |
| Endoplasmic reticulum | Extensive membrane system within the cell; may be rough (rER) studded with ribosomes, or smooth (sER) | Processing and sorting of proteins synthesized on ribosomes (rER), metabolism of fat and steriods |
| Golgi apparatus | System of stacked, membrane-bound sacs | Modification, sorting and packaging of secretory macromolecules |
| Lysosomes | Membrane-bound vesicles containing hydrolytic enzymes | Cells' garbage disposal system |
| Peroxisomes | Membrane-bound vesicles containing oxidative enzymes | Detoxification of certain toxic materials, production of hydrogen peroxide for killing pathogens |
| Ribosomes | Small particles free in cytoplasm or bound to endoplasmic reticulum. | Site of synthesis of proteins for the nucleus, peroxisomes and mitochondria |
| Centrioles | Rod-shaped organelle made by a ring of nine triplets of microtubules | Spindle formation, provide basal bodies for cilia and flagella |
| Microtubules | Hollow tubular structure made by 13 circularly arranged globular dimeric tubulin molecules | Spindle formation, ciliary and flagellar motion and intracellular vesicular transport |
| Intermediate filaments | Made by several tissue specific proteins, such as keratin, desmin and neurofilaments | Mechanical strength and support |
| Microfilaments | Rod-like structure made by protein actin | Muscle contraction and motility in non-muscle cell |
| Glycogen granules | Non-membranous granules present as small clusters | Energy storage |
| Fat droplets | Non-membranous spherical aggregates of lipids of variable size | A storage form of triglycerides and cholesterol |
| Nucleus | Membranous organelle containing chromatin | Chromosomes (DNA) contain the genetic blueprint for all proteins in our body |
| Nuclear envelope | Consists of inner and outer membranes that become continuous around nuclear pores; outer membrane studded with ribosomes | Separates and mediates transport between nucleus and cytoplasm |
| Nucleolus | Dense non-membranous structure in nucleus | rRNA is transcript and produces ribosomes |

## Self Assessment

1. Which organelle is involved in sorting and packaging of proteins within a cell?
   a. Golgi apparatus
   b. Mitochondria
   c. Lysosomes
   d. Endosomes

2. Which of the following is a membranous organelle?
   a. Microtubules
   b. Ribosomes
   c. Centrioles
   d. Nucleus

3. Which organelle is considered as the powerhouse of the cell?
   a. rER
   b. Golgi apparatus
   c. Lysosomes
   d. Mitochondria

4. Microtubules are absent in:
   a. Centrioles
   b. Flagella
   c. Cilia
   d. Microvilli

5. Prokaryotic cell does not possess:
   a. Cytoplasm
   b. Cell wall
   c. Nuclear membrane
   d. All of the above

6. Which organelle has the genetic material?
   a. Ribosomes
   b. Nucleus
   c. Cell wall
   d. Lysosomes

7. Which process is also known as cell eating?
   a. Pinocytosis
   b. Diffusion
   c. Phagocytosis
   d. Active transport

8. Which organelle is called suicidal bags of the cell?
   a. Lysosomes
   b. Nucleus
   c. Mitochondria
   d. Golgi apparatus

9. Mitotic spindle dissociates in which stage?
   a. Prophase
   b. Metaphase
   c. Anaphase
   d. Telophase

10. Crossing over takes place in which substage of meiosis I?
    a. Leptotene
    b. Zygotene
    c. Diplotene
    d. Pachytene

## Answers

1. a,    2. d,    3. d,    4. a,    5. c,    6. b,    7. c,    8. a,    9. d,
10. c

# 4

# Epithelial Tissue and Glands

Epithelial tissue is the basic tissue of our body. In this tissue epithelial cells are arranged in continuous sheets as it covers exterior surfaces as well as lines, both internal closed cavities and tubes that communicate with the exterior. **Epithelial cells line all free surfaces except the joint cavities, and the anterior surface of the iris, which is a bare connective tissue domain.** Epithelial cells rest on a non-cellular basement membrane. The space between adjacent epithelial cells (intercellular space) is narrow (about 20 nm) and contains a small amount of mucopolysaccharide, which is rich in cations (mainly calcium). Epithelial cells are highly regenerative and rapidly replace lost cells by cell division. The epithelium is derived from all three germ layers, i.e. ectoderm, endoderm and mesoderm.

Epithelium is an avascular tissue (no blood vessels), but supplied by nerves. The cells receive their nutrition by diffusion from capillaries of neighboring connective tissue, via the intercellular substances.

## FUNCTIONS OF EPITHELIAL TISSUE

### A. Protection

It protects the underlying tissues of the body against dehydration, chemical or mechanical damage.

### B. Secretion

Epithelial cells invaginate into the underlying connective tissue to form glands, which secrete mucus, hormones and enzymes.

### C. Absorption

In the intestinal tract and in proximal convoluted tubules (PCT) of the kidneys, epithelial cells absorb material from the lumen.

### D. Excretion

Epithelial cells of some part of nephrons of kidney take part in excretion of harmful metabolites.

### E. Selective permeability

Epithelial cells control the movement of materials through the presence of intercellular junctions, thus makes the epithelium selectively permeable.

### F. Transport

Transport of materials occurs along the surface of epithelium by the movements of cilia. Transcellular transport (across the plasma membrane) also occurs in some epithelium, like gaseous exchange in lung alveoli.

### G. Sensory function

Epithelial cells detect external sensations such as cells of taste buds, olfactory cells, and cells of the retina.

## TYPES OF EPITHELIAL TISSUE

Some epithelial cells are one cell thick, and some are more than one cell thick. However, all types of epithelial cells are strongly adherent cells and lie on the basement membrane (Flowchart 4.1). The shape of epithelial cells

**Flowchart 4.1:** The types of epithelium, details of each epithelia are given on the following pages

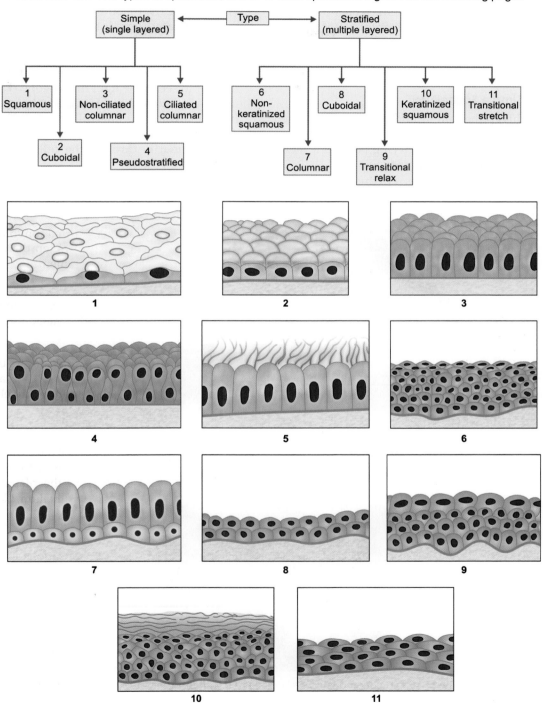

is related to the amount of cytoplasm and organelles present in them, which in turn is related to the metabolic activity of cells. Columnar cells are highly active in comparison to squamous cells as they are having abundant mitochondria and endoplasmic reticulum.

## A. Simple Epithelium

In this epithelium, epithelial cells are arranged in a single layer. All epithelial cells are in contact with the underlying basement membrane. These are of four types:

a. **Simple squamous epithelium:** In this epithelium, epithelial cells are flat. Height

of the cells is very less in comparison to the width (Fig. 4.1A, B). Boundaries of cells are highly serrated and interlocking. When viewed from the top the cells look like pieces on a puzzle board (Fig. 4.2). Cytoplasm is stretched out so thinly that it is difficult to see in the light microscope. The nucleus is flattened and forms a bulging at the cell surface. As the cells are holding together by occluding junctions, the material passes primarily through the cells rather than between them.

i. *Locations:* This epithelium is present in the alveoli of the lungs, parietal layer of

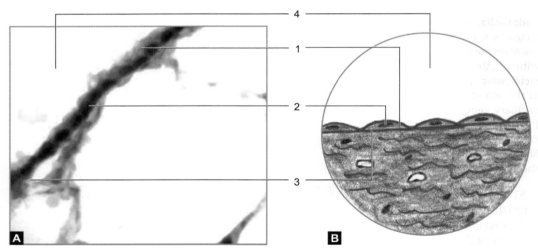

**Fig. 4.1:** Simple squamous epithelial cells (1) with flattened nucleus (2), (A) micrograph, (B) sketch. All epithelial cells rest on the basement membrane (3) on one side and cover the lumen (4) on the other side

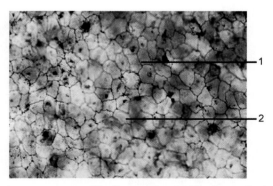

**Fig. 4.2:** Top view of simple squamous epithelium stained with silver nitrate. Intercellular borders (1), epithelial cell (2)

the Bowman's capsule, thin segments of the renal tubules, various parts of the inner ear, posterior surface of the cornea, thyroid follicles (inactive), lining of the heart (endocardium), blood and lymphatic vessels (endothelium), and lining of pleural, pericardial, and peritoneal cavities (mesothelium).

ii. *Functions:* This epithelium allows active transport of fluids and passive transport of gases, such as in the alveoli of the lungs. The cells reduce friction by producing lubricating fluids for movement of viscera.

> **Endothelial cells** of blood vessels produce anticoagulants, which prevent coagulation of blood to maintain normal unobstructed flow of blood. Along with this, these cells also produce von Willebrand's factor, which mediates platelet adhesion to collagen at the site of injury to stop bleeding. In the post-capillary venules of the lymph node paracortex (high endothelial venules) endothelial cells become cuboidal in shape. In the spleen, endothelial cells lining the sinusoids are elongated and fusiform; these are called stave or littoral or rod cells.

b. **Simple cuboidal epithelium:** In this epithelium, epithelial cells are cubical (hexagonal) in shape. Height, width and depth of the cells are approximately equal.

All nuclei are present at the same level (in the center) and they are rounded in shape (Fig. 4.3A, B). Cytoplasm is moderate in amount.

i. *Locations:* This epithelium is present in the glands, ducts, distal tubules in kidney, thyroid follicles (active), covering of the ovary, lens capsule (inner surface), and pigmented epithelium of the retina.

ii. *Functions:* This epithelium mainly participates in secretion and absorption.

c. **Simple columnar epithelium:** In this epithelium, epithelial cells are column like in shape and amount of cytoplasm is more. Height of the cells is more in comparison to the width. All nuclei are present in the base at the same level and they are oval in shape (Fig. 4.4A, B). The epithelium may contain goblet cells or it may have cilia or it may be non-ciliated.

i. *Locations:* Ciliated epithelium mainly lines small bronchi, uterine tubes, and uterus. Non-ciliated epithelium mainly lines digestive tract (from the stomach to the anus) and gallbladder. The goblet cells are present in the small intestine, large intestine, and small bronchi.

ii. *Functions:* This epithelium is adopted for protection, secretion, and absorption. Movements of cilia move the mucus in

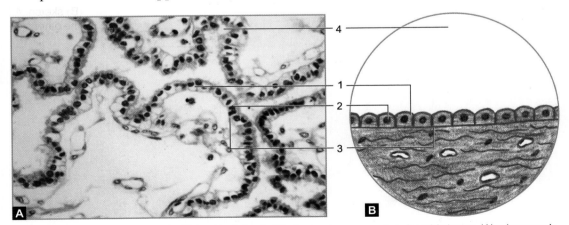

**Fig. 4.3 A, B:** Shows simple cuboidal epithelial cells (1) of ependyma covering choroid plexus, (A) micrograph, (B) sketch. Round nucleus (2), basement membrane (3), lumen (4)

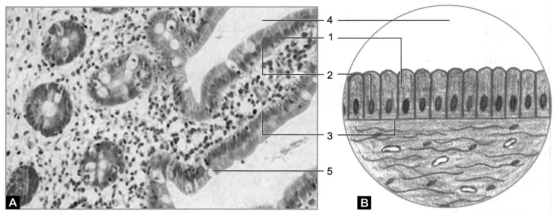

**Fig. 4.4A, B:** Simple columnar epithelium (1), (A) micrograph with goblet cells (5), (B) sketch showing oval nucleus (2), lumen (4) and the basement membrane (3)

the respiratory tract and ovum in the uterine cavity.

d. **Pseudostratified columnar epithelium:** In this epithelium, epithelial cells give the false appearance of stratification. The cells vary in height and only tall cells reach the lumen. Tall cells are broader at their apex and narrow at their base, while small cells are broad at the base and narrow at apex (Fig. 4.5A, B). Small cells probably work as stem cells to replace the lost tall cells. Nuclei are oval and always lie in the broader part of the cell, so the nuclei lie at different levels and epithelium looks stratified. All cells rest on the basement membrane. The epithelium may contain goblet cells or it may have cilia or it may be non-ciliated. At some sites, this epithelium may exhibit stereocilia.

i. *Locations:* Ciliated epithelium is present in most part of the upper respiratory tract. Non-ciliated epithelium mainly lines male urethra (membranous and spongy), ductus deferens, and some parts of the auditory tube. Pseudostratified

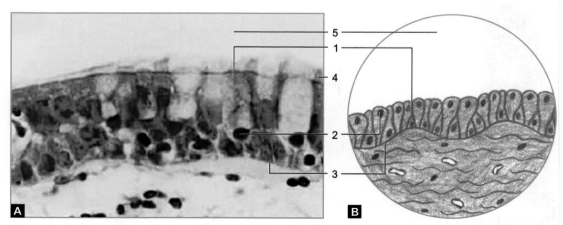

**Fig. 4.5A, B:** Pseudostratified columnar epithelium (1), (A) micrograph of trachea, (B) sketch. Nucleus (2), basement membrane (3), cilia (4) and lumen (5) are clearly visible

epithelium with stereocilia is present in the epididymis.

ii. *Functions:* This epithelium mainly participates in secretion, protection, and absorption.

## B. Stratified or Compound Epithelium

In this epithelium, epithelial cells are arranged in two or more cells thick layer. Except for cells in the basal layer, the cells of stratified epithelium are not in contact with the basement membrane. These are of four types:

a. **Stratified squamous epithelium:** In this epithelium, 3–6 layers of epithelial cells are present. The cells in the deepest layer (basal layer) are cuboidal or columnar in shape. Above this lie 3–4 layers of polyhedral cells. Superficial cells are flat and are continuously sloughed and replaced by cells in the basal layer. Typically, these cells are held together by numerous desmosomes to form strong cellular sheets, which provide protection to underlying tissues against mechanical, microbial, and chemical damage.

This epithelium is further having two types:

i. *Stratified squamous keratinized (cornified):* In this epithelium, epithelial cells of the superficial layer die and lose their nuclei

(Fig. 4.6A, B). These superficial cells are filled with a tough protein called keratin. Keratinized epithelium mainly covers the dry surfaces.

- *Locations:* This epithelium is present in the epidermis of the skin, mucocutaneous junctions of the lips, distal anal canal, outer surface of the tympanic membrane and tip of filiform papillae.
- *Functions:* This epithelium mainly provides protection to the underlying structures. Keratin present in the superficial cells also prevents dehydration of underlying tissues.

ii. *Stratified squamous nonkeratinized:* The superficial cells are live and even nuclei are present in these cells (Fig. 4.7A, B). This epithelium is present on the surfaces which remain moist.

- *Location:* This epithelium is present in the lining of the mouth, esophagus, tongue, vagina, conjunctiva, lacrimal canaliculi, parts of anal canal, external acoustic meatus, eyelids (inner surfaces) and part of the epiglottis.
- *Functions:* This epithelium mainly provides protection to the underlying structures.

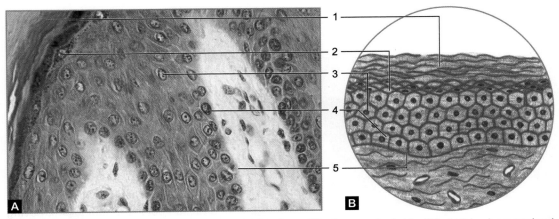

**Fig. 4.6A, B:** Stratified squamous keratinized epithelium, (A) micrograph of skin, (B) sketch, characterized by keratin layers (1) at the top. Squamous cells (2), polyhedral cells (3), basal cuboidal cells (4) are resting on the basement membrane (5)

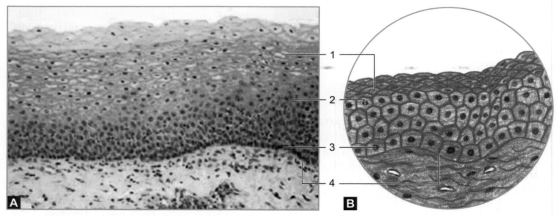

**Fig. 4.7A, B:** Stratified squamous nonkeratinized epithelium of the esophagus, (A) micrograph, (B) sketch, illustrating flat cells (1), polyhedral cells (2), basal cuboidal cells (3) and the basement membrane (4)

Stratified squamous nonkeratinized epithelium even lines some parts of the oral cavity, but the epithelium is considerably thicker and due to considerable abrasion even topmost layer of superficial cells become partially keratinized. This type of epithelium is known as para-keratinized epithelium.

b. **Stratified cuboidal epithelium:** In this epithelium two or more layers of cuboidal cells are present (Fig. 4.8).

i. *Locations:* This epithelium is present in the large ducts of sweat, mammary, and salivary glands.
ii. *Functions:* This epithelium mainly participates in secretion and absorption.

c. **Stratified columnar epithelium:** In this epithelium, basal cells are cuboidal or columnar, while the superficial cells are columnar (Fig. 4.9).

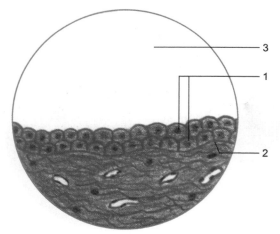

**Fig. 4.8:** Stratified cuboidal epithelium, having two layers of cuboidal cells (1), the basement membrane (2) and lumen (3)

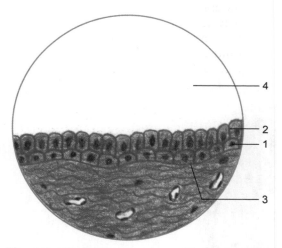

**Fig. 4.9:** Stratified columnar epithelium, having basal layer of cuboidal cells (1), superficial layer of columnar cells (2), the basement membrane (3) and lumen (4)

i. *Locations:* This epithelium is present in the larger ducts of some glands, and fornix of the conjunctiva of the eye.

ii. *Functions:* This epithelium mainly participates in secretion and absorption.

d. **Transitional epithelium (urothelium):** In this epithelium, 4–6 layers of epithelial cells are present. The cells of the deepest layer are cuboidal or columnar in shape and lie on the basement membrane. Above this lie 2–3 layers of polyhedral cells. Superficial cells are transitory when under no tension cells are dome (umbrella) shaped (Fig. 4.10A, B) and under tension superficial cells become flattened. Cells are firmly connected by numerous desmosomes.

i. *Locations:* This epithelium is present in the urinary tract from renal calyces, ureters, urinary bladder to the proximal part of the urethra.

ii. *Functions:* This epithelium allows distension of the urinary tract during urine accumulation and their contraction during emptying process. In addition, the epithelium forms a protective barrier between the cytotoxic effects of urine in the bladder and the underlying tissue fluids.

## GLANDULAR EPITHELIUM

These secretory epithelial cells are derived from invaginations of epithelial cells into the underlying connective tissue. Proteins (pancreas), lipids (sebaceous glands) or complexes of carbohydrates and proteins (salivary glands) are produced, stored and secreted by these epithelial cells. Cells of mammary glands secrete all three substances. Cells of some glands, such as sweat glands, secrete mostly water and electrolytes.

Glands are classified into four types on the basis of their secretory nature:

### A. Exocrine Glands

These glands secrete their products onto the apical surface through ducts.

### B. Endocrine Glands

These are ductless glands, and release their products (hormones) directly into the vascular system (Fig. 4.11A), which even act on distant organs.

### C. Paracrine Glands

These glands are similar to endocrine glands but secrete into the local extracellular space and secretions reach target cells by diffusion (Fig. 4.11B), e.g. enteroendocrine cells of the GIT.

### D. Mixed Glands

These glands have both exocrine and endocrine secretion.

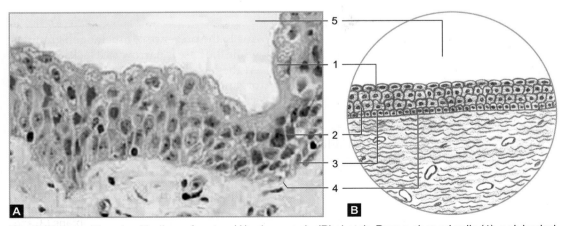

**Fig. 4.10:** Transitional epithelium of ureter, (A) micrograph, (B) sketch. Dome-shaped cells (1), polyhedral cells (2), cuboidal cells (3), rest on the basement membrane (4). Lumen (5) is shown as blank space

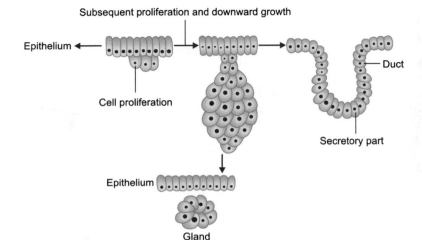

Schematic diagram showing the development of glands

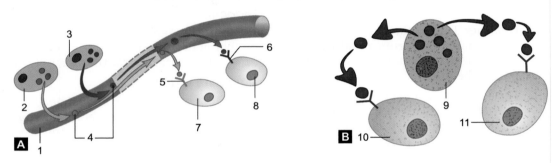

**Fig. 4.11:** Schematic diagram showing (A) endocrine gland pouring their secretion into the blood capillary (1), (B) paracrine gland secrete into the local extracellular space. Endocrine cell A (2), endocrine cell B (3), hormone (4), receptor A (5), receptor B (6), target cell A (7), target cell B (8), signaling cell (9), target cell X (10) and target cell Y (11)

## Classification of Exocrine Glands

The exocrine glands are classified on the basis of number of cells, the nature and mechanism of secretion.

### A. Number of Secretory Cells

a. **Unicellular glands:** In these glands, secretory element is formed of a single cell, which is present in between the other non-secretory cells, e.g. Goblet cells (Fig. 4.12 A, B).

#### Goblet cells

These mucus secreting glands are named so because of their shape like a glass or chalice. They are distended at their apex

due to the presence of mucinogen granules, while the base is narrow as it lacks granules. At the base lie flattened nucleus and other organelles involved in mucinogen synthesis. Their free border bears a few microvilli. Cytoplasm is packed with rER and a few mitochondria are also present. A prominent Golgi apparatus is present in the supranuclear region (Fig. 4.12C).

The protein component of mucinogen is synthesized by rER and then it is passed to the Golgi apparatus where it gets combined with carbohydrate. Finally, it is packaged into membrane-bound secretory granules

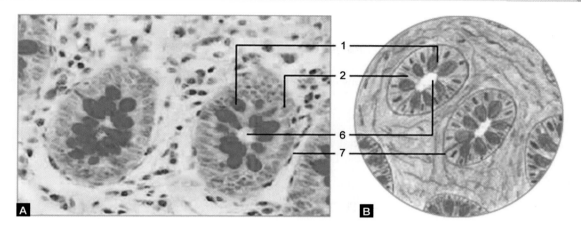

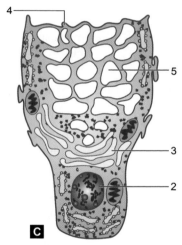

**Fig. 4.12:** Goblet cells (A) micrograph stained by PAS+ Haematoxylin, (B) sketch of PAS+ Haematoxylin stain, (C) fine structure. Goblet cell (1) secrete mucin, which stains magenta in PAS. Nucleus (2), Golgi apparatus (3), microvilli (4), secretory vesicles containing mucus (5), lumen (6), and basement membrane (7)

containing mucinogen. When mucinogen is released by exocytosis, it combines with water to form viscid secretion, called mucus. Goblet cells look empty at their apex by H&E stain, as the mucus gets washed off during tissue processing. Mucinogen granules of Goblet cells can be demonstrated by PAS stain, as carbohydrates look magenta by PAS stain (Fig. 4.12A, B).

i. *Locations:* These cells are present in the intestine and respiratory tract.

ii. *Functions:* These cells produce mucus whose main function is protection and lubrication. These cells also play a role in the immune defense. These cells endocytose IgA secreted by B lymphocytes present in the underlying connective tissue and then discharge them to the surface.

b. **Multicellular glands:** In these glands, secretory element is formed by tubular invaginations from the epithelial surface.

The end piece of the invagination is the secretory element, while the remaining part of the invagination which connects the secretory element to the surface serves as a duct (Fig. 4.13), e.g. surface mucous cells of the stomach and lacrimal gland.

### B. Nature of Secretion

a. **Serous glands:** Cells are pyramidal with a centrally placed rounded nucleus. Lumen is so small that it is hardly visible. Apical cytoplasm is acidophilic due to the secretory zymogen granules and basal cytoplasm is basophilic due to the rER and ribosomes (Fig. 4.14 A). These cells secrete a watery secretion rich in proteins. The lateral cell boundaries are difficult to observe in serous cells, e.g. pancreas and parotid gland.

b. **Mucous glands:** Cells are cuboidal or columnar with a basally placed flattened nucleus. These cells secrete mucus, which is a mixture of glycoproteins. Cytoplasm has an empty, frothy appearance with H&E stain, as mucus gets washed off during tissue processing (Fig. 4.14 B). Lumen is large and can be seen clearly. The lateral cell boundaries are clearly delineated, e.g. sublingual gland.

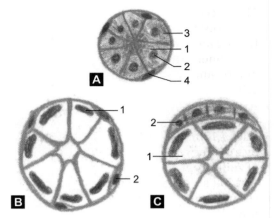

**Fig. 4.14:** (A) Showing single serous acini with apical zymogen granules (1), central nucleus (2), basal basophilic cytoplasm (3) and myoepithelial cells (4)
**Fig. 4.14:** (B) Mucous acini. Flattened nucleus (1) and myoepithelial cell (2) are the characteristic features
**Fig. 4.14:** (C) Illustrates mucous acini (1) capped by half serous acini known as serous demilune (2)

c. **Mixed glands:** Serous and mucous both types of cells are present. Along with these some of the mucous cells may have a cap of serous cells; they are called serous demilunes or crescents of Giannuzzi, or crescents of Heidenhain (Fig. 4.14 C). Small canaliculus from the serous demilune passes between the mucous cells to open into the lumen. Recent studies indicate that the presence of demilune is an artifact of fixation (use of formalin). Due to fixation serous cells swell and they burst out of their position. After sectioning, the cells resembled the common demilune shape. When samples were preserved by quick-freezing in liquid nitrogen and then fixed with osmium tetroxide in acetone, demilunes were not present, e.g. submandibular gland.

For comparison between serous and mucous acini, *see* Table 5 given in Appendix I.

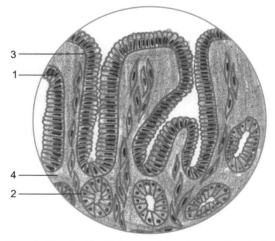

**Fig. 4.13:** Multicellular gastric glands of pyloric region. Nucleus (1), gastric glands (2), basement membrane (3) and lamina propria (4) are seen in the section

### C. Mechanism of Secretion

a. **Merocrine (eccrine) glands:** Secretory granules leave the cell by exocytosis with no loss of other cellular material (Fig. 4.15A).

This mechanism is used by both exocrine and endocrine glands, e.g. digestive enzymes from pancreatic acinar cells, a protein component of milk from the mammary gland, and insulin from pancreatic islet cells.

b. **Apocrine glands:** Secretory vesicles leave the cell with small amount of cytoplasm (Fig. 4.15B). This mechanism is used only by exocrine glands, e.g. the lipid component of milk from the mammary gland, ciliary or Moll's glands (present in eyelids), the ceruminous glands and Clara cells of the lung.

c. **Holocrine glands:** The secretory products accumulate within the cells of the gland itself. These cells then died by programmed cell death or apoptosis. Secretory products as well as cell debris are discharged into the lumen of the glands (Fig. 4.15C). This mechanism is used by exocrine glands only. e.g. sebaceous glands and tarsal (Meibomian) glands of the eyelids.

## D. Shape of Secretory Units

When all secretory cells release their products into a single duct, the gland is known as simple, if the duct system is present, then the gland is known as compound. In simple as well as in compound glands, secretory units may be in the form of a tubule or alveoli. The tubule may be straight, coiled or branched.

a. **Simple straight tubular (Fig. 4.16A):** For example, intestinal glands of Lieberkühn

b. **Simple coiled tubular (Fig. 4.16B):** For example, sweat glands

c. **Simple branched tubular (Fig. 4.16C):** For example, fundic glands of the stomach

d. **Simple alveolar (Fig. 4.16D):** For example, mucus secreting glands of the penile urethra

e. **Simple branched alveolar:** For example, tarsal glands of the eyelids

f. **Simple tubuloalveolar:** For example, minor salivary glands located in the oral cavity

g. **Compound branched tubular (Fig. 4.16E):** For example, Brunner's gland

h. **Compound branched tubuloalveolar (Fig. 4.16F):** For example, submandibular gland

i. **Compound branched alveolar (Fig. 4.16G):** For example, mammary gland.

## EPITHELIAL CELL POLARITY

Most of the epithelial cells display functional and morphological polarity. The cells have three surface domains: Lateral domain, apical domain, and a basal domain. Each domain has some surface modifications or specializations according to the function. Lateral domain represents the membrane present between the adjacent cells. Apical domain is directed

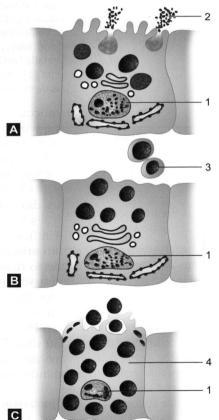

**Fig. 4.15:** Schematic diagram showing different mechanisms of secretion. (A) Merocrine, (B) apocrine, (C) holocrine. Nucleus (1), secretory granules (2), secretory vesicles with small amount of cytoplasm (3), disintegrated cell (4)

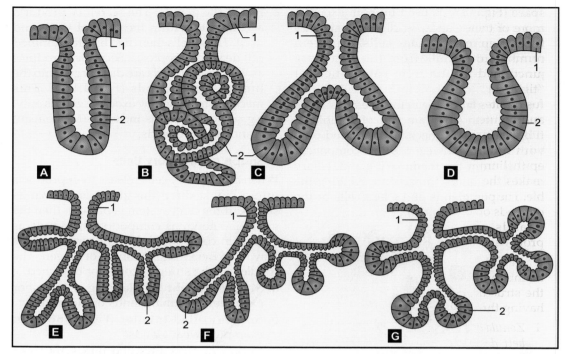

**Fig. 4.16:** Schematic diagram showing different types of glands on the basis of the shape of their secretory unit (A) simple straight tubular, (B) simple coiled tubular, (C) simple branched tubular, (D) simple alveolar, (E) compound branched tubular, (F) compound branched tubuloalveolar, (G) compound branched alveolar. Duct (1), secretory unit (2)

towards the lumen or exterior surface. Basal domain is in contact with the basement membrane.

## A. Lateral Domain

The lateral domain of epithelial cells contains specialized junctions or intercellular links. These links provide adhesion between cells and even restrict movement of materials into and out of the lumen. They are of three types:

a. Tight or occluding junctions
b. Adhering or anchoring junctions
c. Gap or communicating junctions

Some terms are used in conjunction with these three types, according to the shape of the junction. A junction that extends like a belt around the entire boundary of the cell is known as zonula. Instead of this, if the junction is only a strip or a ribbon, it is known

as fascia. If the junction is small, circular, and spot like, it is known as the macula.

a. **Tight junctions (zonula occludens):** These junctions are located near the apical parts of cells in the form of circumferential belt. These junctions are impermeable and prevent the diffusion of material across an epithelium through the intercellular space (paracellular pathway). They mainly maintain the separation of the two tissue compartments by limiting the movements of water and other molecules through the intercellular space. The outer leaflets of the cell membrane of two adjoining cells fuse at various points, giving rise to a pentalaminar sheet. Strands of transmembrane junctional proteins (claudins and occludins) of cells attached them directly to one another, thus sealing off the intercellular space (Fig. 4.17A). The presence of one or more of these fusion sites depends on the type of epithelium. Depending upon the numbers of these fusion sites the tight junctions have been classified either as "tight" or "leaky". Epithelium with a few fusion sites are partially permeable to water and solutes such as epithelium of renal tubules in comparison to the epithelium with numerous fusion sites such as the epithelium of the urinary bladder, which makes the intercellular region impermeable. The permeability of tight junctions also depends on the complexity and number of strands of transmembrane junctional proteins.

b. **Adhering junctions:** These junctions maintain cell-cell adherence and reinforce the structural integrity. These are further having three types:

  i. *Zonula adherens (intermediate junctions or belt desmosome):* These junctions are located just below the zonula occludens and completely surround the cell. The intercellular space of 15–20 nm between the plasma membranes of two adjacent cells is occupied by the extracellular portions of cadherins (mainly E-cadherins). These cadherins are transmembrane linker glycoprotein, which functions in the presence of $Ca^{+2}$. Cadherins of one cell form bond with the adjacent cell. Bundles of actin filaments run parallel to and along the cytoplasmic aspect of the cell membrane. The actin filaments are attached to each other and also linked via anchor proteins (catenin, vinculin, and α-actinin) to the cytoplasmic side of cadherins (Fig. 4.17B). So, these junctions not only join the plasma membranes of adjacent cells, but also link their cytoskeleton.

  ii. *Fascia adherens:* These junctions are similar to zonula adherens, but instead of being a circumferential belt, these are like ribbons. Cardiac muscle cells are joined to each other at their terminal end by a combination of fascia adherens and macula adherens.

  iii. *Macula adherens (desmosomes):* These junctions are in the form of randomly distributed spots over the lateral surface of cells. They provide strong adhesion between the cells and reinforce the structural integrity. Plasma membranes of adjacent cells in this region are very straight and intercellular space is wider (up to 30 nm). On the cytoplasmic side of the membrane of each cell lies a circular attachment plaque, called desmosomal attachment plaque. This plaque is made up of intracellular attachment proteins, mainly desmoplakins and plakoglobins, which are capable of attaching the intermediate filaments. Groups of intermediate filaments are inserted into the attachment plaque, which makes a hairpin turn, and then extend back out into the cytoplasm (Fig. 4.17C). In the region of the attachment plaques, the intercellular space contains filamentous materials of transmembrane linker glycoproteins of the cadherin family. Desmosomes are particularly numerous in epithelium that is subjected to abrasion and physical stress, such as stratified squamous keratinized epithelium.

c. **Gap junctions (nexus or communicating junctions):** These junctions permit the intercellular exchange of molecules with small (less than 1.5 nm) diameters. Certain molecules or ions which are mediating signal transduction move rapidly through gap junctions to allow the cells to act in a synchronized manner rather than as independent units, such as in the heart these gap junctions help in rhythmic contraction. These are broad patches where the plasma membrane comes close to each other leaving a narrow gap. These patches are composed of an ordered arrangement of subunits called connexons, which extend

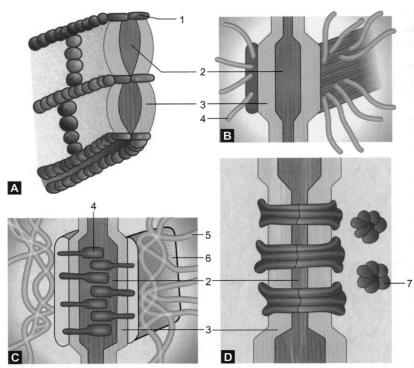

**Fig. 4.17:** Schematic diagram showing specialized junctions present on the lateral domain of the epithelial cells, (A) tight junction, (B) zonula adherens, (C) macula adherens, (D) gap junction. Claudins and occludins (1), intercellular space (2), cell membrane (3), cadherins (4), intermediate filaments (5), attachment plaque (6) and connexons (7)

beyond the cell surface into the gap to keep the opposing plasma membranes approximately 2 nm apart. Each connexon is made up of six transmembrane proteins, known as connexins (Fig. 4.17D). Gap junctions are found in nearly all tissues of the body except skeletal muscle and motile cells such as sperms and erythrocytes.

Cancer cells generally do not have the gap junction. This can explain the uncontrolled growth of cancer cells as the cells cannot communicate their mitotic activity to each other.

### Junctional Complex (Terminal Bar)

It consists of the zonula occludens, zonula adherens, and desmosomes. This complex binds the cell together and controls the passage of materials between them. These structures cannot be determined as separate structures by the light microscope, so they appear as a single, bar-shaped, dark region at the apical regions of adjacent cells (Fig. 4.18).

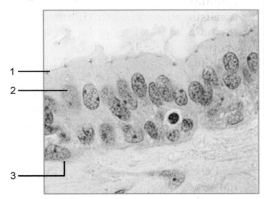

**Fig. 4.18:** Terminal bar (1) present in the epithelium of the epididymis. Nucleus (2) and basement membrane (3)

These can be seen clearly in the apical regions of simple columnar epithelium of the gastro-intestinal tract.

## B. Apical Domain

The apical domain of many epithelial cells contains specialized structures such as cilia, microvilli, and stereocilia which increase the surface area of the cell and move substances or particles stuck to the epithelium. The apical surface of luminal epithelial cells also exhibits nonadhesive property, even in the smallest tubules, such as the apical surface of the small intestine is coated with glycocalyx, which makes the apical surface nonadhesive.

a. **Cilia:** These cylindrical processes are present on the surface of many epithelial cells. They are hair like extensions of the apical plasma membrane containing a core of microtubules, called axoneme. They are of two types:

  i. *Motile cilia:* These cilia are 5–10 µm in length and 0.2 µm in diameter. The axoneme consists of uniformly spaced nine doublet microtubules around two singlet central microtubules (9+2 arrangement). Central singlet microtubules are separated from each other, circular in cross section, and consist of 13 protofilaments. Each of the nine doublets is composed of two subunits. Subunit A consists of 13 tubulin protofilaments and circular in cross section. Subunit B consists of 10 tubulin protofilaments, forms an incomplete circle in cross section, and shares the remaining protofilaments with subunit A. Radial spokes project from subunit A of each doublet inward toward the central sheath surrounding the two singlets. Nexin (an elastic protein) connects the nine doublet microtubules. Each doublet has short arms that consist of dynein ATPase, which splits ATP to provide movement of cilia. Dynein arms extend from the A subunit and interact with B subunit of adjacent doublets, so that

they slide past one another (Fig. 4.19A). At the base of each cilium is a basal body that consists of nine triplet microtubules (Fig. 4.19B) and the central microtubules are absent (9 + 0 arrangement).

These cilia are mainly present on the epithelium which participates in the transportation of secretions or cells or foreign particles on the surface such as in the respiratory system and female reproductive system. Cilia present in respiratory tract move mucus and trapped particulate material toward the oropharynx, where it may be swallowed or expectorated. In the oviduct, cilia transport the fertilized ovum toward the uterus. In the ventricles of the brain, the cilia of ependymal cells move the cerebrospinal fluid. Cilia have a coor-dinated rapid back-and-forth move-ment. The ciliary movement consists of two successive phases: Effective stroke and recovery stroke. The dynein arms of A microtubule move and it forms a temporary connection with adjacent B microtubule (required energy is gene-rated by ATP). Thus the doublet slides

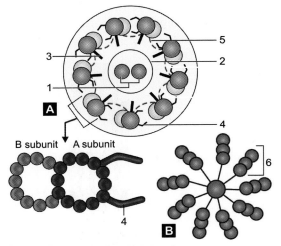

**Fig. 4.19:** Schematic diagram showing a section of (A) cilia, (B) basal body. The central pair of tubules (1), central sheath (2), radial spokes (3), dynein arm (4), nexin (5), triplet microtubules (6)

over each other slightly and cilium which normally remains rigid exhibits a rapid forward movement, called effective stroke. At the same time, the nexin links and radial spokes collect the energy to bring the cilium back to its normal position, called recovery stroke. Such waves of strokes progress in the same direction and affect the adjacent cilia one after another.

ii. *Non-motile cilia:* These are present on most mammalian cells as solitary projection and called primary or sensory cilium. The cilium is 2–3 μm in length and 0.2 μm in diameter. Each cilium consists of nine doublet microtubules and the central microtubules are absent (9 + 0 arrangement). The cilium is non-motile as it is lacking in microtubule associated motor proteins. These cilia work as sensors for mechanical and chemical signals. These cilia are present in epithelial cells of rete-testis, epithelium of bile duct, retinal rods and in vestibular hair cells of the ear. These cilia have no active movements and they only bend because of the flow of fluid.

b. **Microvilli:** These are finger-like cytoplasmic processes, enclosing a core of cytoplasm and are relatively non-motile. The lengths of these processes are 0.5–1 μm and width is 0.08 μm. Each microvillus contains a core of 25 to 30 actin filaments. These filaments are attached to villin at its tip and extend down into the apical cytoplasm (Fig. 4.20A). Here, they interact with a horizontal network of actin filaments, known as terminal web. Terminal web lies just below the base of microvilli and attached to the plasma membrane by spectrin molecules. In some epithelial cells microvilli are arranged regularly and appear as a thickened border on the epithelium, which is known as striated border such as in small and large intestines. In contrast, in some epithelium they are irregularly arranged and appear as brush border, e.g. gall bladder and proximal convoluted tubules. Microvilli are mainly present in the absorptive cells, as they increase the surface area available for absorption.

For comparison between cilia and microvilli, *see* Table 6 given in Appendix I.

c. **Stereocilia:** These are unusually long non-motile microvilli, made up of actin filaments. Erzin, a plasma membrane associated molecule, attaches the actin filaments to the

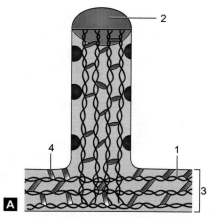
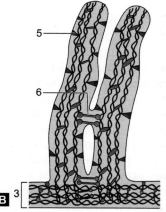

**Fig. 4.20:** Schematic diagram showing fine structure of (A) microvilli, (B) stereocilia. Actin filaments (1), villin (2), terminal web (3), spectrin molecules (4), erzin (5) and α-actinin (6)

plasma membrane. Actin filaments present in the apical cytoplasm and at the stem of the stereocilia are attached to the cross bridges formed by α-actinin (Fig. 4.20B). The villin is absent in the tip of stereocilia. Stereocilia present in the epididymis and vas deferens increase the surface area of the cell for absorption. Stereocilia present in sensory hair cells of ear act as sensory receptors.

For comparison between microvilli and stereocilia, *see* Table 7 given in Appendix I.

d. **Flagella:** These are long thin, motile and whip-like extension. Each male gamete possesses a single flagellum of 70 μm long. Structurally, it is similar to cilia, but the movements of flagella are different from cilia. In a flagellum, the movements start at the base. The part of the flagellum, which is near to the base turns in one direction, which is followed by turning of following parts in opposite directions, so that a wave-like motion of the flagellum is generated.

e. **Glycocalyx:** It is composed of carbohydrate chains that are covalently attached to membrane proteins and/or phospholipid molecules. It varies in appearance (fuzziness) and thickness (up to 45 nm). It is found on the apical portion of microvilli within the digestive tract, especially within the small intestine.

 i. *Functions:*
  • It forms a covering over the plasma membrane and protects it from any external injury.
  • It increases the surface area for absorption and includes enzymes secreted by the absorptive cells that are essential for the final steps of digestion of proteins and sugars.
  • It is used by the body as a type of identification to distinguish between its own healthy cells and transplanted

tissues, diseased cells, and invading organisms. Only identical twins have chemically identical glycocalyx, everyone else is unique.
  • It enables cells to adhere to each other and also guides the movement of cells during embryonic development.

## C. Basal Domain

The basal domain of epithelial cells has three important structures: Basement membrane, basal infoldings, and hemidesmosomes.

a. **Basement membrane:** Epithelial cells rest on a non-cellular basement membrane, which separates it from underlying connective tissue. It is composed of a basal lamina and a reticular lamina (Fig. 4.21). The basal lamina originates from the epithelial cells and consists of an electron-lucent lamina lucida (lamina rara) and an electron-dense lamina densa. Lamina lucida contains laminin glycoprotein and lamina densa is composed of type IV collagen fibers. The reticular lamina originates from the fibroblasts located in the underlying connective tissue and contains fibronectin.

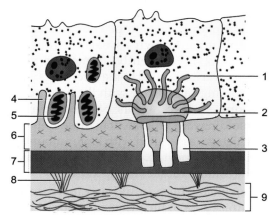

**Fig. 4.21:** Schematic diagram showing structures present on the basal domain of epithelial cells. Keratin filaments (1), attachment plaque (2), integrins protein (3), basal infolding (4), mitochondria (5), lamina lucida (6), lamina densa (7), reticular lamina (8) and anchoring fibrils (9)

By H&E staining basement membrane cannot be distinguished from the underlying connective tissue. To see the basement membrane PAS stain is used, as it stains glycoproteins. With PAS stain, it appears as a well-defined magenta layer. In the alveoli of the lungs and in glomeruli of kidney two epithelial layers adjoin one another through the basal lamina, so it is thickened in comparison to the other places.

*Functions:*

- This membrane provides support to epithelial cells and also forms a selective barrier that regulates the exchange of macromolecules between epithelium and the underlying connective tissue.

- This membrane may exert instructive effects on adjacent tissues, so influence cell polarity, rate of cell division, and influence cellular metabolism.

- This membrane is used by epithelial cells, nerves, and muscle cells as scaffolding during regeneration or wound healing.

b. **Basal infoldings:** In some epithelial cells, basal plasma membrane shows extensive infoldings, known as basal infoldings (Fig. 4.21). Frequently, numerous mitochondria lie parallel to the infoldings; such infoldings are visible with the light microscope and known as basal striations. Infoldings are prominent in those epithelia, which are associated with large amounts of fluid transport, e.g. proximal and distal convoluted tubules of the kidneys.

*Function:* These infoldings increase the surface area of the plasma membrane.

c. **Hemidesmosomes:** These are half of the desmosomes. They are located at the base of the cells. Hemidesmosomes bind the epithelial cells to the subjacent basal lamina. The transmembrane proteins of hemidesmosomes are of integrins instead of cadherin (desmosomes). Attachment plaques (Fig. 4.21) are made up of desmoplakins, but in contrast to desomosomes keratin filaments (tonofilaments) are inserted into these plaques. These filaments allow these junctions to link the cytoskeleton with the extracellular matrix.

## RENEWAL OF EPITHELIAL CELLS

Most of the epithelial cells have a long life span; however, some epithelial cells continuously renewed. This renewal depends on their location and function. Cells lining the small intestine are replaced within 4 to 6 days by regenerative cells in the base of the crypts. The new cells then migrate to the tips of the villi, undergo apoptosis, and are sloughed.

In stratified squamous keratinized epithelium, mitosis takes place within the germinal layer, closest to the basal lamina, which contains the stem cells. Then the cells move towards apical surface, get keratinized and finally, sloughed off. This process is known as terminal differentiation and it takes 28 days.

**Metaplasia:** It is a reversible change in which one adult cell type (epithelial or mesenchymal) is replaced by another adult cell type. This is actually cellular adaptation, in which, cells sensitive to a particular stress are replaced by other cell types that are better able to withstand the adverse environment. It occurs as a response to chronic physical or chemical irritation, such as cigarette smoking that causes the mucus-secreting ciliated simple columnar respiratory epithelial cells (lining the airways) to be replaced by simple squamous epithelium, or a stone in the bile duct that causes the replacement of the secretory columnar epithelium with simple squamous epithelium. If influences that induce metaplastic transformation are persistent, then they may induce cancer transformation in the metaplastic epithelium.

## Summary

| Number of cell layers | Type of cell | Functions | Locations |
|---|---|---|---|
| Simple (single layer) | Squamous | Active transport of fluids, passive transport of gases, and lubrication | Alveoli of the lungs, parietal layer of the Bowman's capsule, lining of the heart (endocardium), blood and lymphatic vessels (endothelium), and lining of pleural, pericardial, and peritoneal cavities (mesothelium) |
| | Cuboidal | Secretion, and absorption | Glands, ducts, distal tubules in the kidney, covering of the ovary, and lens capsule (inner surface) |
| | Columnar | Protection, secretion, and absorption | Ciliated—small bronchi, uterine tubes, and uterus. Non-ciliated—digestive tract (from the stomach to the anus) and gall bladder |
| | Pseudostratified | Protection, secretion, and absorption | Ciliated—most part of upper respiratory tract. Non-ciliated—male urethra (membranous and spongy), and ductus deferens |
| Stratified (multilayered) | Squamous keratinized | Protection | Epidermis of the skin, outer surface of the tympanic membrane, and tip of filiform papillae |
| | Squamous non-keratinized | Protection | Esophagus, tongue, vagina, and conjunctiva |
| | Cuboidal | Secretion, and absorption | Large ducts of sweat, mammary, and salivary glands |
| | Columnar | Secretion, and absorption | Larger ducts of some glands |
| | Transitional | Protection, and allows distention | Urinary tract from renal calyces, ureters, urinary bladder to the proximal part of the urethra |

## Surface modifications of epithelial cells

- **Cilia:** Composed of microtubules; helps in the transport of material across the epithelial surface (motile), acts as sensors for mechanical and chemical signals (non-motile).
- **Microvilli:** Composed of actin filaments; increase the surface area available for absorption.
- **Stereocilia:** Unusually long microvilli; increase the surface area for absorption, act as sensory receptors (in ear).
- **Tight junctions:** Composed of actin filaments and serve as impermeable barrier.
- **Adhering junctions:** Composed of actin filaments and provide mechanical stability.
- **Desmosomes:** Composed of intermediate filaments and help in cell-to-cell attachment.
- **Gap junctions:** Communicating junctions and permit passage of small molecules between neighboring cells.
- **Hemidesmosomes:** Half of the desmosomes and bind epithelial cells to the basal lamina.
- **Basement membrane:** Composed of basal lamina and reticular lamina; supports the epithelial cells and acts as selective barrier.
- **Basal infoldings:** Increase the surface area of the cell membrane.

### Self Assessment

1. Which of the following is a unicellular gland?
   a. Chief cell
   b. Parietal cell
   c. Goblet cell
   d. Myoepithelial cell

2. Which of the following is not a stratified epithelium?
   a. Transitional epithelium
   b. Stratified cuboidal epithelium
   c. Pseudostratified epithelium
   d. Stratified columnar epithelium

3. Which of the following organ is lined by Urothelium?
   a. Kidney
   b. Gall bladder
   c. Trachea
   d. Ureter

4. Microvilli are present on the cells which are involved in:
   a. Secretion
   b. Absorption
   c. Transportation
   d. Neurotransmission

5. Which of the following is a simple coiled tubular gland?
   a. Sweat gland
   b. Gastric gland
   c. Sebaceous gland
   d. Mammary gland

6. Cell junction which is present in the basal domain of cells is:
   a. Desmosome
   b. Tight junction
   c. Hemidesmosome
   d. Gap junction

7. Hair like processes which help in transportation is:
   a. Cilia
   b. Microvilli
   c. Stereocilia
   d. Flagella

8. Columnar epithelium with striated border is present in:
   a. Urinary bladder
   b. Lung alveoli
   c. Small intestine
   d. Large intestine

9. Which one is not a simple epithelium?
   a. Transitional epithelium
   b. Pseudostratified epithelium
   c. Simple columnar epithelium
   d. Simple cuboidal epitelium

10. Epithelium performs all functions EXCEPT:
    a. Protection
    b. Abrasion
    c. Secretion
    d. Absorption

### Answers

1. c,  2. c,  3. d,  4. b,  5. a,  6. c,  7. a,  8. c,  9. a,
10. b

# 5

# Connective Tissue

$C$onnective (supporting) tissue consists of individual cells scattered within an extracellular matrix (Fig. 5.1). Blood vessels and nerves travel through this tissue. Almost all of the connective tissue in the body is formed by mesoderm except in the head region where connective tissue is formed by aggregation of specific progenitor cells, called ectomesenchyme, which is derived from neural crest cells.

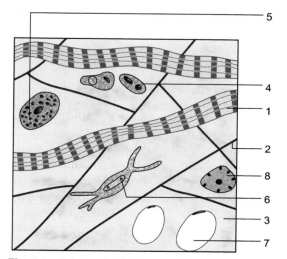

**Fig. 5.1:** Schematic diagram showing components of connective tissue. Collagen fiber (1), elastic fiber (2), ground substance (3), macrophage (4), mast cell (5), fibroblast (6), fat cell (7) and plasma cell (8)

## FUNCTIONS OF CONNECTIVE TISSUE

### A. Support

It provides shape and support to the body and also forms the stroma of the organs.

### B. Transport

It acts as a medium for exchange of nutrients and wastes between the blood and tissues.

### C. Storage

Adipocytes stores fat while ground substance stores water, ions, and inorganic materials.

### D. Repair

It helps in repair of damaged tissue.

### E. Defense

Cells present in it provide the protection against microorganisms.

For comparison between epithelium and connective tissue, *see* Table 8 given in Appendix I.

## EXTRACELLULAR MATRIX

In the matrix, ground substance and the fibers are present. The matrix provides consistency and internal support.

### A. Ground Substance

It is found in all cavities and clefts between the fibers and cells of connective tissues. It is colorless and transparent. It contains a high proportion of water, so it acts as a medium for the transfer of nutrients and waste materials between cells of connective tissue and the bloodstream. It is viscous, so acts as a lubricant and a barrier to the invasion of tissues by foreign agents. Ground substance is always lost during fixation and dehydration in H and E stained sections, so the fibers and cells are visible with empty background.

The ground substance is formed by a complex of anionic macromolecules (glyco-saminoglycans and proteoglycans) and multiadhesive glycoproteins (laminin, fibronectin, chondronectin, and osteonectin) that imparts strength and rigidity to the matrix by binding to receptor proteins (integrins) on the surface of cells and to the other matrix components. The proteoglycans are composed of a core protein associated with the four main glycosaminoglycans: dermatan sulfate, chondroitin sulfate, keratan sulfate, and heparan sulfate. Hyaluronic acid is also a glycosaminoglycans present in the connective tissue, but it is not associated with a core protein.

## B. Fibers

These are long, slender protein polymers present in different proportions in different types of connective tissue. These are synthesized by fibroblast cells and provide strength and support to the connective tissue. Fibers are of three types:

a. **Collagen fibers:** These fibers are found in all connective tissues. These fibers, mostly found in bundles, may be branched or anastomose with neighboring bundles. With H and E stain, collagen looks pink (eosinophilic) due to its positively charged side groups and with Masson's Trichome, it looks green or blue. Upon boiling, collagen fibers get dissolved and converted into gelatin (animal glue), so named collagen, which means "glue producing". With EM collagen fibers are composed of fine collagen fibrils, which exhibit a banding pattern, i.e. the fibrils have closely spaced transverse bands that repeat at every 68 nm distance. The collagen molecule

form, the collagen fibrils and it is composed of three polypeptide chains ($\alpha$ chains) bound together to form a right-handed triple helix. Throughout the body there are 28 types of collagen have been identified on the basis of the combinations of $\alpha$ chains. Collagen molecules are synthesized by the fibroblasts in a variety of tissues such as chondrocytes in cartilage, osteoblasts in bone, and pericytes in blood vessels. Additionally, type IV collagen of basement membrane is produced by the epithelial cells.

Although collagen fibers are flexible, yet have extremely high tensile strength. More than 80% of the collagen in the body is of types I, II, III and IV. Collagen I (most common) is found in the dermis of the skin, organs, bones, dentin, sclera, fascia, aponeurosis, and tendons. Collagen II is found in the hyaline and elastic cartilages. Collagen III is a major component of reticular fibers. Collagen IV is found in the basal lamina of epithelium, glomerulus of the kidney, and lens capsule.

**Birefringence** When a beam of light is thrown on collagen fibers, the light is split into beams that are refracted in different directions. This phenomenon is known as birefringence. This denotes the fact that each collagen fiber is made up of fine fibrils. Relaxed elastic fibers do not show this phenomenon, but when stretched they become birefringent.

b. **Elastic fibers:** These fibers are highly refractive and run singly, but present in bundles in ligamentum flava (connect the laminae of adjacent vertebrae). Fibers branch to form networks and also present in the form of fenestrated lamellae in some arterial wall. These are less widely distributed than collagen and are usually thinner than the collagen fibrils. These fibers are composed of elastin protein surrounded by a network of fibrillin microfibrils. If fibrillin is absent, then elastin is arranged in sheets or lamellae. Elastic fibers require special staining in order to be observed by light microscopy. The Verhoeff-Van Gieson (VVG) stain is commonly used to demonstrate elastic fibers. By this stain elastic fibers appear blue-black to black, while collagen fibers look red. With aldehyde fuchsin (Gomori) stain elastic fibers look purple to black. These fibers do not have a banding pattern like collagen fibers and are resistant to chemical treatment. Elastic fibers are mainly produced by fibroblasts. In the walls of large blood vessels elastic fibers are produced by the smooth muscle cells.

Elastic fibers can recoil elastically after being stretched, thus allow tissue to respond to stretch and distension. These fibers are present in the wall of aorta, lung and the ligamentum nuchae (runs from the external occipital protuberance to the tip of the spine of $C_7$ vertebrae).

c. **Reticular fibers:** These fibers are very delicate and form fine networks instead of thick bundles. Reticular fibers are composed of the type III collagen and are coated with glycoprotein. These fibers are PAS-positive, mainly due to their glycoprotein content. These fibers are not visible by H&E stain, but with silver impregnation looks black and because of their affinity for silver salts, these fibers are called argyrophilic. By silver salts thicker collagen fibers appear yellow or brown. Reticular fibers are mainly produced by the fibroblasts. The other cells that also produce these fibers are: Schwann cells present in the endoneurium, smooth muscle cells present in the blood vessels and the alimentary canal, and reticular cells in the lymphatic tissues.

Reticular fibers provide a supporting framework for the cellular constituents of various tissues and organs. Reticular fibers are particularly abundant in smooth muscle, endoneurium, and in the framework of hemopoietic organs (e.g. spleen, lymph nodes, and red bone marrow) and constitute a network around the cells of parenchymal organs (e.g. liver, and endocrine glands). These fibers are also present in the embryonic tissues and as the development progresses,

the fibers are gradually replaced by the stronger type I collagen fibers.

For comparison among collagen, elastic and reticular fibers, *see* Table 9 given in Appendix I.

## SYNTHESIS OF COLLAGEN FIBERS

Synthesis of collagen fibers by fibroblasts takes place in two different events (Fig. 5.2). These are:

### A. Intracellular Events

mRNA is formed in the nucleus and then move to the rER. With the help of mRNA, amino acids are arranged in sequence to form alpha polypeptide chains. In the rER, proline and lysine amino acids of these chains (vitamin C is required) are converted to hydroxyproline and hydroxylysine. The hydroxylysine then

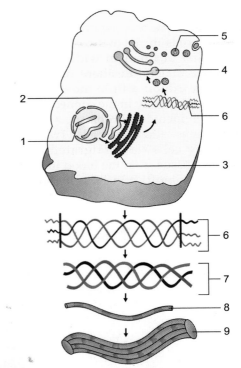

**Fig. 5.2:** Schematic diagram showing steps of synthesis of collagen fibers. DNA (1), mRNA (2), rER (3), Golgi apparatus (4), secretory vesicles (5), procollagen molecule (6), collagen molecule (7), collagen fibril (8) and collagen fiber (9)

joins to the sugar groups. Three polypeptide chains now form the helix, but the terminal ends of these chains remain uncoiled. This molecule is called procollagen, which is then transferred to the Golgi apparatus. In the Golgi apparatus, this procollagen is packaged into secretory vesicles. These vesicles then move to the plasma membrane and exocytosis of procollagen molecules takes place.

### B. Extracellular Events

Various enzymes (procollagen peptidase) secreted by fibroblasts act on uncoiled terminal parts and cleave it. After cleavage the remaining molecule is called collagen molecule, which is then aggregated to form collagen fibrils. These fibrils then assembled to form collagen fiber.

### CONNECTIVE TISSUE CELLS

These cells can be resident or wandering and often these cells are not present in contact with one another but remain widely dispersed within the matrix. Resident or fixed cells are stable, exhibit a little movements and remain permanently in the connective tissue. These cells include fibroblasts, adipocytes, macrophages, and mast cells. Transient or wandering cells have migrated into the connective tissue from the blood in response to specific stimuli. It includes lymphocytes, plasma cells, neutrophils, eosinophils, basophils, and monocytes.

### A. Fibroblasts

These are the predominant cells present in all types of connective tissues. These cells elaborate the precursors of collagen, and elastic fibers and also produce the amorphous ground substance. Two stages of activity (active and quiescent) are observed in these cells (Fig. 5.3A, B). Active fibroblasts are spindle-shaped (fusiform) cells with a few processes. These processes form the bulk of the cytoplasm and are usually difficult to distinguish in H & E stained sections as they blend with collagen fibers. The cytoplasm of these cells is basophilic and nucleus is large euchromatic, and oval. These cells often lie in close association with bundles of collagen fibers. Quiescent fibroblasts (fibrocyte) are small, flattened cells without any cell processes. Their cytoplasm is less basophilic and nucleus is comparatively small, heterochromatic, and flattened. Fibroblast cells may differentiate into other cell types (chondrocytes, osteoblasts, adipocytes) under certain conditions. These cells are very active in wound repair.

### B. Adipocytes

These cells are responsible for the synthesis, storage, and release of fat. The fat in adipocytes

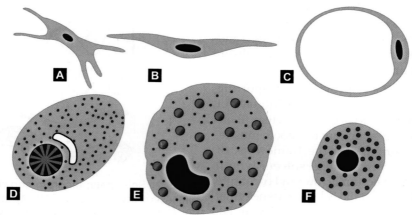

**Fig. 5.3:** Schematic diagram showing cells of connective tissue. (A) Fibroblast, (B) fibrocyte, (C) adipocyte, (D) mast cell, (E) macrophage and (F) plasma cell

is stored in the form of triglycerides, which are the most concentrated form of metabolic energy storage available in our body. In unilocular adipose tissue these cells contain a large lipid droplet (Fig. 5.3C), while in multilocular it contains many small lipid droplets. Multilocular adipocytes contain many more mitochondria but fewer free ribosomes than unilocular adipocytes. Although multilocular adipocytes lack rough ER, they do have smooth ER. In multilocular adipocytes, nucleus is spherical and centrally placed; while in the unilocular adipocytes, nucleus is flattened and peripherally placed. Adipocytes secrete a hormone called leptin, which decreases appetite and body weight. Once mature, fat cells do not divide, but they are comparatively long lived. New fat cells can develop from precursors that persist in adipose tissue.

By H & E stain, the cells look empty as the lipid is washed away by the chemicals like xylene and alcohal. Fat can be stained with Sudan III, which imparts these cells orange color.

## C. Mast Cells

These cells are oval or irregularly shaped connective tissue cells (Fig. 5.3D), between 7 and 20 μm in diameter. In these cells centrally placed, spherical nucleus is present and their cytoplasm is filled with coarse, deeply stained metachromatic granules (metachromasia is a property of certain molecules that changes the color of some basic aniline dyes, e.g. toluidine blue imparts a purple color instead of blue).

Mast cells mediate immediate (type I) hypersensitivity reactions (anaphylactic reactions) by releasing immune modulators. The molecules produced by mast cells act locally (paracrine secretion). Mast cells are particularly numerous near small blood vessels in the skin and mesenteries (perivascular mast cells) and in the connective tissue of the intestinal mucosa and in the lungs (mucosal mast cells). The granules of perivascular mast cells contain the anticoagulant heparin, while granules of mucosal mast cells contain tryptase.

Some secretory products of mast cells are always stored in the granules and they are released upon activation of mast cell. These are called preformed modulators such as tryptase, histamine, heparin, eosinophil chemotactic factor (ECF), and neutrophil chemotactic factor (NCF). Other secretory products are often absent in the resting mast cells, and they are produced and secreted only upon activation such as leukotriene C, tumor necrosis factor-α (TNF-α), and interleukins (IL-3, -4, -5, -6 and -8).

## D. Macrophages (Histiocytes)

These are the principal phagocytosing cells of the connective tissue. These cells process antigenic material before presenting it to the memory lymphocytes, so act as antigen presenting cells (APCs). These cells also secrete a variety of cytokines, which develop local and systemic immune responses. When these cells encounter a large foreign material, the cells coalesce with one another and form multinucleated cells, called foreign body giant cells. These cells also produce substances which participate in the process of healing of wounds. These cells originate in the bone marrow as monocytes; circulate in the bloodstream, then migrate into the connective tissue, where they mature into functional macrophages. Functional macrophages have an eccentric kidney-shaped nucleus (Fig. 5.3E), phagocytic vacuoles, lysosomes, and residual bodies. These residual bodies can be released by exocytosis or may remain in the macrophages, such as injected dyes in tattooing. In certain regions, macrophages have special names, e.g. Kupffer cells in the liver, microglial cells in the central nervous system, Langerhans cells of the epidermis, alveolar macrophages in lung, dendritic cells in lymphatic tissue and osteoclasts in bone.

With conventional staining, macrophages are very difficult to identify unless they show visible ingested material inside their cytoplasm, so they are stained by vital staining. If a colloidal dye such as trypan blue is injected into the loose connective tissue, these cells show the injected dye as accumulations in their cytoplasm.

### E. Plasma Cells

These cells are present in the connective tissue and lymphoid organs. These are oval-shaped cells with round, eccentrically located nucleus (Fig. 5.3F) and cytoplasm is basophilic due to large amounts of rough endoplasmic reticulum. The nuclear chromatin is mostly condensed and distributed like a cart-wheel or clock-face (Fig. 5.4). These cells are derived from B lymphocytes. These cells develop as a result of an immune response and secrete antibodies to provide humoral immunity.

### VARIETIES OF CONNECTIVE TISSUE

### A. Embryonic Connective Tissue

In this tissue, stellate shaped mesenchymal cells interconnected by slender cell processes are present in the amorphous matrix (Fig. 5.5A, B). Mesenchymal cells are characterized by an oval nucleus with prominent nucleoli and generally, the cells are pleuripotent. During development this tissue is present in the embryo and in the umbilical cord (Wharton's jelly) however, in adults, it is present in the dental pulp, the vitreous body of the eye, and

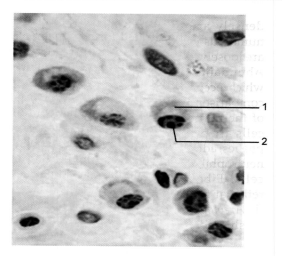

**Fig. 5.4:** Micrograph showing plasma cell (1) with condensed nuclear chromatin (2)

the nucleus pulposus of the intervertebral disc. Embryonic connective tissue gives rise to all adult connective tissue.

### B. Adult Connective Tissue

It is sub-divided on the basis of relative proportion of various cellular and extracellular components into two types: Loosely arranged and densely arranged.

a. **Loosely arranged tissue:** This tissue is more prevalent in the body in comparison to the

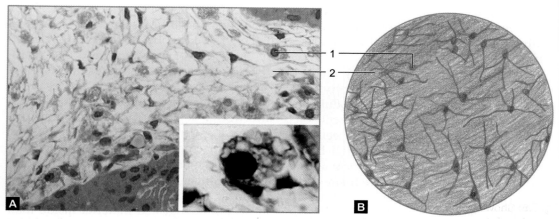

**Fig. 5.5:** Embryonic connective tissue having mesenchymal cells (1) in amorphous matrix (2), (A) micrograph of 60-day fetus (inset), mesenchymal cells at higher magnification, (B) sketch

densely arranged tissue. In this tissue, numerous cells are present, but the fibers are loosely arranged and a few in number. Abundant ground substance is present, which occupies more volume of tissue in comparison to fibers and allows diffusion of the nutrients and wastes. A variety of cells are present, like fibroblast, macrophages, adipocytes, lymphocyte, monocyte, neutrophil, undifferentiated cell, and mast cells. Fibers are collagen, elastic and reticular fibers. This tissue is present in:

i. *Areolar tissue:* In this tissue, spindle-shaped fibroblast cells, adipocytes,

macrophages, mast cells, and abundant ground substance is present. Elastic, fibers, reticular fibers and bundles of collagen fibers are present, but bundles of collagen fibers present here are thin and small in comparison to dense connective tissue (Fig. 5.6A, B, and C). This tissue is highly vascularized, and not very resistant to stress. Areolar tissue is flexible, so allows the tissue to move freely. This tissue works as a passage for the vessels and nerves. Areolar tissue is present in the mesentry, adventitial layer of blood vessels, and lamina propria of gut.

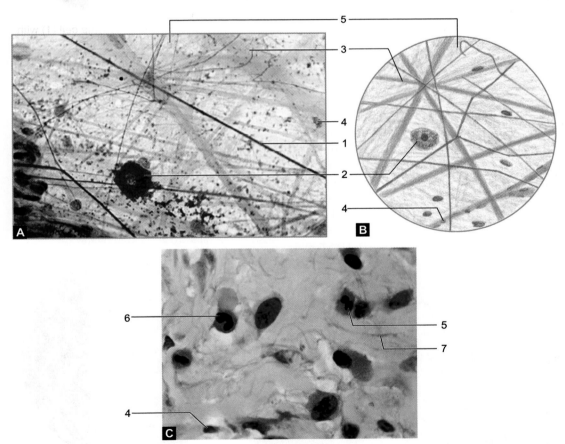

**Fig. 5.6:** Showing loose areolar tissue (A) micrograph of stained with aldehyde-fuchsin + light green stain, (B) sketch of stained with aldehyde-fuchsin + light green stain, (C) micrograph of stained with H and E stain. Aldehyde-fuchsin stains elastic fibers (1) and mast cells (2) as purple, while light green staining stains collagen fibers (3). Fibroblast nuclei (4), eosinophil (5), basophil (6), and pink collagen fibers (7)

ii. *Adipose tissue:* This tissue is honeycomb like in appearance. In this tissue, fat cells (adipocytes) are present. This tissue is of two types:

• **White/unilocular adipose tissue:** In this tissue, fat cells have a rim of cytoplasm around a single central lipid droplet. Flattened nucleus lies in the thickened part of the rim of the cytoplasm. Fat cell looks like signet ring in appearance. As lipid is removed by alcohal and xylene used in routine histology, so the fat cells appear vacuolated in the center (Fig. 5.7A, B). By the use of Sudan III stain fat appears orange in color. Fat cells are spherical when isolated, but are polyhedral in adipose tissue, where they are closely packed. This unilocular tissue is subdivided into incomplete lobules by a partition of connective tissue containing a rich vascular plexus and a network of nerves. Connective tissue contains a finely interwoven network of reticular fibers that supports individual fat cells and binds them together. Adipose tissue mainly stores energy and it also functions as a cushion at some sites (around kidneys and heart). This tissue

is found subcutaneously throughout the body (comprises 20–25% of total body weight) except over the eyelid, penis, scrotum and the entire auricle of the external ear (except for the lobule).

• **Brown/multilocular adipose tissue:** In this tissue, fat cells have a great number of lipid droplets of various sizes, numerous mitochondria and a spherical central nucleus (Fig. 5.8A, B). Fat cells are polygonal and smaller than fat cells of unilocular tissue. This tissue is brown in color due to both the large number of blood capillaries and the numerous mitochondria (containing cytochrome oxidases) in the cells. Brown adipose tissue is more in infants (also in hibernating animals) in comparison to the adults, and it is used to produce heat. The production of heat by brown adipose tissue is directly controlled by the sympathetic nervous system, which releases norepinephrine to promote hydrolysis of lipids. Brown adipose tissue is present in the axilla, between the shoulder blades, around the adrenal glands, in the inguinal region and in the region of the neck.

For comparison between white and brown adipose tissues, *see* Table 10 given in Appendix I.

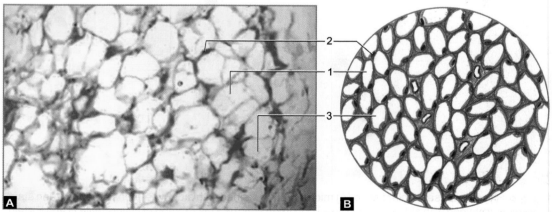

**Fig. 5.7:** White adipose tissue, (A) micrograph, (B) sketch showing single large lipid droplet (1) which compresses the nucleus (2) of adipocyte (3)

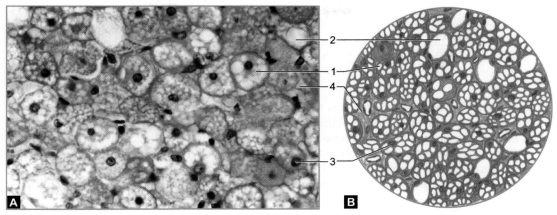

**Fig. 5.8:** Brown adipose tissue from cervix of human neonate, (A) micrograph, (B) sketch, showing multilocular adipose cells (1), but some of the cells are unilocular (2). Adipose nucleus (3), connective tissue (4)

iii. *Reticular tissue:* In this tissue, a very delicate supporting network of reticular (type III collagen) fibers along with reticular cells are present (Fig. 5.9A, B). This tissue is sponge like in appearance. Reticular cells resemble fibroblast and partially cover the reticular fibers as well as ground substance with their cytoplasmic processes. Reticular tissue is present in the liver, pancreas, bone marrow, adrenal glands, spleen, and lymph nodes.

b. **Densely arranged tissue:** In this tissue, cells are few in number, but the fibers are numerous and compactly arranged. Fibers are mainly larger caliber collagen fibers, which provide strength. Ground substance is minimal, so the tissue is poorly vascularized. This tissue is present in:

i. *Dense regular collagenous tissue:* In this tissue, parallel bundles of collagen fibers are present. In between the fibers fibroblast cells are present, which are elongated in the direction of the collagen

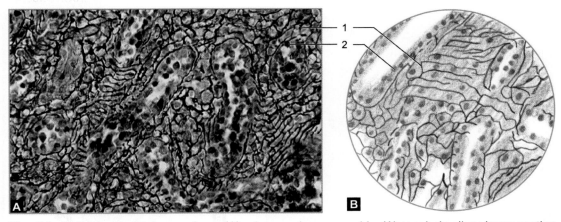

**Fig. 5.9:** Reticular tissue from spleen, (A) micrograph; prepared by Watanabe's silver impregnation technique, (B) sketch. Reticular fibers cannot be demonstrated by H and E stain, so silver impregnation is used and reticular fibers (1) are stained black. Lymphocytes (2) are also seen

fibers (Fig. 5.10A, B). This tissue is present in tendons, ligaments, stroma of the cornea and the aponeurosis of muscles. This tissue is adapted to withstand unidirectional pull transmitted along these fibers without stretching.

ii. *Dense regular elastic tissue:* In this tissue, coarse branched elastic fibers with a few collagen fibers are present. These fibers form a network and fibroblasts are scattered in the spaces present in this network. The elastic fibers are arranged parallel to form fenestrated membranes. This tissue provides flexible support, and reduces pressure on the walls of the blood vessels. This tissue is present in large blood vessels, ligamentum flava of the vertebral column, and the suspensory ligament of the penis.

iii. *Dense irregular tissue:* In this tissue, bundles of collagen fibers form a dense woven network. Among the collagen fibers, there is an extensive network of elastic fibers (Fig. 5.11A, B). This network

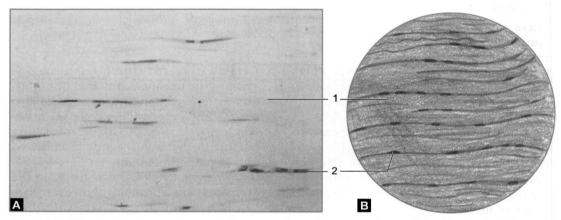

**Fig. 5.10:** Showing tendon made up of dense regular collagenous tissue, (A) micrograph, (B) sketch showing bundles of collagen fibers (1) with fibroblast nucleus (2)

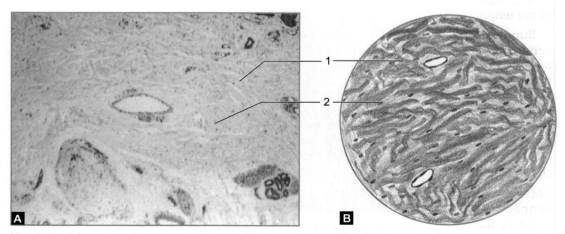

**Fig. 5.11:** Dense irregular connective tissue, (A) micrograph, (B) sketch with irregularly arranged bundles of collagen fibers (1) in between fibroblast nucleus (2) are also seen

facilitates the structure to withstand stress and strain in all directions. The most abundant cells are fibroblasts, which are present in between the bundles of collagen fibers. This tissue is present in the dermis and submucosa of the gut. It forms capsule and trabeculae of the organs such as lymph nodes. This tissue also forms valves of heart and blood vessels, tunica albuginea of testis, sclera, periosteum of bone, and perichondrium of cartilage.

## TENDONS

These are specialized forms of dense regular connective tissue that attaches skeletal muscles to bone. Whole tendon is surrounded by a sheath of dense irregular connective tissue, called epitendineum. In areas subjected to friction, some tendons may also have synovial sheaths. Delicate connective tissue septa made up of dense irregular connective tissue, called endotendineum, divide the tendon into well-organized bundles or fascicles. The blood vessels and nerves travel through the endotendineum. Bundles of collagen fibers are arranged parallel in the fascicles, and tendinocytes (fibroblasts) are squeezed between these bundles. This parallel arrangement allows extreme tensile strength of the tendon.

Bundles of collagen fibers are wavy and separated from one another by a small quantity of intercellular ground substance (Fig. 5.10A, B). But when the tendon is stretched, these bundles become straight. In transverse section, fibroblast cells appear stellate in shape with the cytoplasmic processes extending between the bundles of collagen fibers.

## LIGAMENTS

These are specialized forms of dense regular connective tissue that connects bone to bone at the joints. Most of the ligaments have a parallel arrangement of collagen fibers (Fig. 5.12). However, interwoven

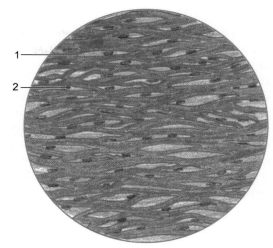

**Fig. 5.12:** Ligament showing bundles of collagen fibers (1) and fibroblast nuclei (2)

with these fibers there are finer collagen fibers along with a variable number of elastic fibers.

For comparison between tendons and ligaments, *see* Table 11 given in Appendix I.

Such arrangement provides a degree of inextensibility to provide the strong support needed at articulating joints. Amount of ground substance is more in the ligaments in comparison to tendons. In some ligaments, elastic fibers are more abundant to bear the strain, such ligaments are known as elastic ligaments, e.g. ligamentum flava, vocal ligaments of the larynx.

## APONEUROSIS

It represents a broad, flat tendon of a muscle and it is dense regular connective tissue. Instead of a parallel arrangement of collagen fibers like tendon, in this collagen fibers are arranged in multiple sheets or lamellae. The bundles of adjacent lamellae cross each other at an angle of 90°. This arrangement is even present in the cornea and is responsible for its transparency.

**Scurvy:** It occurs due to dietary deficiency of vitamin C. It mainly occurs in early childhood and in the very aged. Hemorrhage constitutes the one of the most striking features, as the defect in collagen synthesis results in inadequate support of wall of capillaries and granules. Skeletal changes also occur as there is insufficient production of osteoid matrix by osteoblasts. Resorption of the cartilaginous matrix, then fails or slows, and as a consequence there is cartilage overgrowth. There is delayed healing of wounds because of disturbed collagen synthesis.

**Edema:** It means swelling or fluid retention. It occurs when there is excessive tissue fluid within the loose connective tissue, causing swelling in the affected area. This occurs mainly due to obstruction of venous or lymphatic vessels.

**Inflammation:** It is the complex biological response of vascular tissues to harmful stimuli, such as pathogens, damaged cells, or irritants. It is a protective attempt by the organism to remove the injurious stimuli as well as to initiate the healing process. In the absence of inflammation, wounds and infections would never heal and progressive destruction of the tissue would compromise the survival of the organism.

## Summary

| Types of connective tissue | | | | Structure | Functions | Locations |
|---|---|---|---|---|---|---|
| Embryonic connective tissue | | | | Mesenchymal cells in the amorphous matrix | Give rise to all adult connective tissues | Umbilical cord (embryo), dental pulp, vitreous body, and nucleus pulposus (adults) |
| Adult connective tissue | Loosely arranged | Areolar tissue | | More cells (fibroblasts, adipocytes, macrophages, mast cells) and fewer fibers (collagen, elastic and reticular) | Works as a passage for the vessels and nerves | Mesentry, adventitial layer of blood vessels, and lamina propria of gut |
| | | Adipose tissue | White/ unilocular | Signet ring-like adipocytes | Stores energy and also functions as a cushion for kidneys and heart | Present sub-cutaneously throughout the body except eyelid, penis, scrotum and auricle (except lobule) |
| | | | Yellow/ multilocular | Adipocytes with multiple fat droplets, numerous mitochondria and a central nucleus | Heat production | Axilla, between the shoulder blades, around adrenal glands, in inguinal region and in neck |

*(Contd.)*

*(Contd.)*

| Types of connective tissue | | | Structure | Functions | Locations |
|---|---|---|---|---|---|
| | | Reticular tissue | Reticular fibers with reticular cells | Forms delicate supporting network | Liver, pancreas, bone marrow, adrenal glands, spleen, and lymph nodes |
| | Densely arranged | Regular collagenous | Parallel bundles of collagen fibers with fibroblasts | Adapted to withstand unidirectional pull transmitted along these fibers without stretching | Tendons, ligaments, stroma of cornea and aponeurosis |
| | | Regular elastic | Elastic fibers, few collagen fibers, and fibroblasts | Provides flexible support, and reduces pressure on the walls of the blood vessels | Large blood vessels, ligamentum flava and suspensory ligament of penis |
| | | Irregular | Network of collagen, elastic fibers, and fibroblasts | Facilitates the structure to withstand stress and strain in all directions | Dermis and submucosa |

## Self Assessment

1. Which fibers are found in all connective tissues?
   a. Collagen fibers
   b. Reticular fibers
   c. Elastic fibers
   d. None of the above

2. What color do reticular fibers stain with silver impregnation?
   a. Red color
   b. Orange color
   c. Yellow color
   d. Black color

3. Which of the following cells appears like signet ring?
   a. Mast cell        b. Plasma cell
   c. Fat cell         d. Reticular cell

4. Fibroblasts produce all EXCEPT:
   a. Collagen fibers
   b. Ground substance
   c. Elastic fibers
   d. Fat cells

5. Which of the following connective tissue cells secrete heparin?
   a. Mast cell        b. Plasma cell
   c. Fat cell         d. Fibroblast

6. Which connective tissue is present in the umbilical cord?
   a. Areolar tissue
   b. Adipose tissue
   c. Embryonic tissue
   d. Dense regular connective tissue

7. Which of the following is a dense irregular connective tissue?
   a. Ligament     b. Tendon
   c. Aponeurosis  d. Dermis

8. Which one is the principal phagocytosing cells of the connective tissue?
   a. Fibroblast
   b. Mast cell
   c. Fibrocyte
   d. Macrophage

9. Which of the following is a dense regular connective tissue?
   a. Dermis
   b. Submucosa
   c. Ligament
   d. Perichondrium

10. The tendon is a:
   a. Loose areolar tissue
   b. Dense irregular connective tissue
   c. Dense regular connective tissue
   d. Adipose tissue

## Answers

1. a,    2. d,    3. c,    4. d,    5. a,    6. c,    7. d,    8. d,    9. c,
10. c

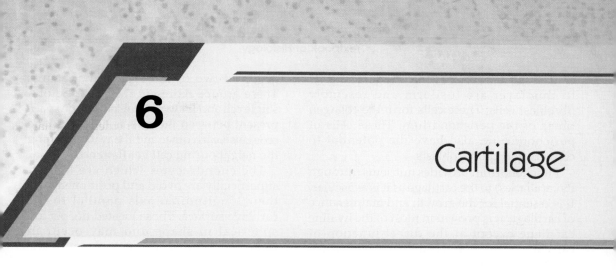

# 6

# Cartilage

C artilage is a firm avascular connective tissue, consists of cells (chondrocytes) and extensive extracellular matrix. Matrix forms more than 95% by volume of cartilage and cartilage even differs from other connective tissues due to the presence of substances in the extracellular matrix. It is nourished by the diffusion of nutrients from capillaries in adjacent connective tissue (perichondrium) or by synovial fluid from joint cavities (articular cartilage). However, in the larger cartilages such as costal cartilages and during the rapid growth of some fetal cartilages, vascular cartilage canals penetrate the tissue at intervals, providing an additional source of nutrients. There is no nerve supply to cartilage.

## FUNCTIONS OF CARTILAGE

### A. Support

It mainly provides support to soft tissues such as in the ear, and nose.

### B. Strength

It is resilient enough to withstand compression forces resulting from locomotion and weight bearing without permanent distortion.

### C. Movements

It helps in sliding movements of joints and also acts as a shock-absorber.

### D. Growth

During early fetal life, most of the human skeleton is cartilaginous, because cartilage can rapidly grow with a considerable degree of stiffness. Subsequently, this cartilaginous skeleton is replaced by bone except at the surfaces of synovial joints, costal cartilages, walls of the nose, larynx, epiglottis, trachea, bronchi and external ear.

Based on the type and amount of the fibers in the matrix, the cartilages are of three types: Hyaline, elastic and fibrocartilage.

## HYALINE CARTILAGE

The bluish-grey most abundant cartilage of the body is known as the hyaline (hyalos means glass) cartilage. All the components of this matrix, i.e. collagen fibers and ground substance have the same refractive indices; therefore, it almost looks transparent like a glass.

### A. Perichondrium of Hyaline Cartilage

The connective tissue layer, which surrounds the cartilage from all sides, is called perichondrium. It consists of an outer fibrous and an inner cellular layer. In an adult cartilage, only fibrous layer of perichondrium is present. Fibrous layer is made up of dense irregular connective tissue containing type I collagen fibers, fibroblasts and blood vessels, lymphatics and nerves. The inner cellular layer is also called chondrogenic layer. The cells in this layer are fusiform and resemble fibroblast cells. These cells form the collagen fibers of the perichondrium. These cells of perichondrium also have the potential to convert into chondroblasts.

Perichondrium provides nutrients (through its capillaries) to the cartilage as it is avascular. It is essential for the growth and maintenance of cartilage. It is present in most of the hyaline cartilage except at the direct junction of cartilage with bone (costal cartilage, which makes direct contact with the rib; an epiphyseal plate of cartilage, which is in direct contact with metaphysis and epiphysis in a developing bone) and in articular cartilage.

## B. Cells of the Hyaline Cartilage

Cartilage is an avascular tissue, so the cells of cartilage are less metabolically active. Two types of cells are associated with cartilage: Chondroblasts and Chondrocytes.

a. **Chondroblasts:** These cells are mainly derived from mesenchymal cells. However, when the growth is initiated, the cells of the inner cellular layer of perichondrium differentiate and also form chondroblasts. These are basophilic cells that contain the organelles required for protein synthesis. Cells contain an extensive Golgi apparatus, abundant rough endoplasmic reticulum, numerous mitochondria, lipid droplets, and glycogen.

Chondroblasts are the precursors of chondrocytes. Chondroblasts secrete matrix and even they become surrounded by this matrix, which is known as a territorial matrix or capsule in small individual compartments called lacunae. Chondroblasts that are surrounded by the matrix are known as chondrocytes.

b. **Chondrocytes:** Chondrocytes are mature cartilage cells, but are still capable of cell division. The matrix surrounding the chondrocytes is distensible, so the chondrocytes divide and form an isogenous

group of two or more cells in a lacuna. These groups represent the offspring of a single cell and known as cell nests. The space present between the cells is limited, so the cells push each other and the wall adjoining the neighbouring cell get flattened.

The chondrocytes which are located superficially are ovoid and positioned with their longitudinal axis parallel to the cartilage surface. Those located deeper are spherical in shape and may occur in isogenous groups. The cytoplasm of the chondrocytes varies in appearance in relation to their activity. Young chondrocytes have a pale-staining cytoplasm with many mitochondria, abundant rER, an extensive Golgi apparatus, secretory granules, and intermediate filaments. Older chondrocytes, which are relatively quiescent, display a greatly reduced complement of organelles, numerous intermediate filaments with an abundance of free ribosomes. Thus, these cells can resume active protein synthesis if they revert to chondroblasts.

**Cartilage cells**, in living tissue, fill the lacunae completely. However, during tissue processing, because of the use of fixatives, cells shrink and become irregular in shape and they retract from their capsule giving a false appearance of a large space (lacunae) between the cell and matrix.

## C. Matrix of Hyaline Cartilage

It is amorphous, solid and firm but somewhat flexible. It allows the tissue to bear mechanical stresses without permanent distortion. The matrix immediately surrounding the chondrocytes is known as territorial matrix or capsule, while the matrix present in between the two cell nest is known as interterritorial matrix. The matrix is basophilic and looks purple with H and E staining. Territorial matrix is more intensely staining because it is poor in eosinophilic collagen, but rich in sulfated glycosaminoglycans, so looks dark purple (Fig. 6.1A, B). Interterritorial matrix looks light purple, as it contains more collagen and less sulfated glycosaminoglycans. The matrix is

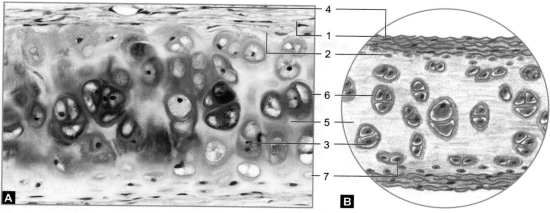

**Fig. 6.1:** (A) Micrograph of hyaline cartilage of trachea, (B) sketch showing outer fibrous (1) and inner cellular layer (2) of perichondrium. Chondrocytes form cell nests (3). Fibroblast nucleus (4), interterritorial matrix (5), territorial matrix (6), chondrocyte in lacunae (7)

intensely metachromatic (cells acquire a color other than that of the dye used) when stained with toluidiene blue, because of the abundance of glycosaminoglycans. The matrix is also PAS positive, because of its glycoprotein content.

a. **Collagen fibers:** The matrix of hyaline cartilage contains mainly type II collagen, but types IX, X, and XI and VI are also present in small quantities. Collagen provides stability and support to the cartilage and constitutes 40% of the dry weight of cartilage.

**Types of collagen** Type II collagen is made up of fine collagen fibrils (10–100 nm in diameter). These fibrils are strong enough to withstand tensile forces. Type IX collagen stabilizes the network of type II collagen fibrils through its contact with intersections of proteoglycan molecules. Type X collagen forms hexagonal network to arrange fibrils of type II, IX, and XI; and type XI collagen regulates the size of type II collagen fibrils. Type VI collagen is mainly present on the periphery of the chondro-cytes and helps in attachment of chondrocytes to the framework of the matrix.

b. **Ground substance:** It is formed by pro-teoglycan, glycoprotein, and water. Most of the proteoglycan is present in the form of aggregates.

**Glycosaminoglycan** molecules (chondroitin 4-sulfate, chondroitin 6-sulfate, and keratan sulfate) joined in a bottle brush configuration to a core protein to form a proteoglycan monomer (Fig. 6.2). The most important proteoglycan monomer present in hyaline cartilage is aggrecan. As many as 80–100 monomers, are bound to hyaluronic acid by link proteins to form large hyaluronate proteoglycan aggregates. These aggregates are bound to thinner collagen matrix fibrils by electrostatic interactions and cross linking glycoproteins and form a framework that resists tensile forces.

In addition to proteoglycan the ground substance also contains a structural glycoprotein; chondronectin, which has binding sites for type II collagen and for glycosaminoglycans. This assists in the adherence of chondroblasts and chondrocytes to the fibrous and amorphous components of the matrix.

Just like connective tissue proper the matrix of cartilage is also highly hydrated and accounts for 80% of weight of cartilage. Most of the water is bound to the aggregates, which accounts for the ability of cartilage to resist forces of compression. However, some of the water is loose enough to allow diffusion of nutrients and waste products.

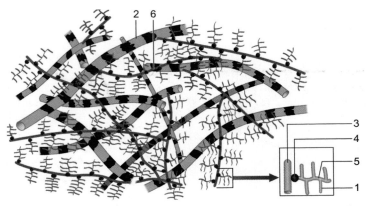

**Fig. 6.2:** Schematic diagram showing the fine structural organization of the hyaline cartilage matrix. Proteoglycan molecule (1), type II collagen fibers (2), hyaluronic acid (3), link protein (4), core protein (5) and glycosaminoglycans (6)

## D. Histogenesis and Growth of Hyaline Cartilage

All cartilages are derived from the mesenchyme. At the site of hyaline cartilage formation the mesenchymal cells aggregate and form a nodule, known as chondrogenic nodule. These cells differentiate and form chondroblasts. The mesenchymal tissue surrounding the chondrogenic nodule forms the perichondrium. Perichondrium is having two layers: Outer fibrous layer and inner cellular layer. The growth of cartilage occurs by the two processes: Appositional and interstitial (Fig. 6.3). Interstitial growth occurs only during the early stages of cartilage formation, in articular cartilage and in the epiphyseal plates of long bones. But, when the cartilage matures, the matrix becomes hard and growth can only take place by the addition of new surface layers, i.e. by appositional growth.

The cells of inner cellular layer of the perichondrium rapidly divide and become rounded by withdrawing their extensions.

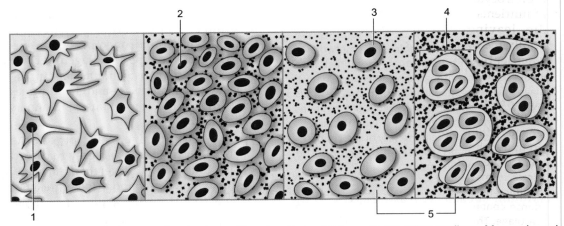

**Fig. 6.3:** Schematic diagram showing appositional and interstitial growth of hyaline cartilage. Mesenchymal cells (1), chondroblasts (2), chondrocytes (3), cell nests (4) and matrix (5)

These cells divide very fast and known as chondroblasts. Chondroblasts secrete matrix and even they become surrounded by this matrix. These chondroblasts are now known as chondrocytes. The production of new matrix increases the mass of cartilage and at the same time, new fibroblasts are also produced to maintain the cell population of the perichondrium. This type of growth is called appositional growth.

Chondrocytes are still capable of cell division and the surrounding matrix is distensible, so they form an isogenous group of two or more cells in a lacuna. These groups represent the offspring of a single cell and known as cell nests. As the cells of an isogenous group manufacture matrix, they are pushed away from each other, forming separate lacunae and thus enlarging the cartilage from within. This type of growth is called interstitial growth.

## E. Calcification of Hyaline Cartilage

With growing age, the matrix of hyaline cartilage calcifies and replaced by bone. Chondrocytes undergo hypertrophy and secrete alkaline phosphatase that provides a calcified matrix. Calcium phosphate is deposited in the matrix, which cuts off the chondrocytes from their only available source of nutrients and oxygen. Thus chondrocytes die, leaving behind empty lacunae and finally the cartilage is replaced by bone. This calcification process is a normal part of endochondral bone formation.

**Regeneration of hyaline cartilage:** In young children, damaged cartilage shows a greater capacity for repair. In adults, regeneration starts from perichondrial activity, which invades the injured area and generates new cartilage. Sometimes in massive injury, perichondrium cannot produce new cartilage, so it produces a scar of dense connective tissue instead of forming new cartilage. The poor capacity of cartilage for repair or regeneration is partly because of avascularity of this tissue.

## F. Effects of Hormones

The functions of chondrocytes depend on a proper hormonal balance. Cartilage growth depends mainly on the hypophyseal growth hormone somatotropin. This hormone does not act directly on cartilage cells but promotes the synthesis of somatomedin C in the liver. Somatomedin C acts directly on cartilage cells, promoting their growth. Growth hormone, thyroxin, and testosterone stimulate growth of cartilage, whereas it is slowed down by cortisone, hydrocortisone and estradiol.

**Articular cartilage** The hyaline cartilage, which covers the end of each bone where it contacts with another bone such as in a movable joint is called articular cartilage. It persists throughout life and is about 2 to 5 mm in the thickness. It is structurally similar to hyaline cartilage, but it does not have the perichondrium on its articular surface as well as on the opposite surface where this cartilage comes in contact with bone. On the surface of this cartilage small, dense, flattened chondrocytes are present, which provide its resistance against pressure and form a smooth surface for the free movements of the joints. The articular cartilage has no capacity to regenerate after damage and even it does not undergo ossification or calcification.

## G. Functions of Hyaline Cartilage

a. **Reduces friction at the joints:** Because of its smooth surface, it provides a sliding area which reduces friction, thus facilitating bone movement.

b. **Movement:** It joins bones firmly but certain amount of movement is still possible between them.

c. **Support:** The hyaline cartilage rings present in the trachea and bronchi prevent their wall from collapsing when air is drawn into the lungs.

d. **Growth:** It is responsible for the longitudinal growth of long bones.

e. **Flexibility:** Hyaline cartilage present in costal cartilage is firm yet flexible enough to permit the rib cage to expand in respiratory movements.

## H. Locations of Hyaline Cartilage

It is most abundant and serves as a temporary skeleton in the fetus until it is replaced with bone through endochondral ossification. It is present in trachea, bronchi, costal cartilages, thyroid cartilage, in the nasal septum, the cartilage of the larynx (cricoid and most of arytenoid), and epiphyseal growth plates (articular cartilage).

## ELASTIC CARTILAGE

This cartilage is almost similar to the hyaline cartilage except that along with type II collagen fibers its matrix and perichondrium (fibrous layer) contains plenty of elastic fibers.

It looks yellow in the fresh state owing to the presence of elastic fibers (elastin). Elastic fibers form a network, which is often so dense that the ground substance is hidden. The fibers are thick and heavily concentrated in the center of the cartilage; while near the perichondrium, the fibers are thin and loosely arranged. Chondrocytes are more abundant and bigger in size and are present singly and in isogenous groups (Fig. 6.4 A, B).

Perichondrium is also present in this cartilage. The matrix is metachromatic and basophilic as that of hyaline cartilage (Fig. 6.5). Although elastic fibers are not stained by H and E stain, yet the matrix does not appear homogenous

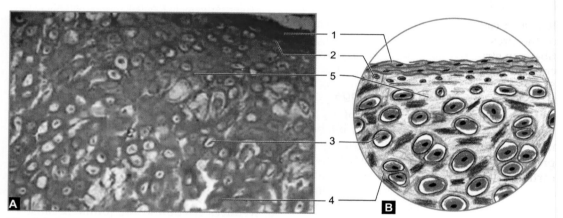

**Fig. 6.4:** Elastic cartilage, (A) micrograph, (B) sketch. Fibrous layer of perichondrium (1), cellular layer of perichondrium (2), chondrocyte in lacunae (3), territorial matrix (4) and interterritorial matrix (5)

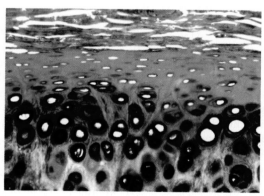

**Fig. 6.5:** Elastic cartilage stained by aldehyde fuchsin or Gomori stain

like hyaline cartilage. The matrix always shows an impression of elastic fibers even if it is stained with H and E stain. The matrix of elastic cartilage does not calcify with aging.

## A. Functions of Elastic Cartilage

It is more flexible than hyaline cartilage because of the presence of elastic fibers. It maintains the shape of the organ and provides support to the organ, with elasticity.

## B. Locations of Elastic Cartilage

It is present in pinna of the ear, epiglottis, lateral part of the external auditory meatus, and medial part of the auditory tube.

### FIBROCARTILAGE

It is also called white fibrocartilage because of the presence of thick bundles of collagen fibers. In structure, it is intermediate of dense connective tissue and hyaline cartilage. Bundles of type I collagen fibers run parallel to each other and are oriented in the direction of functional stress. In between the bundles lie chondrocytes (Fig. 6.6 A, B). Chondrocytes may lie singly, in pairs and in isogenous groups. In comparison to hyaline and elastic cartilage fibrocartilage is less cellular.

Perichondrium is absent in this cartilage. The amount of ground substance is very less and it is usually located immediately around the chondrocytes. The matrix is basophilic, but it shows less metachromasia than hyaline cartilage. The matrix of fibrocartilage contains large amounts of proteoglycan versican produced by the fibroblasts than aggrecan, which is produced by chondrocytes. Like aggrecan, versican can even form proteoglycan aggregates. Calcification of fibrocartilage occurs during repair of bone.

## A. Functions of Fibrocartilage

It provides strength and it is capable of resisting compression and tearing forces.

## B. Locations of Fibrocartilage

It is often present at the sites, where tendons are inserted into the bone and where tendons run in deep groove on bones, the grooves are lined by fibrocartilage. It is also present in the intervertebral discs (annulus fibrosus), pubic symphysis, glenoidal labrum, acetabular labrum, and the menisci of the knee joint. Articular discs of temporomandibular and sternoclavicular joints and triangular articular disc of inferior radioulnar joints are also made up of fibrocartilage.

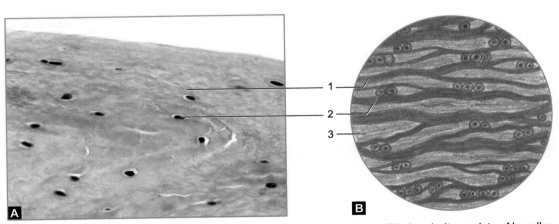

**Fig. 6.6:** White fibrocartilage of intervertebral discs, (A) micrograph and (B) sketch. It consists of bundles of collagen fibers (1). In between bundles lie rows of chondrocytes (2) in the matrix (3)

For comparison between hyaline cartilage, elastic cartilage, and fibrocartilage, *see* Table 12 given in Appendix I.

**Chondroma:** It is a benign cartilaginous tumor, which is encapsulated with a lobular growing pattern. Tumor cells resemble normal cells and produce the cartilaginous matrix (amorphous, basophilic material). Characteristic features of this tumor include the vascular axis within the tumor, which make the distinction with normal hyaline cartilage.

## Summary

| Parameter | Hyaline cartilage | Elastic cartilage | Fibrocartilage |
|---|---|---|---|
| Types of fibers | Type II collagen fibers | Elastic fibers with type II collagen fibers | Type I collagen fibers |
| Chondrocytes | Mainly present in isogenous groups | Present singly, and in isogenous groups | Present singly, in pairs, and in isogenous groups |
| Perichondrium | Perichondrium present in most places except in articular cartilages and at the direct junction of cartilage with bone (costal cartilage, and epiphyseal plate) | Perichondrium present | Perichondrium absent |
| Locations | Trachea, bronchi, costal cartilages, thyroid cartilage, in the nasal septum, cartilage of larynx (cricoid and most of arytenoid), and articular ends of bones | Pinna of the ear, epiglottis, external acoustic meatus and auditory tube | At the sites, where tendons are inserted into the bone and in the intervertebral discs (annulus fibrosus), the pubic symphysis, glenoidal labrum, acetabular labrum, and the menisci of the knee joint |
| Functions | Reduces friction at joints, responsible for longitudinal growth of long bones and provide flexibility to rib cage | Maintains the shape of the organ and provides support to the organ, with elasticity | Provides strength and also capable of resisting compression and tearing forces |

## Self Assessment

1. Which type of cartilage is highly vascular?
   a. Hyaline cartilage
   b. Elastic cartilage
   c. White fibrocartilage
   d. None of the above

2. Which of the following cells produces matrix of cartilage?
   a. Chondroblasts
   b. Chondrocytes
   c. Perichondrial cells
   d. Fibroblasts

3. Which cartilage forms the skeleton of the fetus?
   a. Elastic cartilage
   b. Hyaline cartilage
   c. Fibrocartilage
   d. None of the above

4. Where does cartilage come from?
   a. Ectoderm
   b. Endoderm
   c. Mesenchyme
   d. Connective tissue

5. Which type of cartilage forms the articular surface on bones?
   a. Hyaline cartilage
   b. Elastic cartilage
   c. Fibrocartilage
   d. None of the above

6. Perichondrium is absent in:
   a. Hyaline cartilage
   b. Elastic cartilage
   c. Articular cartilage
   d. None of the above

7. Glenoidal labrum is made up of:
   a. Hyaline cartilage
   b. Elastic cartilage
   c. Fibrocartilage
   d. Articular cartilage

8. Elastic cartilage is present in:
   a. Intervertebral disc
   b. Trachea
   c. Bronchus
   d. Epiglottis

9. Which types of fibers are present in fibrocartilage?
   a. Collagen fibers
   b. Elastic fibers
   c. Reticular fibers
   d. Purkinje fibers

10. Which of the following cartilages has a homogenous matrix?
    a. Hyaline cartilage
    b. Elastic cartilage
    c. Fibrocartilage
    d. All of the above

## Answers

1. d,     2. a,     3. b,     4. c,     5. a,     6. c,     7. c,     8. d,     9. a,
10. a

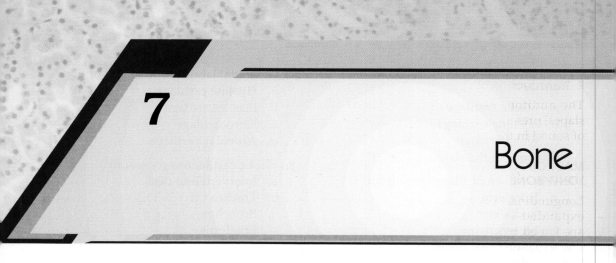

# 7

# Bone

Bone is a rigid and a vascular connective tissue, which originates from mesenchymal cells. Like other connective tissue, it is also made up of extracellular matrix and cells. Bone is the hardest tissue of the body, but if stress is applied to the bone, then it constantly changes its shape, which leads to bone resorption. When tension is applied to the bone, the formation of new bone takes place.

Bone is a special tissue and it is very difficult to study its histological structure because of its hardness. Two methods are employed to prepare the bone for study—decalcification and preparation of ground sections. Decalcification is done by treating the bone with an acid solution to remove the calcium salts. After decalcification, the tissue can be embedded, sectioned, and routinely stained for study. Ground sections are prepared from dry bones, which are handled in the classroom. A dry bone is not covered at its epiphyseal ends by hyaline cartilage. Thin slices of bone are cut with saw, followed by grinding the sections with abrasives between glass plates. When the section is sufficiently thin for study with a light microscope, it is mounted for study. However, both methods have disadvantages. In decalcified sections, osteocytes are distorted by the decalcifying acid bath. In ground sections, the cells are destroyed and the lacunae and canaliculi are filled with debris.

The ground sections are even devoid of periosteum and endosteum.

For comparison between cartilage and bone, *see* Table 13 given in Appendix I.

## FUNCTIONS OF BONE

### A. Support

It forms the supporting framework for the body, such as long bones in the limbs and skull in the face.

### B. Protection

It provides protection to the vital organs such as heart, brain and lungs.

### C. Reservoir

It serves as a reservoir for the calcium and phosphates. Both these ions are stored in the bones and as needed body draw it to maintain the appropriate levels.

### D. Blood Cell Production

Within the medullary cavity of long bones and in cancellous bones lies bone marrow (myeloid tissue), which produces blood cells.

### E. Movements

It forms a strong and rigid endoskeleton to which skeletal muscles are attached to provide movements.

## F. Transduction of Sound

The auditory ossicles (incus, malleus and stapes) present in the ear provide transduction of sound in the middle ear.

## MACROSCOPIC (GROSS) STRUCTURE OF A LONG BONE

Longitudinal section of a long bone has two expanded ends, called epiphyses, which are joined by a long shaft, called diaphysis. The expanded portion of the bone between the epiphysis and diaphysis is called metaphysis. The diaphysis is made up by a thick wall of compact or dense bone enclosing a large central cavity, called marrow cavity or medullary cavity (Fig. 7.1). A thin rim around this marrow cavity is made up by spongy or trabecular bone. The marrow cavity and spaces of spongy bone are covered by a thin membrane, called endosteum. The ends or epiphysis is formed by spongy bone covered with a thin layer of compact bone. The articular surface of the epiphysis (which comes in contact with another bone to form a joint) is covered with articular cartilage. The entire

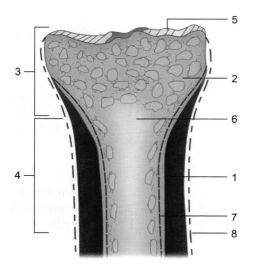

**Fig. 7.1:** Schematic diagram of long bone showing places of compact (1) and spongy bone (2). Epiphysis (3), diaphysis (4), articular cartilage (5), marrow cavity (6), endosteum (7) and periosteum (8)

outer surface of bone, except the area covered by articular cartilage is covered by a membrane, called periosteum.

## SURFACE COVERINGS

The external and internal surfaces of bones are covered by membranes, called periosteum and endosteum respectively. They have osteogenic potential and are essential for growth and repair of bones.

## A. Periosteum

It envelops the outer surface of all bones except on articular surfaces, sesamoid bones, and attachment sites of tendons and ligaments. The periosteum is well vascularized and richly innervated layer made up of an outer fibrous and inner cellular layer. The outer fibrous layer is made up of dense irregular connective tissue, which mainly contains collagen fibers and fibroblasts. The inner cellular layer is composed of fibroblast like cells, called osteoprogenitor (osteogenic) cells, which divide by mitosis and differentiate into osteoblasts.

If an active bone formation is not in progress, then the cellular layer is not well developed and have relatively few cells, called periosteal cells. These cells may convert to osteoblasts under the appropriate stimulus such as in cases of repair of bone after fracture.

Where ligaments and tendons are attached to the bone, bundles of periosteal collagen fibers called Sharpey's fibers, runs at right angle to bone surfaces and are continuous with the collagen fibers of the bone matrix.

## B. Endosteum

It lines all internal cavities within the bone and is composed of a single layer of osteoprogenitor cells, osteoblasts and bone-lining cells. Therefore, it is considerably thinner than the periosteum. Osteoprogenitor cells and bone-lining cells are both flattened in shape and have a similar appearance in the microscope. Because of their location at cavities, they are commonly called endosteal cells.

## BONE MATRIX

Bone matrix contains both organic and inorganic components. If the organic component is removed from the bone by burning the bone, the remaining calcified bone becomes extremely brittle as chalk. If the mineral component is removed by prolonged exposure to acid and chelating agents, bone becomes flexible as rubber. Before calcification the matrix is called osteoid.

### A. The Inorganic (Calcified) Component

It represents about 65% of the dry weight of bone matrix. It mainly consists of calcium and phosphate in the form of rod-like hydroxyapatite crystals $[Ca_{10}(PO_4)_6(OH)_2]$. These crystals are arranged parallel to the collagen fibers and contribute to the lamellar appearance of the bone. Inorganic components enable bone to resist compression. This calcified matrix makes bone impermeable to the diffusion of nutrients, so the bone must be well vascularized.

### B. The Organic Component

It is secreted by osteoblasts and represents about 35% of the dry weight of bone matrix. It mainly consists of type I collagen and to a lesser extent type V collagen are also present. Very small amounts of other collagen such as type III, XI and XIII are also present. Ground substance is minimal and is composed of glycosaminoglycans such as hyaluronan, chondroitin sulfate and keratan sulfate.

Several glycoproteins such as osteonectin, which are responsible for attachment of collagen fibers to hydroxyapatite crystals and sialoproteins such as osteonectin, sialoproteins I and II, which binds bone cells to the extracellular matrix, are also present. Sialoproteins I and II also initiate calcium phosphate formation during the process of mineralization of bone. Bone specific, vitamin K dependent proteins, such as osteocalcin, which captures calcium from circulation and stimulates osteoclasts during remodeling of bone, are also present in the ground substance.

Collagen fibers are arranged in the lamellae, which are soon mineralized by crystals. Collagen fibers within a lamellae are oriented parallel to each other, but the fibers in one lamellae are oriented at an angle to those in an adjacent lamellae. Organic component enables the bone to resist tension.

## BONE CELLS (Fig. 7.2)

### A. Osteoprogenitor or Osteogenic Cells

These cells are derived from embryonic mesenchyme. These cells are present in the

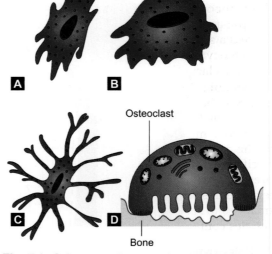

**Fig. 7.2:** Schematic diagram showing bone cells. (A) Osteogenic cell, (B) osteoblast, (C) osteocyte, (D) osteoclast

periosteum, endosteum, and the lining of Haversian and Volkmann's canals. These cells are flattened cells with elongated oval nucleus and are capable of differentiation into osteoblasts, however, at low oxygen tensions, these cells may change into chondrogenic cells.

## B. Osteoblasts

These cells are derived from osteoprogenitor cells and do not undergo mitosis. These cells are present in the innermost portion of the periosteum and in the lining of endosteum. These cells are connected by numerous gap junctions, which facilitate electrical or chemical communication between the cells. Each cell has a single large, oval and euchromatic nucleus.

Osteoblasts are responsible for the synthesis of the organic components of bone matrix. These cells also synthesize high levels of alkaline phosphatase. When osteoblasts are actively involved in the synthesis of matrix, they have a cuboidal to columnar shape and intensely basophilic cytoplasm (due to large amounts of rough endoplasmic reticulum). This newly formed matrix surrounds the osteoblast and now they are known as osteocyte. When they are inactive or quiescent, they become flattened and even their cytoplasm is less basophilic. During this process a space is formed, which is occupied by osteocytes and their extensions and is known as lacuna.

Osteoblasts secrete components of the matrix at the cell surface, producing a layer of non-calcified matrix, which lies in contact with older bone matrix, called osteoid. Deposition of the inorganic components of bone, i.e. calcification of osteoid also depends on the presence of viable osteoblasts. Osteoblasts regulate this calcification process by releasing small, 50 to 250 nm membrane bound matrix vesicles containing alkaline phosphatase.

## C. Osteocytes

These cells are derived from osteoblasts, and do not divide or secrete matrix. These cells comprise 90% of all cells in the mature skeleton. Osteocytes are flat, almond-shaped and have a single, small and heterochromatic nucleus. The size of osteocytes is smaller than the osteoblasts and their cytoplasm is even less basophilic as they contain less rough endoplasmic reticulum in comparison to osteoblasts. Osteocytes lie in lacunae and each lacuna contains only one osteocyte. The cytoplasmic processes of these cells lie in thin, cylindrical canaliculi. The lacunae and canaliculi contain extracellular fluid derived from blood vessels present in the Haversian canal. Processes of adjacent cells make contact through gap junctions and molecules are passed through these junctions from cell to cell.

The canaliculi form an effective exchange connection, i.e. nutrients reach the osteocytes; gaseous exchange occurs between blood and osteocytes and finally, wastes are removed from these cells. In this way, bone tissue depends upon osteocytes for its viability. Osteocytes also play a role in controlling the extracellular concentration of calcium and phosphate, because they are stimulated by calcitonin and inhibited by parathormone (PTH). These cells are present in greatest numbers in young bone and their number gradually decreases with age.

## D. Osteoclasts

These cells are derived from cells in the bone marrow that are also precursors of monocytes. These cells do not undergo mitosis. These cells are multinucleated (up to 50 nuclei), irregularly-shaped giant cells (50–150 μm in diameter). Their cytoplasm is usually acidophilic and has many lysosomes. Osteoclasts are present on internal surfaces as part of the endosteum and on external surfaces as part of the osteogenic layer of the periosteum. In areas of bone undergoing resorption, osteoclasts lie in depressions in the matrix, known as resorption bays or Howship's lacunae. In osteoclasts which are active, the surface-facing bone matrix is highly folded, forming a ruffled border. Surrounding the ruffled border is a clear zone that is devoid of organelles, and contains micro-filaments, which help osteoclasts to maintain contact with the bony surface, and serves to isolate the region of osteolytic activity. Osteoclasts cells have receptors for calcitonin hormone. The acids secreted by ruffled border dissolve the mineral components, while proteolytic enzymes produced by lysosomes destroy the organic osteoid matrix.

### E. Bone-lining Cells

These cells are formed from osteoblasts. These flattened cells are present as a single layer on surfaces where active bone deposition or removal is not taking place. The bone-lining cells present on the periosteal surface are known as periosteal cells, while the cells present on endosteal surface are known as endosteal cells. Processes of adjacent cells make contact through gap junctions. These cells may be responsible for providing nutritional support to the osteocytes.

### TYPES OF BONE

Bone exists in two main forms

### A. Woven Bone (Immature or Primary Bone)

It is the first bone tissue to appear in embryonic development, in fracture repair and other repair processes. It is usually temporary and, is replaced in postnatal life by lamellar bone except near the sutures of the flat bones of the skull, in tooth sockets, and at the insertions of some tendons. In woven bones bundles of collagen fibers are randomly organized along with a low mineral content and a higher proportion of osteocytes than in lamellar bone.

### B. Lamellar Bone (Secondary Bone)

It replaces most of the woven bone and its matrix is more calcified than woven bone and it is even stronger than woven bone. Bone is not a static structure; therefore, lamellar bone is resorbed and reconstructed throughout life. In lamellar bone bundles of collagen fibers are arranged in successive layers or lamellae. The fibers of one lamella course at right angle to those of adjoining lamellae on either side of it. This arrangement gives maximum rigidity and strength. Lamellar bone is further of two types:

a. **Compact (Dense or Cortical) bone:** Structural unit of compact bone is osteon, or haversian system. Each osteon is about 250 μm in diameter and approximately 21 million osteons are present in the adult human skeleton. In the osteon (Fig. 7.3A, B), the lamellae are arranged as concentric cylinders (concentric lamellae) surrounding a central

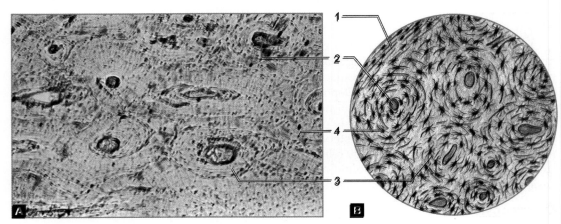

**Fig. 7.3A, B:** Compact bone TS at low magnification. (A) Micrograph, (B) sketch. Circumferential lamellae (1), haversian canal (2), concentric lamellae (3) and osteocyte (4)

haversian canal, which contains nerves, connective tissue and blood vessels.

Most recently formed lamella lies closest to this canal. The number of lamellae in each osteon is highly variable. The average number is 6. Diameter of haversian canal is highly variable, i.e. in the younger person's canal is large, while in the older person's canal is small. In between the lamellae are lacunae, which contain osteocytes (Fig. 7.4).

Canaliculi containing osteocyte cell processes interconnect osteocyte lacunae and also connect these lacunae directly or indirectly to a surface bathed by tissue fluid (Fig. 7.5A, B). Canaliculi bring tissue fluid, together with nutrients and oxygen, to all its osteocytes, enabling them to stay alive in their heavily calcified stone-like environment.

Haversian canals are connected with each other by transverse or oblique Volkmann or perforating canals (Fig. 7.6), which communicate with the marrow cavity and the periosteum. Volkmann's canals are not surrounded by concentric lamellae. Haversian canal supplies the cells of the osteons, while the Volkmann's canal provides communication between osteons.

The long axis of an osteon is approximately parallel to the major axis of stress. In

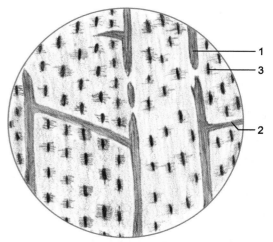

**Fig. 7.6:** Compact bone (LS) showing Haversian canal (1), Volkmann's canal (2) and osteocyte (3)

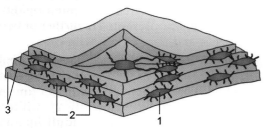

**Fig. 7.4:** Schematic diagram of lamellar bone showing osteocytes (1) present in the lacunae (2) in between the two lamellae (3)

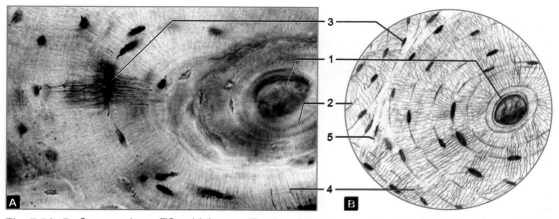

**Fig. 7.5A, B:** Compact bone TS at high magnification, (A) micrograph, (B) sketch. Haversian canal (1), concentric lamellae (2), osteocyte (3), canaliculi (4) and interstitial lamellae (5)

between the osteons, interstitial lamellae are present, which are incomplete or fragmented osteons and left from partial resorption of old osteons during bone remodeling. Haversian canals are not present in interstitial lamellae. The osteons and interstitial lamellae are sharply outlined by a refractile line called the cement line, which consists of a modified matrix with a basophilic zone. Collagen fibers are absent in cement lines and these lines are even not traversed by canaliculi. Lamellae present just beneath the periosteum are known as outer circumferential lamellae, while lamellae present around the marrow cavity are known as inner circumferential lamellae. Compact bone forms diaphysis of long bones. It also forms a thin layer on the external surface of short, flat and irregular bones in which the core is made up of spongy bone.

In the bone, blood that nourishes bone tissue flow from the marrow cavity into and through the bone tissue and comes out through the periosteal veins. Major vessels enter in the compact bone via the Volkmann's canals, while the smaller blood vessels enter through the Haversian canal. Outermost part of the compact bone is supplied by branches of periosteal arteries.

The periosteal vessels communicate with vessels in the Haversian canal through the Volkmann's canal. Lymphatic vessels are absent in bone tissue.

b. **Cancellous (spongy or trabecular or medullary) bone:** It is composed of bony spicules, also called as trabeculae, of varying shapes, numbers and sizes that are oriented along the lines of stress. In the trabeculae lamellae run parallel and osteocyte lies in lacunae in between the lamellae. Osteocytes receive nutrients through diffusion by cell processes that extend to the surface of trabeculae. These trabeculae are less than 0.4 mm in thickness, so blood vessels are not present within the bone tissue (in compact bone, blood vessels are present within the bone tissue, i.e. in haversian and Volkmann's canals). At the margin of trabeculae osteoblasts and osteoclasts are present. Trabeculae gives branches and anastomose with each other to create many interconnecting spaces that are filled with bone marrow (Fig. 7.7 A, B).

Trabeculae receive nutrition from blood vessels in the bone marrow. No true haversian systems are present due to the thinness of the trabeculae. Although spaces present in the spongy bones reduce the weight of the bone, yet provide tremendous

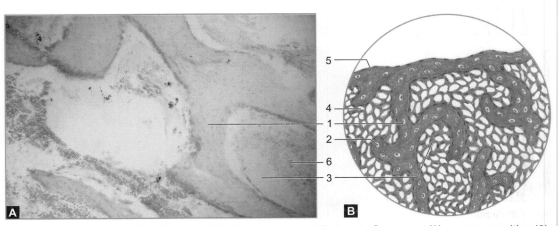

**Fig. 7.7:** Spongy bone with trabeculae (1), (A) micrograph, (B) sketch. Osteocyte (2), marrow cavities (3), fat cells (4), periosteum (5) and blood cells (6)

strength. Spongy bone mainly forms epiphysis of long bones. All short, flat and irregular bones consist of a core of spongy bone. A thin rim around the marrow cavity of the diaphysis of long bone consists of spongy bone.

Bone marrow of the children is red in which blood cells develop, and contain 40% water, 40% fat and 20% protein. In later stages of growth, and in the adult, when the rate of blood cell formation decreased, red bone marrow slowly changes to the yellow bone marrow. Yellow bone marrow is made up mostly of fat cells (80% fat, 15% water, 5% protein). Under the appropriate stimulus, yellow bone marrow can revert to red bone marrow.

For comparison between compact and spongy bones, *see* Table 14 given in Appendix I.

## OSSIFICATION

All bones and cartilages are of mesodermal origin. The process of bone formation is known as ossification. The bone develops in the embryo by two distinct processes: Endochondral ossification and intramembranous ossification. The weight bearing bones, such as vertebrae and bones of the extremities develop from endochondral ossification, whereas the flat bones of the skull develop from intramembranous ossification. Initial bone formation occurs either by endochondral or by intramembranous ossification, but bone formation is always accompanied by bone resorption. The combination of bone formation and resorption is known as remodeling of bone, which occurs throughout life. Remodeling of bone is slower in lamellar bone than in woven bone.

## A. Intramembranous Ossification

In this process, the bone develops from condensation of connective tissue mesenchyme (Fig. 7.8). The frontal and parietal bones, parts of the maxilla, mandible, clavicle, occipital,

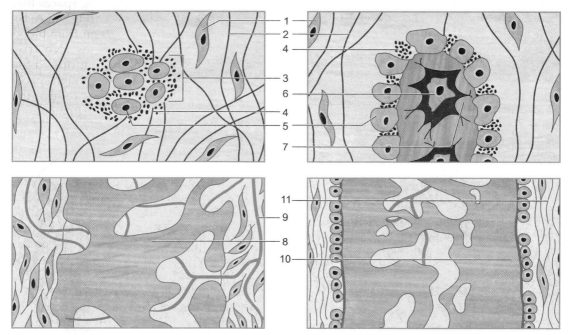

**Fig. 7.8:** Schematic diagram showing the stages of intramembranous ossification of bone. Mesenchymal cells (1), collagen fibers (2), center of ossification (3), osteoid (4), osteoblast (5), osteocyte (6), newly calcified bone matrix (7), trabeculae (8), blood vessel (9), plate of compact bone (10) and fibrous periosteum (11)

and temporal bones are formed by this process. This process also contributes to the growth of short bones and the thickening of the long bones. At the sites where bone is to form, the mesenchyme becomes richly vascularized and show active proliferation to form osteoprogenitor cells. These osteoprogenitor cells enlarge rapidly and differentiate into osteoblasts, which produce bone matrix known as osteoid. The site where osteoblasts first appear in the membrane is known as a center of ossification. As calcification occurs, osteoblasts are surrounded by their own matrix and known as osteocytes. Calcification of the matrix does not kill the osteocyte as they get nutrients and oxygen via canaliculi. Osteoblasts present on the surface of this matrix secrete phosphatatse, which helps in calcification of the matrix. From the center of ossification, osteoblasts proliferate and differentiate in a radiating manner. Osteoblasts form trabeculae of bone and on the surface of these trabeculae, bone formation occurs layer by layer. This process is known as appositional growth and by this process, these trabeculae enlarges and become joined in a trabecular network, giving rise to the woven or immature bone. This woven bone is replaced by lamellar bone through remodeling. The bony tissue between trabeculae differentiates and forms bone marrow. On the surface of bone new bone is added by appositional growth, but due to limited space the trabeculae get thickened and form plates of compact bone.

In the skull bone this compact bone forms outer and inner tables of flat bones. The margins of these flat bones are last to ossify. At birth these parts are soft and known as fontonalles.

## B. Endochondral Ossification

In this process, the bone develops from a cartilage model. All long (except clavicle) and short bones are formed by endochondral ossification. The skeleton of the fetus between 7th and 12th weeks of intrauterine life is mostly formed by hyaline cartilage. This cartilaginous model is covered by a membrane known as perichondrium. This model grows in length due to the continuous division of chondrocytes with secretion of cartilaginous matrix. The cartilage grows in thickness due to the peripheral deposition of matrix by new chondroblasts derived from perichondrium. In the middle of this model a blood vessel penetrates the perichondrium, causing the transformation of chondrogenic cells to osteoprogenitor cells. Osteoprogenitor cells then differentiate into osteoblasts. Then osteoblasts elaborate a thin shell of compact bone deep to the perichondrium that is known as a subperiosteal bone collar (Fig. 7.9). The surrounding perichondrium of bone collar is now known as periosteum.

At the same time with the appearance of the bone collar a few chondrocytes undergo hypertrophy and their cytoplasm becomes vacuolated. Their lacunae enlarge and matrix between these lacunae reduces gradually and form thin trabeculae. These trabeculae then become calcified by the deposition of calcium phosphate. Because of calcification of matrix nutrients cannot reach the chondrocytes and they undergo degenerative changes leading to their death. The periosteal capillaries now grow towards the calcified cartilage. The osteoprogenitor cells present in the developing periosteum migrate along these capillaries and constitute the periosteal bud. These cells then form the bony matrix (osteoid) over the trabeculae of calcified cartilage. The bone formed in this manner is known as cancellous bone. The site where bone first appears in the diaphysis of a long bone is known as a primary ossification center. As the bone formation enlarges towards the ends of the cartilaginous model, the osteoclasts resorbed the bone in the middle portion of the diaphysis and form a cavity, known as medullary cavity. The compact bone of subperiosteal bone collar now encloses this medullary cavity.

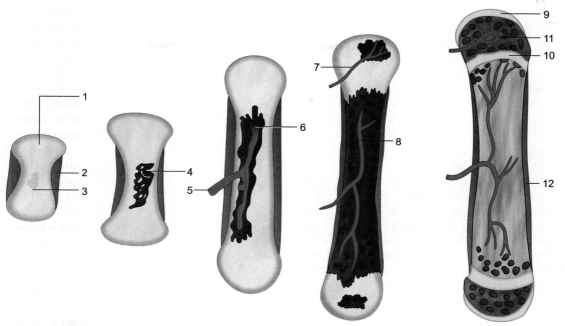

**Fig. 7.9:** Schematic diagram showing the stages of endochondral ossification in a long bone. Hyaline cartilage (1), bone collar (2), primary ossification center (3), degenerating cartilage (4), blood vessel of periosteal bud (5), spongy bone formation (6), epiphyseal blood vessel (7), medullary cavity (8), articular cartilage (9), epiphyseal plate of cartilage (10), spongy bone (11) and compact bone (12)

With the enlargement of this marrow cavity, a distinct zone can be identified at both ends of this cavity, known as the epiphyseal plate of cartilage. This plate of cartilage is responsible for longitudinal growth of bone. It can be divided into 5 zones, starting from the zone most distal to the ossification center and proceeding towards the center, are as follows (Fig. 7.10A, B):

a. **Resting or reserve zone:** This zone consists of small inactive chondrocytes. Proliferation of cells and production of matrix does not take place in this region.

b. **Proliferative zone:** This zone consists of rapidly dividing chondrocytes, which arranged in columns that are parallel to the long axis of the bone. These chondrocytes are larger in size than those in the resting zone.

c. **Hypertrophic zone:** In this zone, chondrocytes are greatly enlarged in size (hypertrophied).

Isogenous groups of cartilages are present in this zone.

d. **Calcification zone:** In this zone, matrix becomes calcified giving a granular appearance, and the cells degenerate.

e. **Ossification zone:** In this zone calcified cartilage is invaded by vascular, osteogenic tissue from the diaphysis. Osteoblasts cover the remnants of calcified cartilage, and form bone on it.

At the time of birth the diaphysis is bony, but the epiphysis or ends of long bones are still cartilaginous. Shortly after birth, secondary centers of ossification develop at the epiphysis. After secondary ossification centers have formed, bone tissue completely replaced cartilage with a sequence of similar events that form the primary center, except a bone collar is not formed. Cartilage remains only in two regions: The articular cartilage, which persists throughout adult life and does not contribute

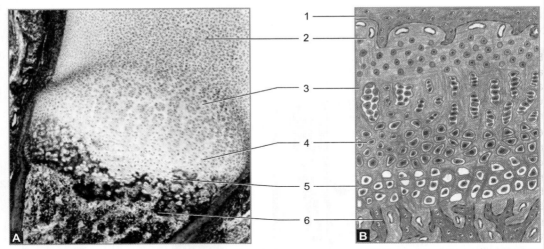

**Fig. 7.10:** Zones of bone growth of human fetal tibia, (A) micrograph, (B) sketch. The bone grows in length at the epiphyseal plate of cartilage. Epiphyseal bone (1), resting zone (2), proliferative zone (3), hypertrophic zone (4), calcification zone (5) and ossification zone (6)

to bone growth in length, and the epiphyseal plate, which connects the epiphysis to the diaphysis. The epiphyseal plate allows the diaphysis of the bone to increase in length until early adulthood. Growth in diameter occurs along with growth in length. In this process, the bone lining of the marrow cavity is destroyed so that the cavity increases in diameter. At the same time, osteoblasts from the periosteum add new osseous tissue around the outer surface of the bone. Initially, ossification of the diaphysis and epiphysis only produces spongy bone, but later on by reconstruction, the outer region of spongy bone is reorganized into compact bone. The epiphyseal plate disappears in adults, so the growth in length of bones becomes impossible in adulthood; although widening may still occur.

## REMODELING OF BONE

The bone formed by both intramembranous and endochondral ossification is woven bone, which is replaced by lamellar bone. Large vascular spaces are enclosed by woven bone, which are lined by osteoprogenitor cells (Fig. 7.11). These cells give rise to osteoblasts, which continue to form longitudinal lamellae

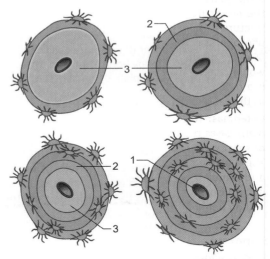

**Fig. 7.11:** Schematic diagram showing remodeling of bone. Haversian canal (1), newly formed lamellae (2) and vascular space (3)

of bone. This results in narrowing of the vascular spaces and form primary osteon. The primary osteons are resorbed by osteoclasts. These newly formed spaces are filled by bony lamellae produced by osteoblasts to form secondary osteon. Remnants of primary osteon form the interstitial lamellae. Remodeling of bone continues throughout life.

**Bone callus:** It is a temporary formation of fibroblasts and chondroblasts at the area of a bone fracture as the bone attempts to heal itself. The cells ultimately scatter and become inactive, lying in the resulting extracellular matrix that is the new bone.

**Osteomalacia (adult rickets):** It is a type of metabolic bone disease in which there is a lack of available calcium or there is a prolonged deficiency of vitamin D. This results in deficient calcification of newly formed bone and decalcification of already calcified bone. This condition may become severe during pregnancy because the calcium requirements of the fetus may lead to calcium loss from the mother.

**Osteoporosis:** It is a skeletal disorder characterized by low bone mass, fewer and thinner bony spicules as well as the presence of horizontal "struts" that do not join to form trabeculae. These changes make the bones fragile and increase susceptibility to fractures. This disease is due to poor calcium/phosphorus ratios, which is seen in persons above 50 years of age. Osteoporosis is more common in women after menopause. After menopause, there is a reduction in estrogen level and is considered as the cause of the osteoporosis.

**Osteomas:** These are rare benign lesions that in many cases represent developmental aberrations or reactive growths rather than true neoplasms. These are composed of a bland mixture of woven and lamellar bone, which may be difficult to distinguish from normal bone. They are not invasive and do not undergo malignant transformation.

## Summary

- Two methods are employed to prepare the bone for study—decalcification (by acid treatment) and preparation of ground sections (by cutting and grinding).
- Functions of bone—supporting framework for body, protection of vital organs, reservoir for calcium and phosphates, production of blood cells by bone marrow, and transduction of sound by auditory ossicles.
- Bone cells—osteoprogenitor cells (capable of differentiation into osteoblasts), osteoblasts (synthesis of collagen and alkaline phosphatase), osteocytes (responsible for the viability of bone tissue), osteoclasts (resorption of bone), and bone-forming cells (may responsible for nutritional support of osteocytes).
- Types of bone—woven and lamellar.
- Woven or immature bone is the first bone tissue to appear in embryonic development and is replaced in postnatal life by lamellar bone except near sutures and insertions of some tendons.
- Types of lamellar bone—compact bone and spongy bone.
- The structural unit of compact bone is haversian system or osteon.
- Spongy bone is composed of bony trabeculae separated by interconnecting spaces of bone marrow.
- The process of bone formation is known as ossification and it is of two types—intramembranous and endochondral.
- In intramembranous ossification, bone tissue develops from condensation of connective tissue mesenchyme, while in endochondral ossification, bone tissue develops from a cartilage model.

### Self Assessment

1. The structural unit of compact bone is:
   a. Sarcomere
   b. Osteon
   c. Volkmann's canal
   d. Haversian canal

2. Which of the following cells secrete component of the matrix?
   a. Osteoblasts
   b. Osteoclasts
   c. Osteocytes
   d. Osteogenic cells

3. Spongy bone is also known as:
   a. Compact bone
   b. Dense bone
   c. Woven bone
   d. Cancellous bone

4. Which cells are responsible for resorption of bone?
   a. Osteoblasts     b. Osteoclasts
   c. Osteocytes      d. Osteogenic cells

5.  All of the following bones are formed by
    intramembranous ossification EXCEPT:
    a.  Frontal bone
    b.  Parietal bone
    c.  Femur
    d.  Mandible

6.  Decalcification of bone is done by:
    a.  Treating the bone with acid
    b.  Treating the bone with alkali
    c.  By smear preparation
    d.  By grinding the sections

7.  Major component of bone matrix is:
    a.  Collagen
    b.  Glycoproteins
    c.  Lipid
    d.  Hydroxyapatite crystals

8.  Which one is not a function of bone?
    a.  Blood cell production
    b.  Support
    c.  Protection
    d.  Lubrication

9.  Which type of bone is made up of bony
    trabeculae?
    a.  Woven bone
    b.  Compact bone
    c.  Cancellous bone
    d.  Cortical bone

10. Haversian system is a characteristic
    feature of:
    a.  Woven bone
    b.  Compact bone
    c.  Cancellous bone
    d.  Trabecular bone

## Answers

1. b,    2. a,    3. d,    4. b,    5. c,    6. a,    7. d,    8. d,    9. c,
10. b

# 8

# Muscle Tissue

Muscle is the contractile tissue of our body, which is primarily designed for movements. Most of the muscles are derived from mesoderm except the arrectores pilorum, muscles of the iris, and myoepithelial cells which are derived from ectoderm. Each

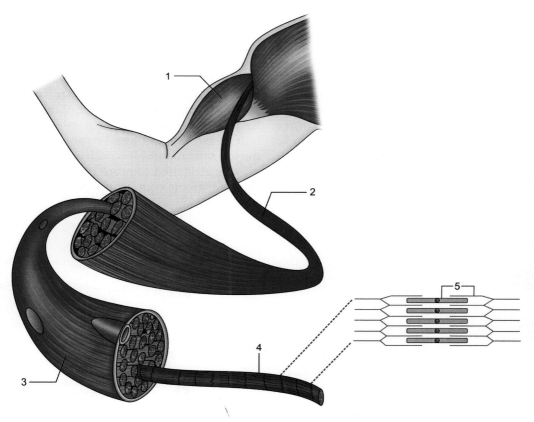

Schematic diagram showing organization of a skeletal muscle (1). Bundles of muscle fibers (2), muscle fiber (3), myofibril (4) and myofilaments (5)

muscle is composed of numerous muscle fibers which are made up of a sarcolemma (cell membrane) enclosing sarcoplasm (cytoplasm). Sarcoplasm contains numerous longitudinal fibrils, known as myofibrils.

Muscles are of three types on the basis of morphological and functional characteristics.

## SKELETAL (STRIATED OR VOLUNTARY) MUSCLE

It is the most abundant type of muscle of our body and comprises about 40% of all body weight. Muscle fibers are long, cylindrical and unbranched (skeletal muscle fibers in tongue are branched). In cross sections, muscle fibers have a polygonal shape with diameter of 10–100 µm. Their length varies greatly; such as in sartorius muscle of front of thigh the fiber length is up to 30 cm and in the stapedius muscle of middle ear the length of fiber is only a few mm. Sarcolemma represents the plasma membrane of the cell, its basal lamina, and the reticular lamina. Sarcoplasm (cytoplasm) contains myofibrils and also contains the usual cell organelles that tend to aggregate near the nuclei. The nuclei of muscle fibers are elongated and lie along the periphery of the fiber (Fig. 8.1A, B), just under its sarcolemma. Each fiber is really a syncytium with hundreds of nuclei along its length. Mitochondria are numerous and substantial amounts of glycogen are also present, which provides energy for the contraction of muscle. Myofibril is the structural and functional subunit of a muscle fiber. Myofibrils extend along the entire length of skeletal muscle fibers and are composed of thin and thick type of myofilaments. Thin myofilaments are composed of F-actin, tropomyosin and troponin; whereas thick myofilaments are composed of myosin II.

The most striking feature of skeletal muscle fibers is the presence of cross striations in them. These striations are due to alternating dark A (anisotropic)- and light I (isotropic)-bands. A-band contains both thin and thick myofilaments, while I-band contain only thin myofilaments. The A-band is bisected by the lighter H-band, which consists of thick myofilaments only. H-band is further bisected by a denser M-band, which represents the areas of cross-connections between myosin filaments. In the middle of I-band a protein disc or Z-line is present. The region between two Z-lines is known as a sarcomere, which is the functional or contractile unit of the muscle. Each sarcomere is made up of an A-band and half of two contiguous I-bands. In resting muscle sarcomere is about 2.5 µm long, but it may be stretched to more than 4 µm and in case of extreme contraction, may be reduced

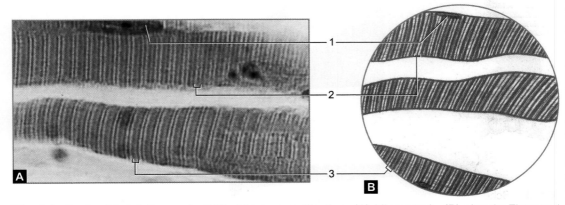

**Fig. 8.1:** Ocular (skeletal) muscle (LS) at high magnification. (A) Micrograph, (B) sketch. Flattened nucleus (1) of muscle fiber is located at the periphery. Cross striations are recognized as I-band (2) and A-band (3)

to 1 µm. Sarcomere is shorter in fast moving muscle (more contractile unit per mm), e.g. digital muscles and biceps.

> When seen with polarizing microscope, the A-band shows birefringence, i.e. they alter the plane of polarized light in two planes, so known as anisotropic or A-band. On the other hand, I-band does not show birefringence, i.e. they do not alter the plane of polarized light, so known as isotropic or I-band.
>
> Z is derived from German word Zwischenschiebe (Zwischen = between, schiebe = disc).
>
> M is derived from German word Mittleschiebe (Mittle = middle).
>
> H is named after Hensen who had first described it.

Myofilaments contain several proteins, in which the four main proteins are F-actin, tropomyosin, troponin, and myosin II. 55% of the total protein of striated muscle is made up by myosin II and F-actin proteins.

> **Myofilaments (Fig. 8.2)** Each F-actin filament is composed of two sub-filaments that are twisted around each other. Each sub-filament is a chain of G-actin molecules. These actin filaments are polar; and each has a head (+) end that extends into the A-band and a tail (−) end that is bound to the Z-line through a protein called α-actinin.

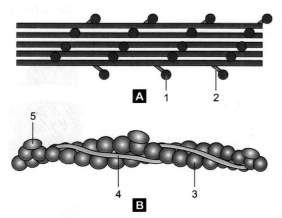

**Fig. 8.2:** Schematic diagram showing myofilaments, (A) thick filament and (B) thin filament. Heads of myosin II (1), tails of myosin II (2), actin filament (3), tropomyosin (4) and troponin (5)

Tropomyosin is in the form of a long fiber that wrapped around actin filament. Troponin is a complex made by several fractions. These complexes are arranged regularly over the actin filament. In a resting muscle tropomyosin and the troponin complex mask the myosin-binding site on the actin molecule.

Myosin II is composed of two heavy and four light chains. Heavy chains are twisted around each other as tails and from each chain a small globular head project at right angles. Light chains are of two types: Essential and regulatory, and one molecule of each type is present in association with each head. Each head has two binding sites; one for ATP and another for actin. The head form transient cross bridges between the thick and thin myofilaments on either side of H-band, i.e. the H-band does not have these globular heads.

Thick and thin myofilaments are aligned precisely by some accessory proteins and these are: Titin, α-actinin, nebulin, desmin, myomesin and tropomodulin.

> **Accessory proteins** Titin supports the thick myofilaments and connect them to the Z-line, thus prevents excessive stretching of sarcomere. α-actinin is present in the region of the Z-lines and it binds the tail ends of actin filaments to the Z-line. Two molecules of nebulin wrap around the entire length of thin myofilament. It attaches the thin myofilament to Z-line and may be responsible for maintaining the length of thin myofilament during muscle development. Desmin is present in intermediate filaments of the cytoskeleton and links myofibrils to each other and also to the cell membrane. Myomesin is present in the region of the M-band and it binds the tail ends of myosin filaments to M-band. Tropomodulin is attached to the free end of thin myofilament and it maintains the length of actin filament.

### A. Organization of Skeletal Muscle

The entire muscle is surrounded by a dense irregular connective tissue sheath known as epimysium (Fig. 8.3), which is continuous with the connective tissue of tendon at

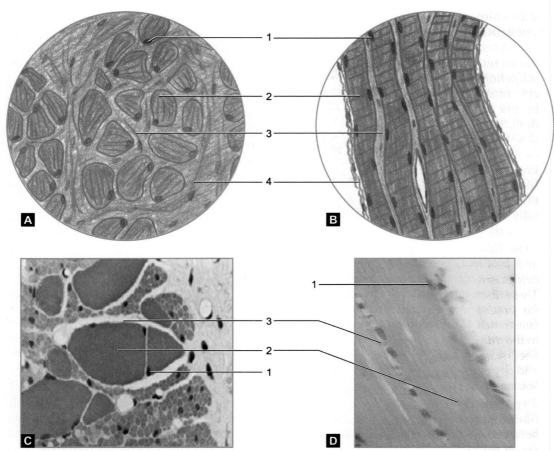

**Fig. 8.3:** Skeletal muscle, (A) sketch of TS, (B) sketch of LS, (C) micrograph of TS, and (D) micrograph of LS with peripheral located nuclei (1) in each muscle fiber (2). Individual muscle fiber is invested by endomysium (3) and bundles of muscle fibers by perimysium (4)

myotendinous junctions. Septa of the epimysium extend inwards and carry the large blood vessels, nerves and lymphatics of the muscle. The bundles or fascicles of muscle fibers are surrounded by the perimysium, but there is no line of demarcation between perimysium and epimysium. The larger blood vessels and nerves travel within the perimysium. Individual muscle fiber is surrounded by endomysium, which is composed of reticular fibers and a basal lamina.

Only small-diameter blood vessels and the fine branches of the nerves are present within the endomysium. The force generated by contraction of a single muscle fiber is transmitted to other muscle fibers through these connective tissue sheaths and thus, the force generated by different muscle fibers gets added together. The amount of connective tissue varies from muscle to muscle and is relatively greater in muscles that are capable of finely graded movements.

## B. Types of Skeletal Muscle Fibers

Skeletal muscle usually consists of three different types of fibers. The differences are due to color, diameter, cytochemical and physiological properties of the fibers.

a. **Type I (red) fibers:** These fibers are of small diameter and have a large number of mitochondria, abundant myoglobin and cytochrome. These fibers are also characterized by the thick Z-line. These fibers are predominant in muscles, where less powerful, slow but prolong contraction is needed such as the muscles of the limbs and back, so known as slow twitch fibers. In these fibers, energy is derived from oxidative phosphorylation (aerobic glycolysis) of fatty acids.

b. **Type IIb (white) fibers:** These fibers are of large diameter and contain less myoglobin and less number of mitochondria in the cytoplasm. Z-line is narrow in these fibers. These fibers contract rapidly and responsible for precise fine movements, so known as fast twitch fibers. White fibers are present in the muscles of eyeball and fingers. These fibers store a considerable amount of glycogen, and depend upon anaerobic glycolysis as a source of energy.

c. **Type IIa (intermediate) fibers:** These fibers have intermediate characteristics between red and white fibers. These fibers are of medium diameter with many mitochondria and high myoglobin content. These fibres are fast twitching and contain large amounts of glycogen in comparison to type I fibers. These fibers are predominant in muscles of legs and depend upon anaerobic glycolysis as a source of energy.

For comparison between red, white and intermediate muscle fibers, *see* Table 15 given in Appendix I.

## C. Motor Innervation

Skeletal muscle fibers are richly innervated through motor neurons that originate in the spinal cord or brainstem. These myelinated motor nerves branch out within the perimysial connective tissue, where each nerve gives rise to several terminal twigs. At the site of innervations, the nerve loses its myelin sheath and forms a dilated termination, known as terminal button that sits within a trough on the muscle surface (Fig. 8.4). This structure is called the neuromuscular junction (motor end plate). At the terminal portion, the axon of the nerve fiber is covered by a thin cytoplasmic layer of Schwann cells. In the axon terminal, numerous mitochondria and synaptic vesicles are present. Synaptic vesicles contain the neurotransmitter acetylcholine. Between the axon and the surface of muscle a space is present, known as the synaptic cleft. At the end plate, the sarcolemma of muscle is thrown into numerous deep folds. Below these folds in the sarcoplasm nuclei, numerous mitochondria, ribosomes, and glycogen granules are present.

A single neuron can innervate one muscle fiber, or it may branch and may be responsible for innervating several to a hundred or more muscle fibers. A single neuron and all the muscles it innervates constitute a motor unit (Fig. 8.5). Muscles which produce fine movements have only a few muscle fibers per motor neuron in their motor units such as in ocular muscles, one neuron only innervates approximately three muscle fibers, while in

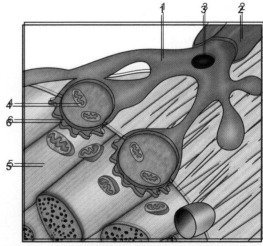

**Fig. 8.4:** Schematic diagram of motor end plate. Axon (1), myelin sheath (2), Schwann cell (3), mitochondria (4), muscle fiber (5) and synaptic cleft (6)

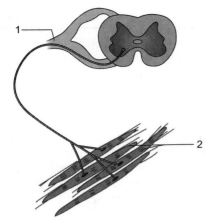

**Fig. 8.5:** Schematic diagram showing motor unit. Spinal nerve (1) and muscle fibers (2)

Intrafusal fibers have two types of muscle fibers: Nuclear bag and nuclear chain fibers (Fig. 8.6A, B). Nuclear bag fibers are much longer and extend beyond the capsule to attach to endomysium of extrafusal fibers, while nuclear chain fibers remain within the capsule.

Each muscle spindle is innervated by the motor as well as sensory nerve fibers. The motor innervation is by axons of gamma neurons located in the spinal cord and brain. The sensory fibers that carry information from the muscle spindle have spiral endings around the middle region of both types of intrafusal fibres. Upon stretching of skeletal muscle, sensory nerves carry information to the central nervous system, which moderates the activity of motor neurons innervating that particular muscle.

case of muscles of back, one neuron innervates hundreds of muscle fibers.

### D. Sensory Innervation

Muscle spindles are highly specialized spindle-shaped stretch receptors located within nearly all skeletal muscles. These receptors are able to measure changes in muscle length as well as the rate of change of muscle length. These receptors contain a few specialized intrafusal muscle fibers (extrafusal fibers form the main bulk of the muscle) bounded by an external capsule made up of connective tissue. Each intrafusal fiber is surrounded by an internal capsule.

### E. Contraction of Skeletal Muscle

Muscle fibers carry their electrical signals for contraction on their sarcolemma. Any time that a muscle fiber has to contract, an electrical signal must run along its sarcolemma. Since the electrical signal does not reach the middle of the muscle fiber because of its large diameter, therefore, it is carried into the cell interior by T (transverse) tubules, which is an invagination of the sarcolemma. The smooth endoplasmic reticulum (sER) present in

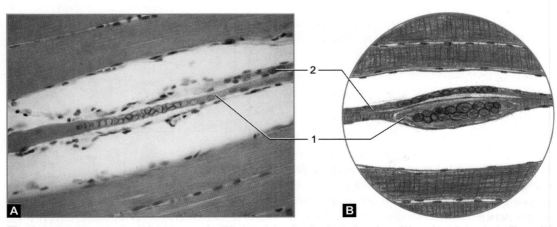

**Fig. 8.6:** Muscle spindle, (A) micrograph, (B) sketch having both nuclear bag (1) and nuclear chain fibers (2)

muscle is known as the sarcoplasmic reticulum (SR) that contains calcium ions required for the contraction of the muscle. The SR surrounds myofilaments and forms a meshwork around each myofibril. At each junction of A- and I- band the SR forms a pair of dilated terminal cisternae, which encircle the myofibrils. One T tubule and two cisternae form the triad (Fig. 8.7). Triad regulates muscle contraction by sequestering calcium ions (leading to relaxation) or releasing calcium ions (leading to contraction) and also allows the nerve impulse to penetrate and reach all parts of the muscle fiber.

Contraction of skeletal muscle fibers is quick, forceful, and usually under voluntary control. It is caused by the interaction of thin actin filaments and thick myosin filaments whose molecular configuration allows them to slide upon one another. In resting sarcomeres, thick and thin myofilaments are partially overlapped. During contraction, each sarcomere shortens and becomes thicker (Fig. 8.8), but both the thick and thin myofilaments retain their original length, because the contraction is the result of an increase in the amount of overlapping between the myofilaments, i.e. it is not caused by shortening of the myofilaments. During contraction, I-band decreases in size as thin myofilaments penetrate the A-band. The H-band diminishes in width as the thin myofilaments completely overlap the thick myofilaments. Width of A-band remains unchanged.

In many cases the contraction of skeletal muscle may not be strictly voluntary, e.g. in sneezing or coughing, respiratory movements, maintenance of posture.

## SMOOTH (NON-STRIATED OR INVOLUNTARY) MUSCLE

These muscle fibers are 10–20 µm in diameter and range in length from 20 µm in blood vessels to 500 µm in the uterine wall during pregnancy. Each muscle fiber is spindle shaped and possesses a single elongated nucleus, which is located in the widest portion of the fiber. Each fiber is enclosed by a basal

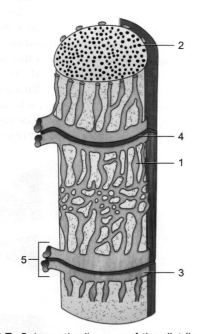

**Fig. 8.7:** Schematic diagram of the distribution of the sarcoplasmic reticulum (1) around the myofibrils (2) of skeletal muscle. Terminal cisternae (3), T tubule (4), Z-line (5), and triad (5)

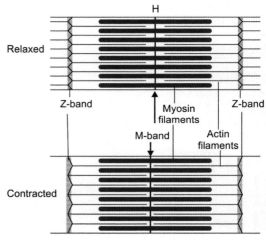

**Fig. 8.8:** Schematic diagram showing arrangements of myofilaments in contracted and resting stage

lamina and a network of reticular fibers. Smooth muscle fibers make close contact with each other through abundant gap junctions, which allow for rapid ionic communication between the smooth muscle fibers.

Thin myofilaments, which contain actin, tropomyosin and two actin binding proteins; caldesmon and calponin. Thick myofilaments contain myosin II, but it is different from myosin II present in skeletal muscle fibers. Myofilaments are not organized into myofibrils. Myofilaments overlap as in striated muscle and form a crisscross reticulum throughout the sarcoplasm. In the cytoplasm of smooth muscle dense bodies are present, which link thin myofilaments and intermediate filaments of the cytoskeleton to the cell membrane. These dense bodies are similar to the Z-lines of skeletal muscles. A rudimentary endo-plasmic reticulum is present; it consists of a closed system of membranes, similar to the sarcoplasmic reticulum of striated muscle. Sarcolemma of smooth muscle invaginates and form flask-shaped caveolae. Beneath the plasma membrane, and often in close proximity to sER cytoplasmic vesicles are present. These caveolae and vesicles may be functional analogues to the T tubule system of skeletal muscle.

Smooth muscle fibers are arranged in layers in such a way that near the central wide portion of a fiber, thin tapering end of neighbouring fibres are placed (Fig. 8.9A, B). There is minimal connective tissue between adjacent fibers.

In cross (transverse) sections (TS), the fibers of smooth muscles are of different diameter. The nucleus is even not present in all sections, i.e. it is only present in the fibers showing largest diameter (Fig. 8.10A, B).

It is innervated by autonomic nerves. The degree of innervation in a particular bundle of smooth muscle depends on the function and the size of that muscle. Extensive neuromuscular junctions are not present in the smooth muscle such as those in skeletal muscle.

## A. Types of Smooth Muscle Fibers

These are of two types:

a. **Visceral (single-unit) smooth muscle:** It is present in the form of sheets in the wall of hollow organs, e.g. digestive tract. It is minimally innervated and its contraction spreads are facilitated by large numbers of gap junctions such as peristaltic waves of contraction in the intestine. It is specialized for slow and prolonged contraction.

b. **Multi-unit smooth muscle:** It is richly innervated and gap junctions between neighbouring fibers are a few or absent. It is specialized for precise and graded contraction, e.g. iris of the eye.

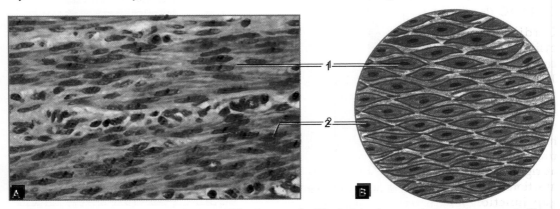

**Fig. 8.9:** LS of smooth muscle: Rectum, (A) micrograph, (B) sketch shows spindle shape muscle fibers (1) with a single elongated nucleus (2)

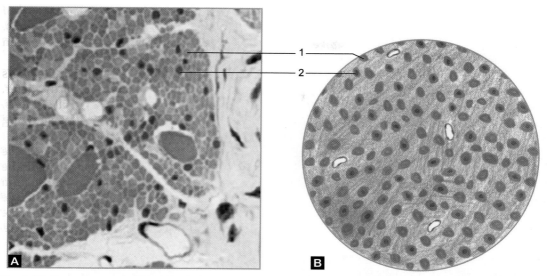

**Fig. 8.10:** Smooth muscle (TS) (A) micrograph, (B) sketch. Individual muscle fiber (1) with single nucleus (2)

## B. Contraction of Smooth Muscle

T tubules are absent in smooth muscle fibers. These muscle fibers are slowly contracted, but are more capable of sustained contractile activity than contraction of skeletal muscle. The contraction is not under voluntary control. The entire fiber, or only a portion of the fiber, may contract at a given instant. Contraction of smooth muscle may be produced by voluntary effort such as in passing urine.

## CARDIAC (INVOLUNTARY) MUSCLE

Cardiac muscle fibers are short, thick, cylindrical branched fibers with one or two central oval nuclei. Fibers are approximately 15 μm in diameter and from 85 to 100 μm in length. Fibres are joined serially end to end by intercalated discs (Fig. 8.11). The disc crosses the fibers in step-like pattern, so have transverse and longitudinal parts. The transverse part runs across the muscle fibers at right angles and possesses three types of junctions: Fascia adherens, desmosomes, and gap junctions. The longitudinal part is continuous with the transverse part and has desmosomes and numerous large gap junctions.

These intercalated discs are better visible by silver stains.

In cardiac muscle the myofibrils are relatively few. At places, the myofibrils merge with each other. Even large numbers of mitochondria are present among its myofibrils. Sarcoplasm is more abundant than the skeletal muscle fibers. As a result of these factors, the myofibrils and cross striations of cardiac muscle are not as distinct as those of skeletal muscle. Around the nucleus clear zone of non-fibrillar perinuclear sarcoplasm is present, which is devoid of cross striations. Each cardiac muscle fiber does not receive direct innervation like skeletal muscle fibers. Sarcoplasm is abundant in cardiac muscle fibers. In cardiac muscle mitochondria are more abundant than in the skeletal muscle, and occupy 40% or more of the cytoplasmic volume, reflecting the need for continuous aerobic metabolism in heart muscle. Because the oxygen requirement of cardiac muscle fibers is high, they contain an abundant supply of myoglobin.

The cardiac muscle fibers are very close to the red (type I skeletal) muscle fibers. Like red fibers, cardiac muscle fibers also have

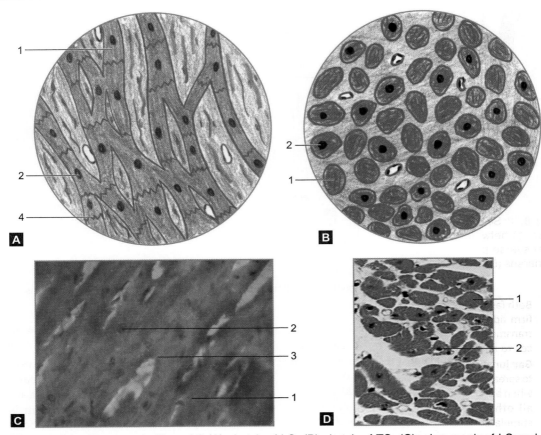

**Fig. 8.11:** Cardiac muscle fibers (1) (A) sketch of LS, (B) sketch of TS, (C) micrograph of LS and (D) micrograph of TS exhibits single central nucleus (2), branching (3) and intercalated disc (4)

significant amounts of glycogen and myoglobin. Around the cardiac muscle fibers rich density of the capillary network is present. Cardiac muscle fibers contain a red brown pigment, known as lipofuscin (wear and tear pigment), which is derived from turnover of cell material within lysosomes. With aging, this pigment accumulates in the human heart and may be responsible for the brown color of the cardiac muscle.

Cardiac muscle fibers of the atria are somewhat smaller than those of the ventricles. These fibers also contain granules (especially in the muscle fibers of right atrium) containing atrial natriuretic peptide, which inhibits the contraction of smooth muscles present in the wall of blood vessels and thereby functions to lower blood pressure. This peptide acts on renal tubules and decrease their capabilities to conserve sodium and water. This hormone, thus opposes the actions of aldosterone and antidiuretic hormone, whose effects on kidneys result in sodium and water conservation.

**Intercalated disc** (Fig. 8.12) Transverse portions of intercalated disc is thick, while longitudinal portions are thin.
- **Fascia adherens:** It is the site of attachment of actin filaments to sarcolemma and occurs at the level of I-band.
- **Desmosomes:** It may also be present between fascia adherens.

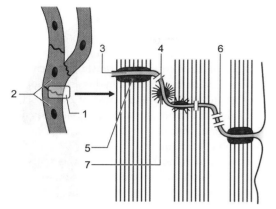

**Fig. 8.12:** Schematic diagram showing intercalated disc (1) between two cardiac muscle fibers (2). Transverse part (3), longitudinal part (4), fascia adherens (5), gap junction (6) and desmosome (7)

Both fascia adherens and desmosomes provide firm adhesion to actin filaments and help in transmission of force of contraction from one cell to another.

- **Gap junctions:** It allows muscle action potential to spread from one muscle fiber to another. Thus, when a single fiber of the network is stimulated all other fibers in networks also become stimulated. In this way cardiac muscle fiber acts as a syncytium.

### Contraction of Cardiac Muscle

T tubules are larger and are located at the level of the Z-lines, rather than at the junction of A- and I-band. T tubule of cardiac muscle is associated with one terminal cistern, forming diads (Fig. 8.13).

Cardiac muscle fibers even need calcium ions for their contractions just like skeletal muscle fibers. The sarcoplasmic reticulum, which stored calcium ions is not so developed, so these fibers import the calcium from outside for contraction. Cardiac muscle differs from skeletal and smooth muscles in that it possesses an inherent rhythmicity as well as the ability to contract spontaneously. The rate of this rhythmicity can be modified by autonomic nerves that supply it.

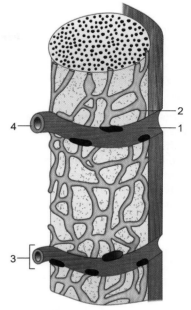

**Fig. 8. 13:** Schematic diagram of the distribution of the T-tubule system (1) and sarcoplasmic reticulum (2) in cardiac muscle. Diad (3), and Z-line (4)

For comparison between skeletal, smooth, and cardiac muscle fibers, *see* Table 16 given in Appendix I.

### MYOEPITHELIAL CELLS

These are stellate cells forming a meshwork around the ducts and acini like an octopus. In cross section, these cells appear as spindle shaped. These cells are modified muscle cells with multiple processes. When the myoepithelial cells contract, they expel the contents of acini and ducts. These cells are of ectodermal origin. These cells are innervated by autonomic nerves.

**Hypertrophy:** It is an increase in the size of cells and consequently an increase in the size of the organ. It can be physiologic or pathologic and is caused either by increased functional demand or by specific hormonal stimulation, e.g. skeletal muscle can undergo hypertrophy in response to increased demand, because in the adult they cannot divide to generate more cells to share the work.

**Hyperplasia:** It is characterized by an increase in cell number in an organ or tissue. It can be physiologic or pathologic. It usually occurs in the uterus during pregnancy.

**Rigor mortis:** It is one of the recognizable signs of death that is caused by a chemical change in the muscles after death, causes the limbs to become stiff and difficult to move and manipulate. This postmortem rigidity is due to the buildup of lactic acid, which causes the actin and myosin filaments of the muscle fibers to remain linked until the muscles begin to decompose. The facial muscles are first to undergo rigor mortis.

**Myasthenia gravis:** It is an acquired autoimmune disorder of neuromuscular transmission chara-cterized by muscle weakness. In this acetylcholine receptor in the motor end-plates of the muscles are damaged. Extraocular and eyelid muscles are affected first, followed by the muscles of necks and limbs. Although in histological sections muscles appear normal, but a few clumps of lymphocytes may be found around small blood vessels and degenerating muscle fibers may be present.

## Summary

| Parameter | Skeletal muscle | Smooth muscle | Cardiac muscle |
|---|---|---|---|
| Shape | Long, cylindrical and unbranched | Spindle shaped and unbranched | Short, cylindrical and show branching |
| Nuclei | Multinucleated, elongated and peripherally located | Single, elongated and centrally located | Single, oval and centrally located |
| Intercalated disc | Absent | Absent | Present (fascia adherens, desmosomes and gap junctions) |
| Striations | Cross striations are present | Striations absent | Less prominent cross striations are present |
| Control of contraction | Voluntary | Involuntary | Involuntary |
| Contraction | Quicker and faster | Slow and sustained | Rhythmic contraction |
| Location | Limbs, tongue | Walls of respiratory and digestive tracts | Heart |

### Self Assessment

1. Sarcomere is defined as region between two:
   a. I-bands
   b. A-bands
   c. H-bands
   d. Z-lines

2. Which organelle is more in red skeletal muscle fibers in comparison to white skeletal muscle fibers?
   a. Ribosome
   b. Mitochondria
   c. Lysosome
   d. rER

3. Cross striations are best seen in:
   a. Skeletal muscle
   b. Smooth muscle
   c. Cardiac muscle
   d. Involuntary muscle

4. Intercalated disc is a characteristic feature of which muscle?
   a. Skeletal muscle
   b. Smooth muscle
   c. Cardiac muscle
   d. All of the above

5. Which is not a feature of smooth muscle?
   a. Spindle-shaped cell
   b. Striations
   c. Single central nucleus
   d. Involuntary

6. Branched muscle fibers are present in which muscle?
   a. Skeletal muscle
   b. Smooth muscle
   c. Cardiac muscle
   d. All of the above

7. During contraction of skeletal muscle sarcomere shortens as:
   a. Thick myofilaments contracts
   b. Thin myofilaments contracts
   c. I-band decreases in size
   d. I-band increases in size

8. In the skeletal muscle centre of triad is present:
   a. At the junction of A- and I-band
   b. At the Z-lines
   c. In the middle of A-band
   d. In the middle of I-band

9. Caveolae is present in:
   a. Skeletal muscle
   b. Smooth muscle
   c. Cardiac muscle
   d. All of the above

10. Which of the following pigments accumulates with aging in the cardiac muscle?
    a. Melanin
    b. Lipofuscin
    c. Rhodopsin
    d. None of the above

## Answers

1. d,   2. b,   3. a,   4. c,   5. b,   6. c,   7. c,   8. a,   9. b,
10. b

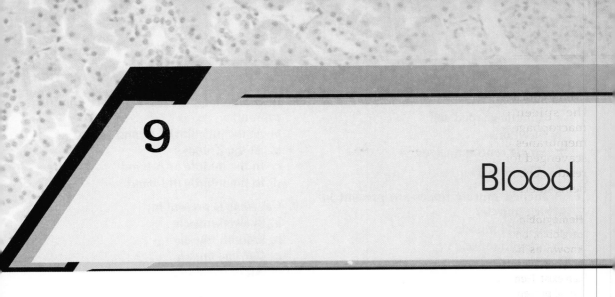

# 9

# Blood

Blood is a special form of connective tissue, having suspension of cells (blood cells) in a liquid called plasma. The cells present in the blood are: Erythrocytes, leukocytes and platelets. The relative volume of cells and plasma in the blood of adults is approximately 45% and 55%. In this 45% volume of cells, leukocytes and platelets constitute only 1% of the blood volume. Blood is a bright to dark red, viscous and slightly alkaline (pH 7.4) fluid. In an adult, the blood is about 1/7th of the body weight and this corresponds to 5–6 litres. Blood carries oxygen, carbon dioxide, nitrogen and nutritive substances, e.g. amino acids, sugars and mineral salts. It even carries hormones, enzymes and vitamins. It performs the defence of the organism by means of the phagocytic activity of the leukocytes. It also helps to regulate body temperature, and to maintain the acid–base and osmotic balance of the body fluids.

## PLASMA

It is a slightly alkaline fluid, with a typical yellowish color. It consists of 91% water, 9% protein and other solutes are 1%. The proteins are numerous and diverse, including albumin (maintains the correct proportion of blood to tissue fluid volume), immunoglobulins (involved in immunological defence mechanism), blood clotting factors, antiproteases and transport proteins. Other solutes in plasma are: Electrolytes, nutrients, gases, nitrogen substances, hormones and enzymes. These solutes help in maintenance of homeostasis of our body. Plasma forms the extracellular fluid of connective tissue and its electrolyte composition is even similar to the extracellular fluid. However, the concentration of some proteins in the extracellular fluid is much lower in comparison to the plasma.

## ERYTHROCYTES (RED BLOOD CELLS: RBCs)

These are the smallest and most numerous (about 4–6 millions/mm$^3$) blood cells. These cells have the shape of a biconcave lens with a diameter of 7.8 μm, thickness of 2.6 μm at its edge and 0.8 μm in the center. The cells are rich in protein hemoglobin, which is able to bind in a faint manner to oxygen. Therefore, these cells are mainly responsible for providing oxygen to the tissues and partly responsible for recovering $CO_2$ produced as waste. Mature RBCs lack nucleus and other typical cell organelles. The lack of nucleus allows more room for hemoglobin and the biconcave shape raises the surface and cytoplasmic volume ratio. These characteristics make more efficient diffusion of oxygen by these cells. The cytoskeleton of erythrocytes is flexible so it allows these cells to deform rapidly, so they can pass through small capillaries. The mean life span of erythrocytes is about 120 days. After that time they develop surface "senescence" markers and get engulfed in the spleen or bone marrow or liver by macrophages. The hemoglobin and plasma membranes of RBCs are broken down and scavenged for re-usable components, and the residue becomes the iron containing pigment hemosiderin.

**Hemoglobin** It consists of four polypeptide chains of globin, bound to an iron containing porphyrin known as haem. Depending on the particular polypeptides present, several types of hemoglobin can exist. Hemoglobin HbA is the major hemoglobin (96%) present in adults. In adults, small amounts of $HbA_2$ is also present. Fetal erythrocytes have nucleus and also contain a different form of hemoglobin known as HbF (fetal hemoglobin). However, production of HbF falls very rapidly after birth.

## LEUKOCYTES (WHITE BLOOD CELLS: WBCs)

These are less numerous than red blood cells. The density of the leukocytes in the blood is 5000–7000/mm³ and divided in two categories: granulocytes and lymphoid cells (agranulocytes) (Fig. 9.1). On the basis of granules, granulocytes are further divide into neutrophil, eosinophil (acidophil) and basophil. The lymphoid cells are lacking in granules, have a compact nucleus and a transparent cytoplasm. The lymphoid cells are further divided in lymphocytes and monocytes. Granulocytes will never divide again, as they lost their capacity of the division during their differentiation. On the contrary, lymphoid cells have the potential for further division. Usually, the shape of the nucleus of various kinds of leukocytes is different. It can show

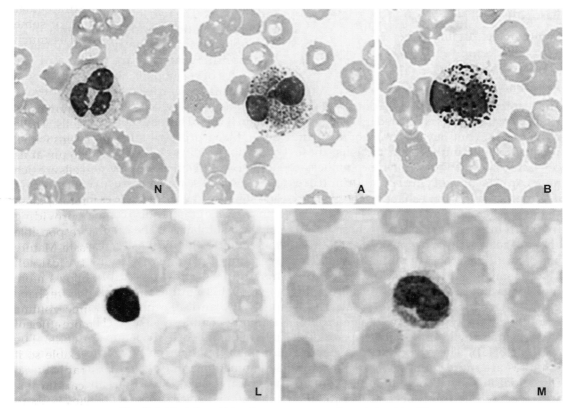

**Fig. 9.1:** Peripheral blood-smear preparation stained by Giemsa

multiple lobes or may be indented or kidney-shaped (reniform). These cells are responsible for the defence of the organism. These cells do not function within the bloodstream, but use it as a way of travelling from one region of the body to another. These cells adhere to receptors on the endothelial cells of blood vessels through their surface proteins. Upon reaching at their target, these cells leave the bloodstream by migrating between the endothelial cells of the blood vessels (diapedesis) and enter in the connective tissue spaces to perform their function. These cells will die in the tissues, i.e. they do not re-enter in the blood.

Each type of leukocyte is present in the blood in different proportions:

**Neutrophil:** 50–70%

**Eosinophil:** 2–4%

**Basophil:** 0.5–1%

**Lymphocyte:** 20–40%

**Monocyte:** 3–8%

## A. Neutrophils

The diameter of these cells is about 10–12 μm. Nucleus of these cells is divided into 2–5 lobes connected by a fine nuclear strand or filament. Because of this multi-lobed nucleus, these cells are also known as polymorphonuclear neutrophils or polymorphs. Immature neutrophils have a band-shaped or horseshoe-shaped nucleus and are known as band cells. In the females, Barr body, which is an appendage like a little drumstick is present at one of the nuclear lobes of the neutrophil. The cytoplasm of neutrophils contains three types of granules. The primary or azurophilic granules are large and spheroidal. These granules are the lysosomes of the neutrophil and contain acid hydrolases and myeloperoxidase (antibacterial). The secondary or specific granules are more numerous, smaller and ellipsoidal in shape. These granules contain substances that upon secretion into the extracellular spaces stimulate an inflammatory reaction. Tertiary granules are associated with adhesion of leukocytes to other cells and their phagocytosis.

Neutrophils are very active in phagocytosing bacteria and are present in large amount in the pus of wounds. Once a neutrophil makes contact with a bacterium, the neutrophil attaches to the bacterium and then engulfs it (phagocytosis) within a phagosome. Phago-cytosed bacteria are killed within phagolysosomes by the generation of toxic, reactive oxygen compound produced by a process known as respiratory burst. Besides this process, bacteria can be killed by bacteriolytic enzymes and antimicrobial peptides.

## B. Eosinophils

These are quite rare in the blood. These are 10–14 μm in diameter and have a sausage-shaped nucleus, which is darkly staining and bi-lobed. The two lobes are connected by a thin chromatin strand. The cytoplasm of eosinophils contains two types of granules. Azurophilic granules are a few and are lysosomes of eosinophils, which contain acid hydrolases. Specific granules contain a crystalline body, which contains major basic protein (MBP). The matrix of granules contains other three proteins such as eosinophilic cationic protein (ECP), eosinophil-derived neurotoxin (EDN) and eosinophil peroxidase (EPO). All these proteins are toxic to parasites and some RNA viruses. Besides these four proteins, specific granules also contain histaminase and aryl sulphatase. The eosinophil counters the action of many mast cell mediators by secreting degradative enzymes, including histaminase and aryl sulphatase, which destroy histamine and leukotrienes respectively and also phagocytose antigen–antibody complexes. These cells are present in large numbers in the lamina propria of the intestinal tract and at other sites of chronic inflammation. An elevated eosinophil count is typical in allergic reactions and in parasitic infestations, which support both these putative functions.

## C. Basophils

These are the rarest leukocytes. These are approximately 0.5 µm in diameter. Their cytoplasm is very rich in granules which take a dark purple color. The nucleus is bi- or tri-lobed, but pale staining. The nucleus is often obscured by the basophilic granules. The cytoplasm of basophils contains two types of granules. Azurophilic granules are a few and are lysosomes of eosinophils, which contain acid hydrolases. Specific granules secrete anti-coagulant and vasodilatory substances such as histamine, heparin sulphate, and serotonin. The basophils are functionally related to mast cells. These cells have a phagocytic capability, but their main function is secreting substances which mediate the immediate hypersensitivity reaction.

## D. Lymphocytes

These are quite common in the blood, but besides being present in the blood, these cells are also present in the lymphoid tissues and organs, as well as in the lymph circulating in the lymphatic vessel. Generally, these are smaller than the other leukocytes but larger than red blood cells. These cells are 8–10 µm in diameter. Large, spheroid, darkly stained nucleus leaves only a narrow rim of cytoplasm with a few small granules. Peripheral rim of cytoplasm stains light blue. Most lymphocytes circulating in the blood are in a resting state and can be activated following antigenic stimulation.

## E. Monocytes

These are the biggest leukocytes and 12–15 µm in diameter. They have a great reniform or horseshoe-shaped nucleus, in some cases nucleus is even bi-lobed. The cytoplasm is transparent, but with an appearance of "ground glass". The cytoplasm contains a moderate number of small, scattered azurophilic granules, but specific granules are absent. Monocytes after attaining maturity in the bone marrow, enter the blood circulation where they stay for 24–36 hours. Then they migrate into the connective tissue, where they become macrophages and move within the tissues. Macrophages after activation release cytokines and also coordinate inflammatory and defensive reactions. In response to large foreign particle, macrophages fuse with one another, forming foreign body giant cells that are large enough to phagocytose the foreign particle.

## PLATELETS OR THROMBOCYTES

Like the erythrocyte, the platelet was once part of a cell, but in its maturation, it loses its true cellularity. Platelets are small, membrane bound cytoplasmic fragment which is derived from a pre-existing precursor cell of the bone marrow, i.e. a very large megakaryocyte. In the course of its differentiation, the megakaryocyte develops fissures in its cytoplasm, and literally falls apart; the membrane bound cytoplasmic fragments thus formed are known as platelets. Platelets are round to oval, biconvex discs with a diameter of 2–4 µm and nucleus is absent in these cells. There are between 2,50,000 and 4,00,000 platelets per mm$^3$ of blood are present, each with a life span of 10 days. The granules present in the platelets is of 2 types: α- and γ-granules. These cells have a central zone that is slightly basophilic (granulomere), and a pale, homogeneous periphery (hyalomere). Hyalomere contains a circumferential bundle of microtubules and cytoplasmic filaments, which help in maintenance of shape of platelets. Platelets continuously monitor the vascular system and in case of damage to the endothelial lining of the vessel, the platelet adheres to the damaged site, release granules and initiate the clotting process.

## BONE MARROW

It is a gelatinous, vascular connective tissue, which is found in the medullary cavity of long bones and in the spaces between the trabeculae of spongy bones. It contains sinusoids and numerous cells that are responsible for hemopoiesis. It constitutes almost 5% of the total body weight. It is of two types: Red bone marrow named due to the presence of blood-forming cells; and yellow bone marrow, whose color is produced by the presence of a great number of fat cells. In newborns, bone marrow is generally red, however, as the child grows, most of the bone marrow changes gradually into the yellow bone marrow. The yellow bone marrow, however, retains its hemopoietic potential and when necessary, such as after severe blood loss, it can revert to red bone marrow. In adults, red marrow is present in the epiphysis of long bones and in flat, irregular, and short bones.

## PRENATAL HEMOPOIESIS

Formation of blood cells is known as hemopoiesis. It includes development of RBC (erythropoiesis), WBC (leukopoiesis) and platelets (thrombopoiesis). It begins in early embryonic life and divided into four phases: Yolk sac, hepatic, splenic and myeloid.

Yolk sac phase of hemopoiesis begins in three weeks after gestation in the mesoderm of the yolk sac, where mesenchymal cells aggregate into clusters known as blood islands. Cells present at the periphery of these islands gives rise to the vessel wall and the remaining cells become erythroblasts, which latter on forms erythrocytes. In the 6th week, hemopoietic centers develop in the liver (hepatic phase) and along with RBC some WBC also develops.

The splenic phase begins during the second trimester and both hepatic and splenic phases continue until the end of gestation. Myeloid phase (hemopoiesis in the bone marrow) begins by the end of the second trimester.

After birth, hemopoiesis takes place only in the red bone marrow and lymphatic tissues, however, both liver and spleen can form new blood cells in emergencies.

## POSTNATAL HEMOPOIESIS

All blood cells arise from a single type of stem cell in the bone marrow, called pluripotent stem cell (PPSC). The pluripotent stem cell is not only capable of differentiating into all blood cell lineages, but it is also capable of self-renewal. These stem cells proliferate and form one cell lineage that will become lymphocytes [colony-forming unit-lymphocyte (CFU-Ly) cells] and another lineage that will form the myeloid cells that develop in bone marrow [colony-forming unit-granulocyte, erythrocyte, monocyte, megakaryocyte (CFU-GEMM) cells]. These colony forming unit cells are responsible for the formation of various progenitor cells. Lymphoid cells migrate from the bone marrow to the thymus, lymph nodes, spleen and other lymphoid structures, where they proliferate.

The progenitor cells form by colony-forming unit cells are unipotent (committed to a single cell line) or bipotent (committed to two cell lines). These cells have only limited capacity for self-renewal. These progenitor cells give rise to precursor cells, which are incapable of self-renewal. These precursor cells have specific morphological characteristics and they can be regarded as the first cell of a particular cell line. These cells only produce mature blood cells.

## ERYTHROPOIESIS (ERYTHROCYTE FORMATION)

This process yields about 1 trillion erythrocytes daily in a normal adult. It begins with the formation of burst-forming unit-erythroid (BFU-E) from CFU-GEMM cells. These cells have a high rate of mitotic activity and responds to high concentrations of erythropoietin, a hormone that stimulates erythropoiesis. These cells form a colony-forming unit-erythroid (CFU-E) cells, which can even respond to low concentrations of erythropoietin and gives rise to the first histologically recognizable erythrocyte precursor, the proerythroblast. Proerythroblast is a large cell (14–19 μm) with basophilic cytoplasm and chromatin is loose and lacy, and nucleoli are clearly visible. These cells give rise to the basophilic erythroblast, which have a strongly basophilic cytoplasm and a condensed nucleus that has no visible nucleolus. The basophilia of proerythroblast and basophilic erythroblast is caused by the large number of polyribosomes involved in the synthesis of hemoglobin. During the next stage, polyribosomes decrease and areas of the cytoplasm begin to be filled with hemoglobin. At this stage, staining causes several colors to appear in the cell, so the cell is called polychromatophilic (Gr. *polys,* many; *chroma,* color; *philein,* to love) erythroblast (12–15 μm). In the next stage, the nucleus continues to condense and no cytoplasmic basophilia is evident, resulting in a uniformly acidophilic cytoplasm, so the cell is called ortho-chromatophilic erythroblast (8–12 μm). After this stage, a number of cytoplasmic protrusions form in the cell and expels its nucleus covered with a thin layer of cytoplasm. The expelled nucleus is engulfed by macrophages. The remaining cell still has a small number of polyribosomes and is called reticulocyte (7–8 μm), which soon loses its polyribosomes and becomes a mature erythrocyte.

## GRANULOPOIESIS

Neutrophils originate from CFU-GEMM cells, which differentiate into the bipotential colony-forming unit-granulocyte, monocyte in the

**Flowchart 9.1:** Showing differentiation of a pluripotent hematopoietic stem cell into the myeloid stem cell line

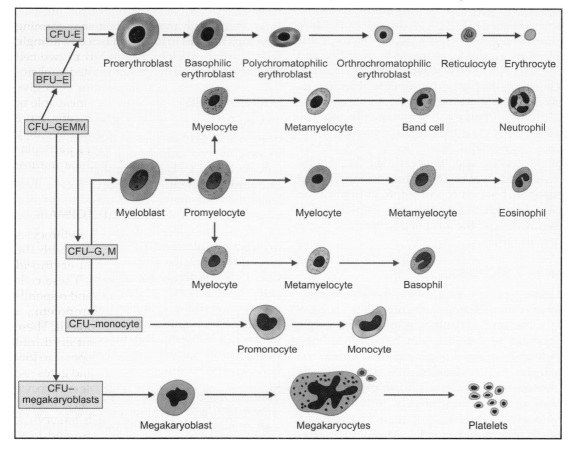

presence of cytokines and growth factors. Eosinophils and basophils also originate from CFU-GEMM cells, which differentiate into colony-forming unit-eosinophils to form eosinophils and colony-forming unit-basophils to form basophils. Microscopically, the precursors of these three cells cannot be differentiated from one another until the cells reach the myelocyte stage in which specific granules arise.

Myeloblast is the first recognizable precursor cell of eosinophil, basophil and neutrophil. It has a large, spherical nucleus with 3–5 nucleoli. It measures about 14–20 μm in diameter. The cytoplasm stains intensely basophilic. The myeloblast matures into a promyelocyte (L. pro, before, + Gr. myelos, marrow, + kytos, cell), which is having a basophilic granular cytoplasm and it will give rise to eosinophil, basophil, and neutrophil. The promyelocyte then differentiates into myelocyte, in which specific granules gradually increase in quantity and eventually occupy most of the cytoplasm. These eosinophilic myelocyte, basophilic myelocyte and neutrophilic myelocyte continue to divide and give rise to metamyelocyte. The metamyelocyte is the stage at which three cell lines can be clearly identified by the presence of numerous specific granules. The meta-myelocyte gives rise to mature eosinophil and basophil, but neutrophil before its maturation pass through an intermediate stage in which its nucleus has the form of a curved rod (band or stab cell).

## MONOCYTOPOIESIS

Monocytes originate from CFU-GEMM cells, which differentiate into the bipotential colony-forming unit-granulocyte, monocyte in the presence of cytokines and growth factors. Colony-forming unit-granulocyte, monocyte will give rise to colony-forming unit-monocyte (monoblasts), which will form promonocyte. Half of the promonocyte will form the monocyte, while half of them remain as a reserve progenitor cells. Monocytes after

attaining maturity in the bone marrow, enter in the blood circulation where they stay for 24–36 hours. Then they migrate into the connective tissue, where they become macrophages and move within the tissues.

## PLATELET FORMATION

These cells originate from CFU-GEMM cells, which differentiate into colony-forming unit-megakaryocyte in the presence of cytokines and growth factors. With further development it forms megakaryoblasts, which is a large cell with basophilic cytoplasm and a large nucleus. These cells undergo endomitosis, whereby the cell does not divide; instead, it becomes larger and the nucleus becomes polyploidy. These cells are stimulated to differentiate and proliferate by thrombopoietin and they form megakaryocytes (Gr. megas, big; karyon, nucleus; kytos, cell). With maturation megakaryocyte develops fissures in its cytoplasm and literally falls apart; the membrane bound cytoplasmic fragments thus form are known as platelets.

## LYMPHOPOIESIS

The multipotential stem cell colony-forming unit-lymphocyte divides in the bone marrow to form the two unipotential progenitor cells, CFU-LyB and CFU-LyT, neither of which is immunocompetent. The CFU-LyT cells then leave the bone marrow and travel to thymus where they complete their differentiation. In birds, the CFU-LyB cell migrates to a diverticulum attached to the gut, known as the bursa of Fabricius (thus B cell). Here the CFU-LyB cells divide and give rise to immuno-competent B lymphocytes. A similar event occurs in mammals, but in the absence of a bursa this development of immunocompetence occurs in a bursa-equivalent location, such as bone marrow, gut-associated lymphatic tissue (GALT), and spleen.

**Artificial blood** Karl Landsteiner, who got Nobel Prize in 1930, gave the idea of artificial blood. Blood can be produced artificially by three different procedures: Synthetic production, chemical isolation, and recombinant biochemical technology. Several companies working on the production of a safe and effective artificial blood substitute. However, various substances suffer from certain limitations such as hemoglobin-based products only last up to 30 hours, even they do not mimic blood's ability to fight diseases.

## Summary

Cells present in the blood are as follows.

| Cells | Diameter (μm) | Nucleus | Cytoplasm | Functions |
|-------|---------------|---------|-----------|-----------|
| Erythrocyte | 7–8 | Absent in this biconcave disc-like cell | Pink, because of acidophilia of hemoglobin | Transports hemoglobin that binds $O_2$ and $CO_2$ |
| Eosinophil | 10–14 | Sausage shaped and deeply stained bi-lobed | Specific granules containing crystalloid body are present | Phagocytoses of antigen–antibody complexes and parasites |
| Basophil | 0.5 | Bi-lobed or tri-lobed, pale stained | Granular, dark purple color | Secretes anti-coagulant and vasodilatory substances |
| Neutrophil | 10–12 | 2–5 lobes connected by fine filament | Ellipsoidal-specific granules are present | Present in large amounts in the pus of wounds |
| Lymphocyte | 8–10 | Large spheroidal, deeply stained | Agranular, light blue color | Circulate in blood in resting state and can be activated upon antigenic stimulation |
| Monocyte | 12–15 | Reniform or horse-shoe shaped | Transparent having ground glass appearance | Gives rise to macrophages |
| Platelet | 2–4 | Absent in this oval, biconvex disc-like cell | Central slightly basophilic granulomere, peripheral homogenous hyalomere | In case of damage to the endothelial lining of the vessel, initiate the clotting process |

## Self Assessment

1. Which cells contain protein hemoglobin?
   a. Erythrocytes
   b. Basophils
   c. Eosinophils
   d. Platelets

2. The shape of erythrocyte is:
   a. Biconcave        b. Biconvex
   c. Concavo-convex   d. Oval

3. Blood cells, which are involved in phagocytosing bacteria at sites of infection is:
   a. Basophils        b. Eosinophils
   c. Neutrophils      d. Platelets

4. Red bone marrow is present in adults in:
   a. Epiphysis of long bones
   b. Diaphysis of long bones
   c. Vertebrae
   d. Ribs

5. Basophils:
   a. Contain bi-lobed nucleus
   b. Functionally related to mast cells
   c. Mediate immediate hypersensitivity reactions
   d. All of the above

6. Eosinophils possess:
   a. Spherical nucleus
   b. Granules with crystalloid body
   c. Metachromatic granules
   d. All of the above

7. Blood platelets in humans:
   a. Possess nuclei
   b. Tri-lobed nucleus
   c. Have a life span of 120 days
   d. None of the above

8. Development of RBC is known as:
   a. Erythropoiesis
   b. Leukopoiesis
   c. Thrombopoiesis
   d. All of the above

9. After birth, hemopoiesis can take place at which site?
   a. Red bone marrow
   b. Kidney
   c. Thymus
   d. Yellow bone marrow

10. Which leukocytes can be considered as an APC?
    a. Monocytes
    b. Basophils
    c. Neutrophils
    d. Platelets

## Answers

1. a,     2. a,     3. c,     4. a,     5. d,     6. b,     7. d,     8. a,     9. a,
10. a

# 10

# Cardiovascular System

The cardiovascular system consists of a pump; the heart, and an extensive system of tubes; the blood vessels, which make up a closed circular system. The vessels that leave the heart are called arteries and that return blood to the heart are called veins. The vascular system transports oxygen and nutrients to the tissues, carries carbon dioxide and waste products from the tissues, and circulate hormones from the site of synthesis to their target cells.

Customary, vascular system is having two parts: Macrovasculature and microvasculature. Macrovasculature includes the vessels, which are more than 0.1 mm in diameter and this includes arteries, large arterioles and veins. Microvasculature includes the vessels, which are less than 0.1 mm in diameter and this includes arterioles, capillaries, and postcapillary venules. Microvasculature is visible only with a microscope, but it is important as being the site of interchanges between the blood and the surrounding tissues.

## HEART

The heart is a muscular pump, which maintains the unidirectional flow of blood. It has four chambers: Right atrium, right ventricle, left atrium and left ventricle. The chambers are arranged to support two separated circulations: The pulmonary circulation, which carries blood to and from the lungs; and the systemic circulation, which distributes blood to and from all of the organs and tissues of the body. The right atrium receives venous blood from the systemic circulation via superior and inferior vena cava and delivers it to the right ventricle through the right atrioventricular valve (tricuspid valve). As the ventricles contract, blood from the right ventricle is pumped out into the pulmonary trunk, a large vessel that bifurcates into the right and left pulmonary arteries to deliver deoxygenated blood to the lungs for gaseous exchange. Oxygenated blood is returned to the left atrium from the lungs via the four pulmonary veins and then through the left atrioventricular valve (bicuspid or mitral valve) it passes into the left ventricle. Contraction of left ventricle expels the oxygenated blood from it into the aorta, which gives many branches to distribute blood to the tissues of the body (Fig. 10.1).

## A. Layers of the Heart Wall

The heart is lined with three layers. From inner to outer side these are: Endocardium, myocardium and epicardium.

a. **Endocardium:** It provides a smooth surface for all the chambers of the heart. It consists of an inner layer of endothelial cells (simple squamous epithelium), which cover all surfaces including valves and lies on a basement membrane. Beneath the basement

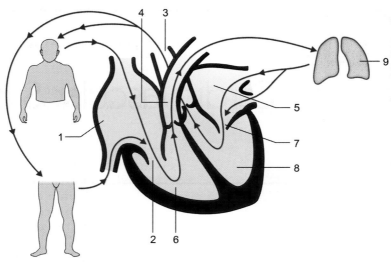

**Fig. 10.1:** Schematic diagram of the heart in relation to the blood circulatory system. The pulmonary circulation is shown on the right and the systemic circulation on the left. Right atrium (1), tricuspid valve (2), aorta (3), pulmonary trunk (4), left atrium (5), right ventricle (6), mitral valve (7), left ventricle (8) and lungs (9)

membrane lies a subendothelial connective tissue layer made up of dense connective tissue and a few smooth muscle fibers. Beneath that the subendocardial layer of loose connective tissue is present, containing Purkinje fibers, small blood vessels and nerves. This layer binds endocardium to the underlying cardiac muscle. Endocardium is continuous with the tunica intima of the blood vessels entering and leaving the heart. This layer is thick in the atria especially in the left atrium, and thin in the ventricles.

b. **Myocardium:** It is the thickest middle layer of the heart, which is composed of cardiac muscle fibers. Some cardiac muscle fibers attach the myocardium to the fibrous cardiac skeleton. Variation in the thickness of the myocardium depends on the function of each chamber, so it is thicker in ventricles than the atria. It is even thicker in the left ventricle than right ventricle, as the left ventricle works at a high pressure and pumps oxygenated blood throughout the systemic circulation, whereas atria and right ventricle works at a relatively low pressure. Cardiac muscle fibers are arranged in complex spirals in the atria and ventricles. In the atria, bundles of cardiac muscle form a network, known as musculi pectinati, while in ventricles isolated bundles of muscle form the trabeculae carneae. Cardiac muscle fibers contract through intrinsically generated action potentials, which are then passed on to neighboring muscle fiber by gap junctions, so the heart beat is myogenic. Specialized cardiac muscle fibers in the atria produce several peptides including atrial natriuretic peptide, atriopeptine, cardiodilatin, and cardionatrine that maintain fluid and electrolyte balance and also decrease blood pressure (Fig. 10.2).

c. **Epicardium:** It is the outermost layer of the heart and constitutes the visceral layer of the pericardium. The epicardium is reflected back at the great vessels entering and leaving the heart as the parietal layer of pericardium. It is composed of simple squamous epithelium (mesothelium) and fibroelastic connective tissue (subepicardial

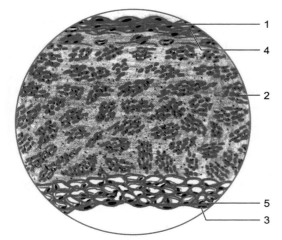

**Fig. 10.2:** Wall of heart is having three layers. From inner to outer side these are: Endocardium (1), myocardium (2) and epicardium (3). Subendocardial layer (4) and subepicardial layer (5)

layer). Mesothelial cells secrete pericardial fluid, which is present in between the parietal and visceral layers of pericardium and provides lubrication as well as reduces friction. Subepicardial layer contains the coronary vessels, nerves and adipose tissue that cushion the heart in the pericardial cavity. The epicardium is thinner in the ventricles than in the atria.

### B. Cardiac Skeleton

It is composed of dense fibrous connective tissue, which provides a structural framework for the heart. It is present in the form of four fibrous rings, two fibrous trigones connect the rings, and the membranous part of interventricular and interatrial septa. The rings surround the two atrioventricular orifices, the aortic orifice and opening of the pulmonary trunk. These rings are known as annulus fibrosus and these rings provide attachment sites for leaflets of all four valves. The right and left fibrous trigones are thickened areas of connective tissue between the aortic ring and right and left atrioventricular rings, respectively.

Membranous part of the interventricular septum is devoid of cardiac muscle; it is made up of dense connective tissue.

### C. Cardiac Valves

These are present between the atria and ventricles [atrioventricular valves (bicuspid and tricuspid)] and at the openings of the aorta and pulmonary trunk (semilunar valves). Although present at different locations, yet they are similar in structure. They are attached to the annulus fibrosus, the connective tissue of which extends into each valve to form its core. The valves are covered on both sides by extensions of the endocardium. The atrioventricular valves are thicker than the semilunar valves. Apart from the aorta and pulmonary trunk no other artery is equipped with valves. Valves open and close to allow the blood to flow through the openings and prevent backflow of blood.

### D. Conducting System

This system initiates and coordinates the contraction of the heart and consists of the sinoatrial (SA) node, atrioventricular (AV) node, atrioventricular (A-V) bundle of His, and Purkinje fibers. The nodes and A-V bundle and its branches are specialized cardiac muscle fibers that are smaller than the normal. The Purkinje fibers are specialized cardiac muscle fibers that are larger than the normal.

a. **Sinoatrial (SA) node:** It is located in the epicardium at the junction of the superior vena cava and the right atrium. It is the pacemaker of the heart. It initiates the impulse that spread along the cardiac muscle fibers of the atria as well as transfer it to the atrioventricular node.

b. **Atrioventricular (AV) node:** It is located on the right side of the interatrial septum, above the tricuspid valve, just under the endocardium. From here impulse travels rapidly along the A-V bundle of His (Fig. 10.3).

c. **Atrioventricular (A-V) bundle of his:** It is a band of connective tissue that extends

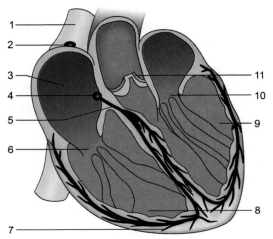

**Fig. 10.3:** Schematic diagram of the conducting system of the heart. Superior vena cava (1), SA node (2), right atrium (3), AV node (4), AV bundle (5), tricuspid valve (6), Purkinje fibers (7), right ventricle (8), left ventricle (9), mitral valve (10) and aortic valve (11)

from the AV node to the interventricular septum. It divides into right and left bundle branches and then into subendothelial branches, called Purkinje fibers. Fibers from the A-V bundle passes down into the interventricular septum to conduct the impulse to the cardiac muscle, thus producing a rhythmic contraction.

d. **Purkinje fibers:** It is the thickest specific cardiac muscle fibers involved in the impulse conducting system. It transmits impulses to the cardiac muscle fibers located at the apex of the heart. In these cells, sarcoplasm is poorly developed. Abundant mitochondria and glycogen granules are present in these cells, which do not disappear even after starvation. Glycogen granules are mainly accumulated in the central parts of the fibers and as they lost during tissue preparation; the fibers look empty in the center. These fibers do not show typical intercalated disc, but diffuse desmosomes and gap junctions are seen. Myofibrils are a few, branched and relatively irregular (Fig. 10.4A, B).

## COMMON STRUCTURES OF BLOOD VESSELS

Blood vessels are tubular structures having three concentric layers (tunics). From inner to outer side tunics are—tunica intima, tunica media and tunica adventitia. These layers are analogus to the endocardium, myocardium and epicardium. There is a gradual transition in the size and wall thickness from one type of vessel to another, so there is no clear-cut point at which one type of vessel ends and other types begins.

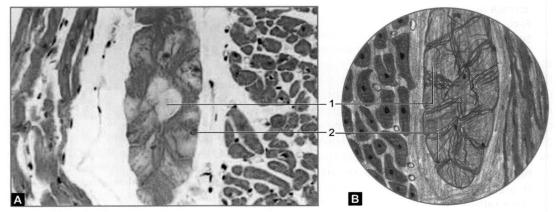

**Fig. 10.4:** Purkinje fibers present in human heart, (A) micrograph, (B) sketch, Purkinje fiber (1), Nucleus of Purkinje fiber (2)

## A. Tunica Intima

It lines the lumen and it is composed by a thin layer of endothelial (simple squamous epithelium) cells and subendothelial layer. The endothelial cells rest on a basement membrane. These elongated, flattened cells are arranged in such a way that their long axis is approximately parallel to the long axis of the vessel. These cells are joined by tight junctions, but some gap junctions and desmosomes are also present.

Subendothelial layer lies immediately beneath the endothelial cells. It is composed of loose connective tissue and a few scattered smooth muscle cells, both arranged longitudinally. Beneath the subendothelial layer is an internal elastic lamina that is especially well developed in muscular arteries. The internal elastic lamina is composed of elastin and it separates the tunica intima from the tunica media. It is a fenestrated sheet, which permits the diffusion of substances into the deeper regions of the arterial wall to nourish the cells there. In larger arteries, which must stretch considerably, the tunica intima is often highly folded when the artery is relaxed.

### Functions of Endothelium

- It forms a selective permeable barrier between blood present in the lumen and in vessel wall.
- It produces anticoagulant normally, but upon damage to these cells they produce factor VIII. Factor VIII promotes platelets adhesion to subendothelial collagen, as well as blood coagulation. This factor is stored in the Weibel-Palade bodies present in the cytoplasm of endothelial cells.
- It alters the blood flow by secreting vasoconstrictors [endothelins, angiotensin-converting enzyme (ACE)] as well as vasodilators (prostacyclin, nitric oxide).
- It secretes type IV collagen, laminin and proteoglycans for the synthesis of basal lamina.
- It breaks down the lipoproteins to form cholesterol and triglycerides, which are used as substrates for the synthesis of steroid hormones.

- It facilitates passage of lymphocytes through the walls of vessels under the influence of certain stimuli such as by cytokines.
- It proliferates to provide new cells during the period of increasing size of blood vessel.
- It also produces growth inhibitors such as heparin (Fig. 10.5).

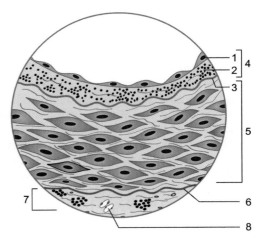

**Fig. 10.5:** Schematic diagram showing common structures of blood vessels. Endothelium (1), subendothelial connective tissue (2), internal elastic lamina (3), tunica intima (4), tunica media (5), external elastic lamina (6) and tunica adventitia (7) with vasa vasorum (8).

## B. Tunica Media

It is the middle layer of the vessel wall and formed by concentric cell layers of smooth muscle fibers. In between the layers of smooth muscle, elastic fibers, type III collagen and ground substance (proteoglycans) are also present. These collagen and proteoglycans are secreted by the smooth muscle fibers. Ground substance is more in the arteries. The amount and arrangement of smooth muscles and elastic fibers depend on the mechanical factors represented by the blood pressure and the metabolic factors represented by the needs of body tissues. Contraction and relaxation of smooth muscle fibers alter the size of the lumen. In this way it influences blood flow in the vessels and blood pressure. Elastic fibers are present in the form of fenestrated lamellae (lamina). Fenestrations of the elastic lamellae allow diffusion of substances. An external elastic lamina, which is more delicate than the internal elastic lamina separates the tunica media from tunica adventitia. Tunica media is thicker in arteries as compared to similar sized veins.

## C. Tunica Adventitia

It is a layer of loose connective tissue that consists of fibroblasts, type I collagen fibers and some elastic fibers. Collagen fibers are arranged longitudinally and prevent undue elongation of the vessel wall during systole. Elastic fibers are not arranged in the form of lamellae. Often, surrounding connective tissue elements blends with the adventitial connective tissue and form an indistinct boundary between tunica adventitia and surrounding tissues. The adventitial layer of large arteries and vein contains small vessels known as vasa vasorum and network of autonomic nerves known as nervi vascularis. Tunica adventitia is thicker in veins as compared to similar sized arteries.

---

**Vasa Vasorum** In the tunica adventitia of larger blood vessels, small vessels are present and these are known as vasa vasorum. The wall of larger blood vessels is very thick, so the nourishment via diffusion alone is not sufficient. Thus, the nourishment to the tunica intima and inner half of the tunica media is supplied via diffusion; while the rest of the wall, i.e. outer half of tunica media and tunica adventitia is supplied by vasa vasorum. Vasa vasorum enter into the vessel wall through the tunica adventitia and branch profusely to form a network. Vasa vasorum are more frequent in veins than in arteries.

---

## SPECIFIC STRUCTURES OF BLOOD VESSELS

## A. Arteries

These vessels conducts blood away from the heart to the tissues and organs. In its initial portions, these vessels resist changes in blood pressure, while at termination these regulates the blood flow. Arteries have thicker walls and smaller diameter in comparison to their corresponding vein. The arteries branch repeatedly between large arteries to the capillaries and due to this branching, the total cross-sectional area of vascular system increases 800 times in comparison to the aorta. With each branching, the rate of flow of blood decreases gradually and this slow flow provides sufficient time for exchange of substances through capillaries. Arteries always carry oxygenated blood except the pulmonary and umbilical arteries, which carry deoxygenated blood. Arteries are classified into three types on the basis of diameter, wall thickness and dominant component of tunica media.

a. **Elastic (conducting) arteries:** These large vessels conduct blood from the heart to the muscular artery. These have thick, strong walls to cope with the sudden high pressure produced during diastole. The subendothelial connective tissue layer is larger in these arteries and along with collagen and elastic fibers it contains numerous smooth muscle fibers. Tunica media is thickest and contains 50 or more (the number increases with age) concentric elastic lamellae made up of elastin. The lamellae are fenestrated, i.e. they have holes in them, thus allowing passage of nutrients diffusing from the blood in the aortic lumen out into the tissues of the wall (Fig. 10.6A, B).

In between the lamellae along with matrix some collagen and smooth muscle fibers are present. Fibroblasts are not present in the tunica media. Matrix, collagen fibers, and elastin are produced by smooth muscle fibers. Presence of prominent elastic fibers in the tunica media allows it to expand during contraction (systole) and to recoil during relaxation (diastole) of the heart. The internal and external elastic lamina is not clearly visible, as the tunica media also

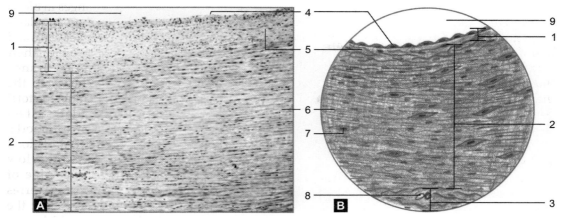

**Fig. 10.6:** Elastic artery, (A) micrograph of aorta, (B) sketch. Elastic fibers (6) form the bulk of tunica media (2). Tunica intima (1), endothelial cells (4), subendothelial tissue (5), smooth muscle fibers (7), tunica adventitia (3), lumen (9) and vasa vasorum (8) are seen in the section

contained many elastic laminas. The adventitial layer is relatively thin and contains abundant vasa vasorum.

Aorta, pulmonary trunk and their main branches all are of elastic type.

b. **Muscular (distributing) arteries:** These arteries are of smaller diameter (0.5–10 mm) and distribute blood to an organ or tissue. Tunica intima is thinner in these arteries in comparison to the elastic arteries. With the decreasing size of the vessel, subendothelial layer decreases in thickness. In some muscular arteries subendothelial layer is so thin that basement membrane of endothelial cells appears to make direct contact with the internal elastic lamina. Media is thickest and consists of 10–40 concentric layers of smooth muscle fibers. Interspersed within the layers of smooth muscle fibers are elastic fibers, type III collagen fibers, and chondroitin sulfate, all secreted by the smooth muscle fibers. Contraction of muscle fibers pushes the blood towards smaller blood vessels. Fibroblasts are not present in the tunica media. The internal and external elastic lamina is clearly visible. The adventitial layer is relatively thinner in comparison to elastic artery and contains vasa vasorum and nervi vascularis (Fig. 10.7A, B).

Brachial artery, ulnar artery, femoral artery, popliteal artery, coronary artery, umbilical artery, arteries located in the brain all are of muscular type.

c. **Arterioles:** Small arteries having diameter less than 100 μm are known as arterioles. Their luminal diameters usually equal the wall thickness. The tunica intima consists of a continuous endothelium and a very thin subendothelial layer. Media is composed of 1–5 layers of smooth muscle fibers. The internal elastic lamina is lacking except in the largest arterioles. The adventitia is relatively thin and shows no external elastic lamina (Fig. 10.8).

Arterioles having a diameter less than 50 μm are known as terminal arterioles. Arterioles play a major role in regulation of blood pressure. They control the blood flow through capillaries. The change in the diameter of arterioles (vasoconstrictor or vasodilator) can also significantly alter the blood pressure.

For comparison among elastic artery, muscular artery, arteriole and metarteriole, *see* Table 17 given in Appendix I.

**Metarterioles** These are narrow vessels, which arise from the terminal arterioles and give rise to capillaries. These are surrounded by incomplete

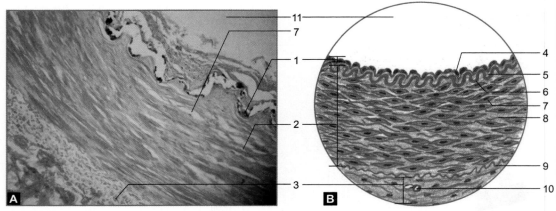

**Fig. 10.7:** Muscular artery, (A) micrograph, (B) sketch showing all three layers, i.e. tunica intima (1), tunica media (2) and tunica adventitia (3). Internal elastic lamina (6), external elastic lamina (9), lumen (11), endothelial cells (4), subendothelial connective tissue (5), smooth muscle fibers (7), elatsic fibers (8) and vasa vasorum (10)

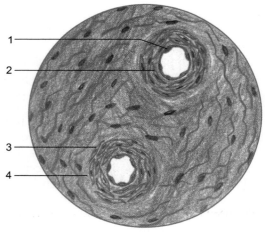

**Fig. 10.8:** Showing arteriole with tunica intima (1). Tunica media (2) comprises 2–3 layers of smooth muscle fibers (3). Tunica adventitia (4) is thin

and venules that bypass the capillary bed. The structures of the arteriole and venule forming this anastomosis are similar to those of an artery and vein, respectively, whereas the intermediate segment has a thickened tunica media. The luminal diameters of these vessels, however, vary with the physiological condition of the organ. When these anastomotic channels are closed, the blood passes through the capillary bed. These anastomosis works as a thermoregulator at the surface of the body. When these shunts are closed, blood passes through the capillary bed, which results in severe heat loss. On the contrary, when these shunts are open, blood flow through the capillary bed is reduced, which results in conservation of heat. These anastomotic channels are numerous in the skin of finger tips, lips, nose and in the erectile tissue of the penis and clitoris (Fig. 10.9).

rings of smooth muscle fibers. The slight thickening of the smooth muscle at the origin of a capillary is known as precapillary sphincter. Precapillary sphincter opens and closes every few seconds and thus, regulates the flow of blood through the capillary bed as per the need of the tissue.

**Arteriovenous Anastomosis (A-V Shunts)** These are direct vascular connections between arterioles

## B. Capillaries

These tubes like blood vessels have the smallest diameter (less than 10 µm), which are composed of a single layer of endothelial cells resting on a basal lamina. These vessels are large enough to allow the passage of red blood cells in a single profile. However, in many capillaries the lumen is so narrow that the red blood cells fold on themselves to pass through

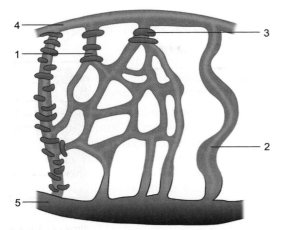

**Fig. 10.9:** Schematic diagram showing metarterioles (1) and arteriovenous anastomosis (2). Precapillary sphincters (3), arteriole (4) and venule (5)

the vessel. Endothelial cells contain pinocytic vesicles. Smooth muscle fibers are not present. Occasionally pericytes or Rouget cells are present, which are non-contractile and phagocytic in function. These cells stimulate the endothelial cells to sprout for the growth of new capillaries.

---

**Pericytes** These cells have long primary processes that are located along the long axis of the capillary and from which secondary processes arise to wrap around the capillary, forming a few gap junctions with the endothelial cells. Pericytes share the basal lamina of the endothelial cells. Pericytes possess a small Golgi complex, mitochondria, rER, microtubules, and filaments extending into the processes. These cells also contain tropomyosin, isomyosin, and protein kinase, which are all related to the contractile process that regulates blood flow through the capillaries. Pericytes are pleuripotent stem cells derived from mesenchyme, which can give rise to endothelial cells, fibroblasts or smooth muscle fibers in blood vessels; if the need arises.

---

The lumen of small capillaries may be encircled by a single endothelial cell, while larger capillaries may be made up of portions of 2 or 3 endothelial cells. Capillaries exhibit selective permeability, permitting the exchange of gases and metabolites between the blood and tissues. They form capillary beds interposed between arterioles and venules. Capillaries are absent in epithelial cells, epidermis, hairs, nails, cornea and articular hyaline cartilage.

Capillaries are classified into three types

a. **The continuous (somatic) capillaries:** In these capillaries, the endothelial cells form a continuous tube (Fig. 10.10A). Numerous pinocytic vesicles are present except in the central nervous system (CNS). In CNS capillaries contain only a limited number of pinocytic vesicles, which is partly responsible for the formation of blood–brain barrier. Exchange of materials occurs through the pinocytic vesicles, but the exchange of macromolecules is restricted. These types of capillaries are present in connective tissue, muscle, brain, skin and lung.

b. **The fenestrated (visceral) capillaries:** These capillaries are highly permeable, so these are mainly present in areas engaged

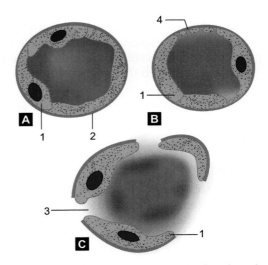

**Fig. 10.10:** Schematic diagram showing the types of capillaries (A) continuous, (B) fenestrated, (C) sinusoid. Endothelial cells (1), basal lamina (2), pores (3) and diaphragm (4)

in transport of fluids. In this type, the endothelial cells have many circular pores or fenestrations (80–100 nm in diameter), which are closed by thin diaphragm (Fig. 10.10B). The diffusion of substances takes place through these pores. These types of capillaries are present in the pancreas, endocrine glands, intestinal villi, gall bladder, and kidney. In the renal glomerulus, fenestrations are larger and diaphragm is absent. At some locations, fenestrated capillaries help to produce important blood filtrates, e.g. CSF in the choroid plexus, and aqueous humor in the ciliary body.

c. **The discontinuous (sinusoidal) capillaries:** These capillaries are wider and more irregular, so the blood flow is sluggish through these capillaries. Some of the lining endothelial cells are phagocytic. Basal lamina may be deficient or absent (Fig. 10.10C). The endothelial cell does not create any barrier for exchange of materials. These types of capillaries are present in the liver and in hematopoietic organs such as the bone marrow and spleen. Structural variations are present in these capillaries according to the sites. In liver, Kupffer cells and Ito cells are closely associated with the endothelium of these capillaries. In the spleen, sinusoids are wider and endothelial cells are spindle-shaped with gaps between the neighboring cells.

For comparison among continuous capillary, fenestrated capillary and sinusoid, *see* Table 18 given in Appendix I.

## C. Veins

These vessels return blood to the heart. The caliber of veins is larger in comparison to accompany artery, but their walls are thinner, because of reduction of elastic and muscular components. The connective tissue components in veins are more prominent than in the arteries. Their lumen is generally collapsed. The tunics of veins are not well defined as the tunics of the arteries. Tunica media is thin in veins in comparison to the same size artery, but the tunica adventitia is thick. The venous blood contains less oxygen, so the vasa vasorum are more prevalent in the walls of veins than the arteries. These are classified as larger veins, medium to small sized veins and venules.

a. **Large veins:** These veins possess valves that are extensions of tunica intima and serve to prevent backflow of blood. Their diameter is more than 10 mm. These have an enodothelium and thick subendothelial layer. Tunica media is relatively thin and contain circularly arranged smooth muscle fibers, collagen fibers and a few fibroblast cells. Although only a few major vessels have a well-developed smooth muscle layer, most large veins are without a tunica media. Exceptions are the pulmonary veins and superficial veins of the legs, which have a well-defined muscular wall. Adventitia is thick and contains vasa vasorum. It is made up of longitudinally oriented smooth muscle fibers along with usual collagen fibers, elastic fibers and fibroblasts. Elastic laminas are not present. The vena cava and pulmonary veins are large veins and even these veins possess cardiac muscle in the tunica adventitia for a short distance as they enter the heart. Internal jugular, brachiocephalic, portal, splenic, renal, and superior mesenteric veins are also large veins (Fig. 10.11).

b. **Medium to small sized veins:** In these veins tunica intima is thin and subendothelial tissue is inconspicuous. Presence of valves is the main feature of these vessels. Elastic laminas are not present. Media is thin in comparison to same size artery and made with a few layers of circularly arranged smooth muscle fibers with collagen and elastic fibers. Adventitia forms the main bulk and contains vasa vasorum (Fig. 10.12).

　　Most of the veins (except main venous trunks of the thorax and abdominal cavity) are small to medium size.

c. **Venules:** These are thin walled vessels, which permit exchange of fluid and cells

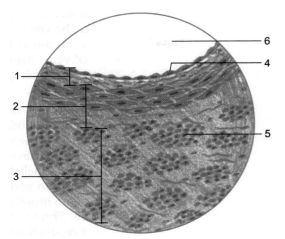

**Fig. 10.11:** Large vein having thick adventitia (3) with longitudinally oriented smooth muscle fibers (5). Tunica media (2) is thin. Tunica intima (1), lumen (6) and endothelial cells (4) are also seen

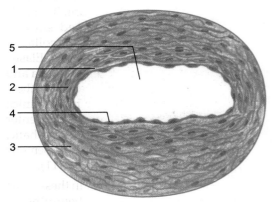

**Fig. 10.12:** Medium size vein. Tunica intima (1), tunica media (2), tunica adventitia (3) and endothelial cells (4) cover the lumen (5)

through their walls. The diameter of these vessels is larger than the capillaries. In venules, leukocytes leave the bloodstream to enter the tissue spaces by passing through the intercellular junctions and this process is called diapedesis. Venules can be categorized as muscular venules (50–100 µm), collecting venules (30–50 µm) and postcapillary venules (10–30 µm). In muscular venules tunica media is present and made

up by 1–3 layers of smooth muscle fibers. Adventitia is present and thicker. Postcapillary venules only have tunica intima made up by endothelial cells and an outer sheath of collagen fibers (Fig. 10.13).

In the post-capillary venules of lymph node paracortex (high endothelial venules) endothelial cells become cuboidal in shape. These venules detect and isolate lymphocytes by type-specific receptors on their luminal surface.

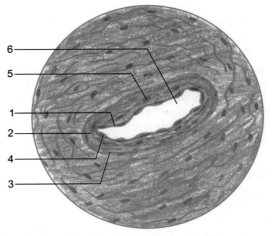

**Fig. 10.13:** Venule with tunica media (2) made up by smooth muscle fibers (5), tunica intima (1), tunica adventitia (3), lumen (6) and endothelial cells (4) are also seen

d. **Valves of veins:** It is having two leaflets, which are composed of a thin connective tissue with a network of elastic fibers of the tunica intima. Veins which are more than 2 mm in diameter have valves. Valves are especially abundant in the veins of the extremities, but they are generally absent from the veins of the thorax and abdomen. Valves are commonly located immediately distal to sites where tributaries join veins. Valves help to overcome the force of gravity by preventing backflow of blood.

For comparison between arteries and veins, *see* Table 19 given in Appendix I.

**Atherosclerosis:** It comes from the Greek words *athero* (meaning gruel or paste) and *sclerosis* (hardness). In this condition, deposit of fatty substances, cholesterol, cellular waste products, calcium and other substances build up in the inner lining of an artery. This build up is called plaque. It usually affects large and medium-sized arteries. Plaques can grow large enough to significantly reduce the blood flow through an artery. But most of the damage occurs when they become fragile and rupture. Plaques that rupture cause blood clots to form that can block blood flow or break off and travel to another part of the body. If either happens and blocks a blood vessel that feeds the heart, it causes a heart attack (myocardial infarction). If it blocks a blood vessel that feeds the brain, it causes a stroke (cerebral thrombosis).

**Aneurysm:** When the media of an artery is weakened by an embryonic defect, disease, or lesion, the wall of the artery may balloon out. An aneurysm that grows and becomes large enough can burst, causing dangerous even often fatal, bleeding inside the body. Arterial aneurysm is more common than venous aneurysm.

**Infarction:** If the arterial supply or the venous drainage is blocked, then specific areas of certain organs become necrotic (death of tissues from a lack of metabolites). These infarcts commonly occur in the heart, kidneys, and cerebrum.

**Clotting:** When blood vessels are cut or damaged, the loss of blood from the system must be stopped before shock and possible death occur. This is accomplished by solidification of the blood, a process called coagulation or clotting. A blood clot consists of a plug of platelets enmeshed in a network of insoluble fibrin molecules. Platelet aggregation and fibrin formation both require the proteolytic enzyme thrombin. Clotting also requires calcium ions and about a dozen of other proteins (clotting factors). Most of these circulate in the blood as inactive precursors. They are activated by proteolytic cleavage becoming, in turn, active proteases for other factors in the system. The precursors of clotting factors are synthesized in the liver and then processed in the blood.

## Summary

| Type | Tunica intima | Tunica media | Tunica adventitia | Functions |
|---|---|---|---|---|
| Elastic artery | Endothelium, subendothelial connective tissue with smooth muscle fibers | 50 or more elastic lamellae with collagen and smooth muscle fibers | Loose connective tissue thinner than media with vasa vasorum | Conduct blood from heart |
| Muscular artery | Endothelium, very thin subendothelial tissue | Many layers of smooth muscle fibers with less elastic fibers | Thinner than elastic artery with vasa vasorum | Distribute blood to the tissues and organs |
| Arteriole | Endothelium, very thin subendothelial tissue | 1–5 layers of smooth muscle | Very thin connective tissue layer | Resist and control blood flow to capillaries |
| Capillaries | Endothelium with occasional pericytes | None | None | Exchange metabolites by diffusion to and from cells |
| Venules | Endothelium, subendothelial connective tissue with scattered smooth muscle fibers | 1–3 layers of smooth muscle fibers | Present and thicker than media | Site of exit of leukocytes from bloodstream |

(Contd.)

(Contd.)

| Type | Tunica intima | Tunica media | Tunica adventitia | Functions |
|------|---------------|--------------|-------------------|-----------|
| Medium to small size veins | Endothelium, inconspicuous subendothelial tissue | Few layers of smooth muscle fibers | Thicker than media with vasa vasorum | Carry blood to larger veins |
| Large veins | Endothelium, thin subendothelial tissue | Thin with layers of smooth muscle fibers | Thick and with vasa vasorum | Return blood to heart |

## Self Assessment

1. Vasa vasorum provide a functional analogous to which of the following?
   a. Valves
   b. Arterioles
   c. Endothelium
   d. Coronary arteries

2. Internal and external elastic lamina are most prominent in which vessels?
   a. Elastic arteries
   b. Aretrioles
   c. Large veins
   d. Muscular arteries

3. Pericytes are:
   a. Phagocytic cells
   b. Modified endothelial cells
   c. Pleuripotent cells
   d. Cuboidal cells

4. Fenestrated capillaries are present in:
   a. Kidney          b. Spleen
   c. Lung            d. Brain

5. The process of migration of leukocytes from blood to tissues is known as:
   a. Exocytosis      b. Endocytosis
   c. Diapedesis      d. Diffusion

6. Elastic artery is characterized by:
   a. Presence of elastic fibers in tunica media
   b. Well-defined internal and external elastic lamina
   c. Well-defined internal elastic lamina
   d. Presence of smooth muscle fibers in tunica media

7. Muscular artery is characterized by:
   a. Presence of elastic fibers in tunica media
   b. Presence of smooth muscle fibers in tunica adventitia
   c. Presence of smooth muscle fibers in tunica media
   d. Presence of elastic fibers in tunica intima

8. Precapillary sphincter is present in:
   a. Terminal arteriole
   b. Venule
   c. Metarteriole
   d. All of the above

9. The proportion of tunica media to the tunica adventitia in the artery is:
   a. 1:1             b. 1:2
   c. 2:1             d. 1:3

10. The proportion of tunica media to the tunica adventitia in the vein is:
    a. 1:1            b. 1:2
    c. 2:1            d. 1:3

## Answers

1. d,    2. d,    3. c,    4. a,    5. c,    6. a,    7. c,    8. c,    9. c,
10. b

# 11

# Lymphatic System

The lymphatic system is a closed system of vessels which begin blindly in the tissue spaces in and around the blood capillaries. The lymphatic vessels transport lymph, which carry the large substances that cannot be carried in the blood vessels. These substances are the particulate matter, large molecules, abnormal cells and cells responsible for the immune responses in the body. Lymphatic drainage is a one-way flow, not a circulation (Fig. 11.1). Cells of this system has the ability to differentiate between "self" (the organism's own molecules) and "non-self" (foreign substances). This system provides the second and the third lines of defence against foreign substances. The first line of defence is the skin, which covers surfaces of the body. Lymphatic tissues are distributed throughout the body and serves as sites where lymphocytes proliferate, differentiate and mature.

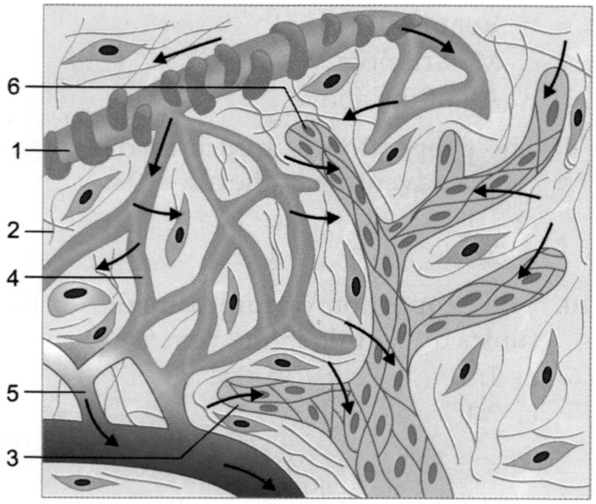

For comparison between blood and lymph, *see* Table 20 given in Appendix I.

## COMPONENTS OF THE LYMPHATIC SYSTEM

- Cells of lymphatic system
- Lymphatic nodules
- Lymphatic vessels
- Lymphoid organs

## CELLS OF LYMPHATIC SYSTEM

These are of two types:
A. Fixed cells
B. Free cells

### A. Fixed Cells

These are the reticular cells, which are responsible for the formation and maintenance of reticular fibers. Reticular fibers are composed of type III collagen. Reticular cells and fibers form a structural meshwork that allows fluid to pass through it while providing delicate, non-distensible support for cells suspended within it. In the thymus,

Fig. 11.1: Schematic diagram showing association of blood capillaries (1), tissue (2) and lymphatic capillaries (3). Arteriole (4), venule (5), endothelial cells of lymphatic capillaries (6)

epithelioreticular cells form the structural meshwork within the tissue.

## B. Free Cells

These cells lie in the network form by reticular cells and reticular fibers. The main cells are lymphocytes but macrophages and antigen-presenting cells (APCs) are also present in variable numbers. These cells possess different types of unique molecules on the surface of their cell membrane. These specific molecules are called cluster of differentiation (CD) molecules. These CD molecules can be visualized by immunohistochemical methods using monoclonal antibodies. These CD molecules are designated by numbers according to an international system, which provides numbers as per their expressed antigens at their different differentiation stages.

a. **Lymphocytes:** These cells account for 20–40% of leukocytes. The life span of lymphocytes ranges from a few days (short-lived) to many years (long-lived). Long-lived lymphocytes play a significant role in the maintenance of immunological memory. The lymphocytes have large nucleus, which occupies most of the volume of the cell, leaving only a thin crescent of cytoplasm. There are three classes of lymphocytes: T lymphocytes, B lymphocytes, and natural killer (NK) cells. The precursors of all these cells originate in the bone marrow. T and B cells require special surface determinants for their activation, while NK cells lack the surface determinant characteristics. About 80% of all circulating lymphocytes in normal blood are T-cells.

   i. *T Lymphocytes*: These lymphocytes have a long lifespan and are involved in cellular immunity, in which they interact with and destroy foreign or "non-self" cells. These cells are produced in the bone marrow, and through the blood circulation leave the bone marrow and reach the thymus where they undergo intense proliferation and differentiation

or die. After their final maturation, T-cells leave the thymus and are distributed throughout the body in connective tissues and lymphoid organs. Their activation, subsequent proliferation and functional maturation are under the control of APC cells. Cellular immunity is mediated by T lymphocytes. T-cells express CD2, CD3, CD4, CD5, CD7 and CD8 markers and T-cell receptors (TCRs).

The major T-cell subgroups are the helper, suppressor, killer, and memory cells.

- *Helper (CD4$^+$) cells*: These cells are necessary in the initial antigen responses. These cells interact with B cells to stimulate their proliferation and their differentiation into plasma cells, to promote activation of macrophages, activation of cytotoxic lymphocytes, and induction of an inflammatory reaction.

- *Suppressor (Regulatory) cells*: These cells work as inhibitory cells by influencing the activities of other cells in the immune system and play a role in determining the duration of the immune response. The immune response has potentially good as well as harmful effects and should be modulated to prevent a hyper immune response; T-suppressor cell serves this purpose. These cells depress antibody production by depressing the conversion of B-lymphocytes into plasma cells, i.e. the antagonistic effect to helper cells.

- *Killer (Cytotoxic or CD8$^+$) cells*: These cells are the effector cells of the thymus-dependent system. These cells kill target cells in a similar fashion to that of natural killer cells.

- *Memory cells*: These cells only become effector cells if the body is exposed to the same antigen at some future date. The vaccines work on this basis.

   ii. *B Lymphocytes*: These lymphocytes mature and become functional in the bone marrow and after leaving the bone marrow, enter the blood circulation to populate connective tissues, epithelia, lymphatic nodules and lymphoid organs. In birds B cells were first identified, they become immunocompetent in a diverticulum of the cloaca, known as the bursa of Fabricius (hence named "B" cells). These cells are involved with humoral immunity.

When B cells come in contact with any foreign antigen, they differentiate into plasma cells. These plasma cells secrete the antibodies against the same foreign antigen. These antibodies are known as immunoglobulin, which are divided into five major classes: IgG, IgA, IgM, IgD and IgE. In most cases, the activation of B cells requires the assistance of T-helper lymphocytes. Not all activated B cells, however, become plasma cells; some remain B memory lymphocytes, which react rapidly to a second exposure to the same foreign antigen. B cells express CD9, CD19 and CD20 markers.

iii. *Natural killer cells*: These cells are 5–15% of the total circulating lymphocyte population. Their name derives from the fact that they attack virus-infected cells, transplanted cells and cancer cells without previous stimulation. The cytoplasm of these cells has small granules, which contain special proteins such as perforin and proteases known as granzymes. Upon release in close proximity to a cell scheduled for killing; perforin forms pores in the cell membrane of the target cell through which the granzymes and associated molecules can enter, inducing apoptosis or cell death.

b. **Macrophages:** These are enlarged monocytes (white blood cells) that engulf microbes and cellular debris. These cells vary in diameter from 10 to 20 μm and possess an oval kidney or horseshoe-shaped nucleus. The cytoplasm is abundant and basophilic and contains ingested material. When macrophages come in contact with any foreign antigen their size increases. These activated macrophages then become phagocytic to lyse engulfed microbes.

c. **Antigen-presenting cells (APCs):** These cells are a group of very diverse cell types and found in most of the tissues. This group includes dendritic cells of lymphatic follicles, Langerhans cells of the epidermis and some macrophages. These cells phagocytose and process antigens and then present the antigen to T lymphocyte, inducing their activation.

## LYMPHATIC NODULES

Lymphatic nodules (follicles) are circumscribed masses of densely packed lymphocytes (mostly B cells) contained in a meshwork of reticular cells. These nodules are considered as the basic structural unit of lymphoid tissue. Each nodule may contain a light staining pale central area, termed germinal center. This center is an active site of lymphocyte production and contains large euchromatic lymphoblasts and plasmoblasts. Besides these, follicular dendritic cells (FDC) are also present in the germinal center. These cells may have a role in maintaining an initial immune response. The center is surrounded by darkly stained zone (corona) of densely packed small, newly formed lymphocytes (Fig. 11.2).

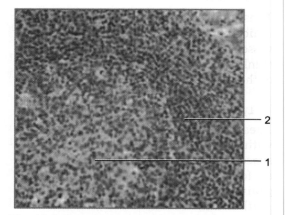

**Fig. 11.2:** Lymphatic nodules with germinal center (1) and corona (2)

The germinal center, only develops when a nodule is exposed to antigen. Nodules with germinal centers are called secondary nodules, while primary nodules lack germinal centers. The size of the germinal center is proportional to the immunological response.

The distribution of nodules in the tissues varies from single (solitary) to many in groups (Payer's patches in the ileum) or ring form (appendix). Solitary nodules may exist anywhere in the mucosa of all open tracts, known as mucosa associated lymphoid tissue (MALT). The best examples of these accumulations are those associated with the mucosa of the gut: Gut-associated lymphoid tissue (GALT), the genitourinary tract, bronchus-associated lymphatic tissue (BALT) and the tonsils. Lymphatic nodules also form prominent structural components of lymphatic organs such as lymph nodes and spleen.

## Functions of Lymphatic Nodule

It filters the lymph and provides immunological surveillance for the fluid of the layer/organ in which it is located, e.g. tissue fluid in the lamina propria, lymph in lymph nodes and blood in the spleen. Lymphatic nodules detect specific antigens and cause proliferation of antigen-specific B lymphocytes.

## LYMPHATIC VESSELS

These vessels begin as lymph capillaries, which drain into larger collecting lymph vessels and finally into two large lymphatic trunks. Lymph nodes are present in the course of the lymphatic vessels.

## A. Lymphatic Capillaries

These are the smallest lymphatic vessels without valves, which begin in the tissue spaces as blind-ended sacs. Lymph capillaries are found in all regions of the body except the brain, spinal cord, cornea, internal ear, epithelium, cartilage and bone marrow. They are especially numerous in the loose connective tissue under the epithelium of the skin and mucous membranes. These are wider and their wall consists of a thin endothelium, but a continuous basal lamina and pericytes are not present. Cell junctions are not present between adjacent endothelial cells. These cells may overlap and intercellular clefts are present between cells, so that the tissue fluid can enter into the lymph capillaries, but the reverse flow of lymph back to the tissue spaces is prevented through these clefts. Externally, these endothelial cells are surrounded by a small amount of collagenous connective tissue. Fine filaments (5–10 nm in diameter) run perpendicularly from the collagen bundles and attach to the outer surface of the endothelium as anchoring filaments, which maintain the patency of the capillary (Fig. 11.3), i.e. the lymph capillaries cannot collapse during increased pressure of tissue fluid. The excess of tissue fluid, containing particulate matter and colloidal material, is absorbed through lymphatic capillaries because these are more permeable than blood capillaries.

For comparison between blood and lymphatic capillaries, *see* Table 21 given in Appendix I.

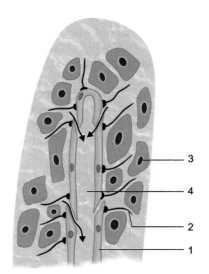

**Fig. 11.3:** Schematic diagram showing details of a lymphatic capillary. Endothelium (1), anchoring filament (2), tissue cell (3) and lymph (4)

## B. Collecting Lymphatic Vessels

The walls of these vessels have three coats. From inner to outer side these are: tunica intima, tunica media and tunica adventitia. These layers are not as clearly demarcated as in the blood vessels. Tunica intima is made up of an endothelial cell layer, which is surrounded by a longitudinally arranged thin network of elastic fibers. Folds of tunica intima form valves, which are more in number in comparison to veins and prevent backflow of lymph. Proximal to the valves the walls of lymph vessels are dilated, so the lymph vessels are beaded in appearance. Tunica media is made up of circularly arranged smooth muscle fibers. In between the smooth muscle fibers a few elastic fibers are also present. Tunica adventitia is thickest and consists of longitudinally arranged bundles of collagen, elastic and some smooth muscle fibers. Contraction of surrounding skeletal muscles causes lymph to move.

## C. Lymphatic Trunks

The collecting lymph vessels finally form two large lymphatic trunks: Thoracic duct and right lymphatic duct. The structure of these two trunks is similar and has three tunics. Tunica intima is made by a continuous layer of endo-thelial cells beneath which a subendothelial layer of fibroelastic tissue with some smooth muscle fibers are present. Tunica media is the thickest and form by circularly arranged smooth muscle fibers. In between the smooth muscle fibers abundant collagenous connective tissue and a few elastic fibers are also present. In between the tunica intima and tunica media a thin internal elastic lamina is present. Tunica adventitia is thin and made up of longitudinally arranged bundles of collagen fibers, elastic fibers and occasional smooth muscle fibers. It finally merges in the surrounding connective tissue.

All the lymph collected from the entire left side of the body, the digestive tract and the right side of the lower part of the body flows into the thoracic duct. The thoracic duct empties into the left subclavian vein. The lymph in the right side of the head, neck, and chest are collected by the right lymph duct and empties into the right subclavian vein.

**Lymph** Normally lymph is said to be colorless but because of the presence of the fat molecules (chylomicrons) which are absorbed from the small intestine, it appears to be milky white (especially after a heavy fatty meal), hence the lymph is also called the chyle. Lymph is rich in larger protein molecules, fat molecules, and lymphocytes.

## LYMPHOID ORGANS

Thymus, and fetal bone marrow is referred as primary or central lymphoid organs; which store, release and confer competence of the lymphocytes that populates the secondary or peripheral organs, but do not participate directly in defense. Secondary lymphoid organs are lymph nodes, spleen, tonsils, MALT and skin; where lymphocyte responds to antigenic challenge.

Spleen is responsive to blood-borne antigens, whereas the lymph nodes protect the organism from antigens which come from tissues via the lymphatic system. In contrast, the mucosal system protects the organism from antigens entering the body directly through mucosal epithelial surfaces.

## A. Lymph Nodes

These are widely distributed in chains or groups throughout the body along the course of lymphatic vessels and they are concentrated in some regions such as axilla, groin and mesenteries. Size of lymph nodes ranges from 1 mm to more than 2 cm. The lymph node is kidney-shaped and convex all around except in an indented region, the hilum. It is covered by a capsule, which is formed by densely packed collagen fibers, a few elastic and smooth muscle fibers. The capsule is usually surrounded by adipose tissue and sends trabeculae into its interior. Just beneath the capsule a subcapsular (marginal) sinus is present, which is formed by a loose network of macrophages, reticular cells and reticular fibers. Afferent lymphatic vessels enter at multiple points on the convex surface of the node. At the hilum arteries and nerves enter, while the veins and the efferent lymphatic vessel leave the node. It is the only lymaphatic organ which has both afferent and efferent lymphatic vessels. Both sets of vessels have valve to provide unidirectional flow of lymph through the node.

The space enclosed by a capsule and trabeculae is filled with an intricate network of reticular fibers with reticular cells. The most common cells of lymph nodes are lymphocytes, macrophages, plasma cells and reticular cells. Follicular dendritic cells are also present within the lymphoid nodules. The different arrangement of the cells and a network of reticular cells creates two regions, an outer cortex and an inner medulla. The cortex is missing at the hilum.

a. **Cortex:** In the outer part of the cortex lymphocytes are organized in the form of nodules, which may be in the form of primary nodules or secondary nodules. In the deeper part of the cortex (paracortex) lymphocytes are diffusely arranged. In the outer part of cortex mainly B lymphocytes are present, while in the paracortex T lymphocytes are present. In between the nodules and trabeculae cortical sinuses are present (Fig. 11.4A, B).

b. **Medulla:** In the medulla lymphoid tissue is organized in the form of lymphoid strands, or medullary cords, containing B lymphocytes, T lymphocytes, abundant macrophages, and numerous plasma cells. These cords are separated by dilated, capillary like structures, called medullary lymphatic sinuses. These sinuses contain reticular cells and macrophages.

c. **The flow of lymph:** Afferent lymphatic vessels cross the capsule and pour lymph in the subcapsular sinus. From here it passes in the cortical sinuses that run parallel to the trabeculae and reach in the medulla, where they drain into medullary

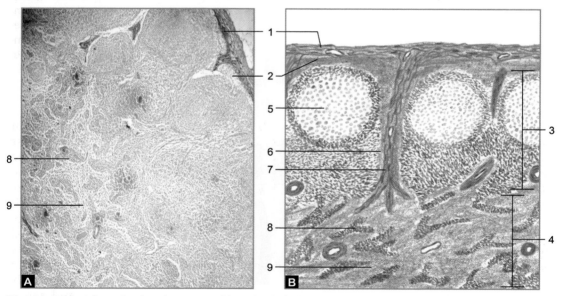

**Fig. 11.4:** Lymph node showing several lymphatic follicles (5) with germinal center in the cortex (3), (A) micrograph, (B) sketch. Medulla (4) consists of medullary cords (8) separated by medullary lymphatic sinuses (9). Capsule (1), subcapsular sinus (2), cortical sinuses (6), and trabeculae (7) are also seen

sinuses. From these it collects in the efferent lymphatic vessels present at the hilum (Fig. 11.5).

d. **Blood circulation in lymph node:** The arteries enter the substance of lymph nodes at the hilum. Then they run through the medulla within trabeculae and become smaller as they repeatedly branch. Eventually, they lose their connective tissue sheath, travel within the substance of medullary cords and form the medullary capillary beds. These small branches of the arteries continue in the medullary cords until they reach the cortex. Here they form a cortical capillary bed, which is drained by postcapillary venules. Blood from postcapillary venules drains into larger veins, which exit the lymph node at the hilum.

In the deeper part of the cortex, the venules have a special appearance and known as post-capillary venules. In these venules, endothelial lining is made by cuboidal epithelium rather than squamous and these are known as high endothelial venules (HEV) (Fig. 11.6).

The cells lining the HEVs are specialized endothelial cells, which are having a high

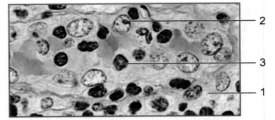

**Fig. 11.6:** High endothelial venule (1) present in the deeper part of the cortex and lined by cuboidal endothelial cells (2). Lymphocytes (3)

concentration of water channels. The lymph entering through the afferent lymphatic vessels is drawn into the deeper cortex by rapid resorption of interstitial fluid through these water channels. Along with these channels these cells also possess receptors for lymphocytes, which help lymphocytes to stop and attach to these venules. These venules are the site where lymphocytes leave the vascular supply by migrating between the endothelial cells in a manner similar to that of neutrophils (diapedesis). B cells migrate to the outer cortex, whereas most of the T-cells remain in the deeper cortex.

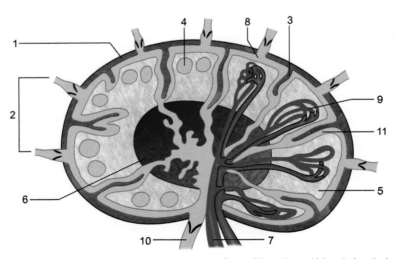

**Fig. 11.5:** Schematic diagram of lymph node showing the flow of lymph and blood circulation. Capsule (1), afferent lymphatic vessels (2), trabeculae (3), lymphatic nodules (4), cortex (5), medulla (6), efferent arteriole (7), subcapsular sinus (8), capillary bed (9), efferent lymphatic vessel (10) and trabecular sinus (11)

e. **Functions of the lymph node:**
  i. It is a filter for lymph before its return to the thoracic duct. The lymph passes through the sinuses slowly, which gives the macrophages that lies in the sinuses more time to phagocytose foreign particulate matter. The network of reticular fibers also obstructs the foreign bodies.
  ii. It maintains and produces T and B cells and possesses memory cells (especially T memory cells). Antigens delivered to the lymph nodes by antigen presenting cells are recognized by T-cells and an immune response is initiated.
  iii. B lymphocytes mature to form plasma cells in lymph nodes, which produce antibodies.
  iv. Through lymph nodes, re-circulation of B and T lymphocytes takes place. The circulating lymphocytes may enter the lymph node through post-capillary venule and pass via the efferent lymphatics in lymph.

## B. Tonsils

These are incompletely encapsulated large aggregation of lymphatic nodules. These are present in the lamina propria of the mucosa of the initial portion of the digestive tract.

Depending on their location, tonsils are:
a. Palatine tonsils
b. Pharyngeal tonsil
c. Lingual tonsils
d. Tubal tonsils

a. **Palatine tonsils:** These are paired, ovoid masses (1–2.5 cm in diameter) of lymphoid tissue, which are located laterally at the junction of the oral cavity and oropharynx between the palatoglossal and palato-pharyngeal arches. They lie in the connective tissue of the mucosa and are covered on their free surface by a stratified squamous nonkeratinized epithelium. Each tonsil has 10–20 epithelial invaginations that are known as tonsillar crypts. Secondary crypts may branch from these crypts (Fig. 11.7A, B). Just beneath the epithelium lies aggregation of lymphatic nodules, many with prominent germinal centers within the diffused lymphoid tissue. A layer of dense connective tissue underlies the tonsil and forms its capsule. This capsule usually acts as a barrier against spreading tonsillar infections. Tonsils do not possess afferent lymphatics. Instead, dense plexuses of fine lymphatic vessels surround each nodule and form efferent lymphatics which pass towards the capsule and drain in upper deep cervical lymph nodes.

b. **Pharyngeal tonsil:** It is a single tonsil located in the posterior wall of the nasopharynx. It is covered by ciliated pseudostratified columnar epithelium typical of the respiratory tract with patches of stratified squamous epithelium. Instead of crypts, it has shallow, longitudinal infoldings called pleats. Ducts of seromucous glands open into the base of the pleats. The parenchyma of the pharyngeal tonsil is composed of lymphoid nodules, some of which have germinal centers. Its capsule is incomplete and thinner than the capsule of the palatine tonsils. Hypertrophied pharyngeal tonsils resulting from chronic inflammation are called adenoids.

c. **Lingual tonsils:** They are located on the dorsum of the posterior one-third of the tongue and are covered by a stratified squamous nonkeratinized epithelium. Each tonsil has a deep crypt and ducts of mucous glands open into the base of these crypts. The parenchyma of the lingual tonsil is composed of lymphoid nodules, which frequently have germinal centers. Its capsule is very delicate.

d. **Tubal tonsils:** These are sometimes considered as a separate tonsillar group. Each tubal tonsil lies around the pharyngeal orifice of the pharyngotympanic (auditory) tube and constitutes a lateral extension of

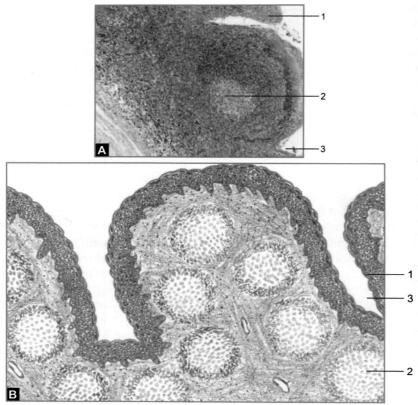

**Fig. 11.7:** Section of palatine tonsil, (A) micrograph, (B) sketch having collection of lymphatic follicles (2) with germinal centers just below the stratified squamous nonkeratinized epithelium (1). Tonsillar crypts (3) can also be seen in the figure

the pharyngeal tonsil. The tubal tonsil is covered by ciliated columnar epithelium.

### Function of Tonsils

They have no afferent vessels and even they do not contain lymphatic sinuses for filtration of the lymph, so they do not filter lymph. They react to the foreign antigen by formation of lymphocytes and rising an immune response. Tonsils are known to be frequent portals of infection.

### C. Thymus

It is situated in the superior mediastinum and extending over the great vessels of the heart. It is the only lymphatic organ, which is well developed and relatively large at birth, whereas spleen and lymph nodes are underdeveloped. The thymus is most active during childhood, reaching a weight of about 30 to 40 gm. At puberty, it undergoes progressive involution and is partially replaced by fat and connective tissue. Thymus does not filter lymph and blood. It is covered by a capsule of loose connective tissue and consists of two lobes joined by connective tissue. Each lobe contains many lobules (2 mm), which are incompletely separated from each other by septa. Through the septa travels the blood vessels, lymphatics and nerves. A lobule is composed of an outer cortex and inner medulla, in which medulla sends a projection to join with the medulla of adjacent lobules (Fig. 11.8A, B). The supporting parenchyma within a lobule is formed by the epithelioreticular cells, which are stellate in shape like reticular cells, but differ from them in origin and function. These cells are of endodermal origin, rather than the usual mesodermal origin and cells, even do not form fibers like typical reticular cells. These epithelioreticular cells are usually joined with similar adjacent cells by desmosomes.

The cortex is densely packed with thymocytes, i.e. the developing T lymphocytes. These cells mature in the cortex, then migrate into the medulla where they enter the blood stream for transport to secondary lymphoid organs. In addition to the thymocytes and epithelioreticular cells; the cortex also houses macrophages. These macrophages are responsible for phagocytosis of incompetent T-cells. The cortex lacks lymphatic nodules. The cortex is richer in small lymphocytes than the medulla so it stains more darkly.

Three types of epithelioreticular cells are present in the thymic cortex.

a. **Type I cells:** These cells are located at the boundary of the cortex and the connective tissue capsule as well as between the cortical parenchyma and the trabeculae. These cells form occluding junctions with each other, completely isolating the thymic cortex from the remainder of the body.

b. **Type II cells:** These cells are located in the midcortex. These cells have long, wide, sheath-like processes that form desmosomal junctions with each other. Their processes form a cytoreticulum that subdivides the thymic cortex into isolated areas of the developing T-cells.

c. **Type III cells:** These cells are located at the boundary of the cortex and medulla. Occluding junctions are present between sheath-like cytoplasmic processes of adjacent cells. Like type I cells, these cells also form a barrier between cortex and medulla.

The medulla has fewer thymocytes, but the epithelioreticular cells are predominate and prominent in comparison to the cortex.

Three types of epithelioreticular cells are present in the thymic medulla.

a. **Type IV cells:** These cells are present between cortex and medulla in close association with type III epithelioreticular cells of the cortex.

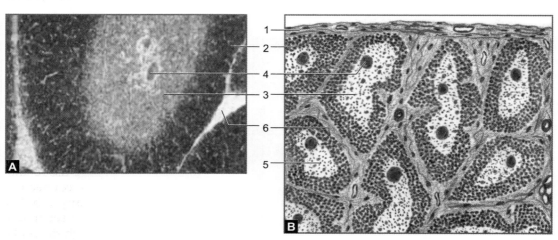

**Fig. 11.8:** Thymus at low magnification, (A) micrograph, (B) sketch. It consists of many lobules having an outer cortex (2) and inner medulla (3). In the medulla lie Hassall's corpuscles (4) and reticular cells (5). Capsule (1), and connective tissue septa (6)

These cells assist type III cells to form the barrier between cortex and medulla.

b. **Type V cells:** These cells are present throughout the medulla. Like type II cells, the processes of adjacent cells are joined by desmosomes to form a reticulum, thus these cells isolate areas for lymphocytes.

c. **Type VI cells:** These cells form the most characteristic feature of the thymic medulla. These cells coalesce around each other, forming a whorl-shaped thymic corpuscles (Hassall's corpuscles) around a central degenerated homogenous mass (Fig. 11.9A, B). The diameter of Hassall's corpuscles is 20–500 μm. The functions of Hassall's corpuscles are not well understood, but it is believed that these corpuscles produce interleukins (IL-4 and IL-7) that play a role in lymphocyte maturation. They stain pink with eosin and increase in size as well as in numbers with aging. Afferent lymphatics, germinal centers and significant numbers of reticular fibers are absent in the thymus. The few lymphatic vessels present in the thymus are all efferent; they are present in the walls of the blood vessels, in the connective tissue of the septa, and in the capsule. These vessels end in the brachiocephalic, parasternal and tracheobronchial lymph nodes.

Within the thymus gland, the maturation and selection of T-cells includes positive selection and negative selection of T-cells. Only a small number (10%) of lymphocytes generated in the thymus gland reach maturity. As maturation progresses in the cortex, the APCs present self and foreign antigens to the T-cells. Lymphocytes which are unable to recognize foreign and self-antigen die and are eliminated by macrophages (negative selection). The lymphocytes which recognize the foreign antigens (positive selection) only survive. Then these lymphocytes leave the cortex and enter in the medulla, from where they enter into the blood stream.

a. **Blood-thymic barrier:** The thymus receives numerous small arteries, which enter the capsule and are distributed throughout the organ via the trabeculae between adjacent lobules. Branches of these vessels do not gain access to the cortex directly; instead, from the trabeculae they enter at the corticomedullary junction, where they form capillary beds that penetrate the cortex. The capillaries of the cortex are invested by a sheath of type I epithelioreticular cells. The endothelium of capillaries is not fenestrated and the basal lamina is very thick. This prevents most of the circulating antigens from

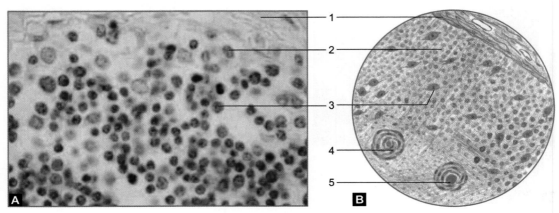

**Fig. 11.9:** Thymus at high magnification showing a part of thymic lobule, (A) micrograph, (B) sketch. Hassall's corpuscles (4) are masses of epithelioreticular cells around a central homogenous mass (5). Capsule (1), lymphocytes (2), and epithelioreticular cell (3)

reaching the thymic cortex and thus forms a blood–thymus barrier. This barrier consists of:

  i. Capillary endothelium with pericytes and its basal lamina,

 ii. The basal lamina of epithelioreticular cells and

iii. Epithelioreticular cells.

The barrier is not found in the medulla and it prevents antigen contamination of developing and programmed T lymphocytes.

b. **Functions of the thymus**

  i. The developing T-cells mature in the cortex of the thymus.

 ii. It secretes thymosin, thymic humoral factor and thymopoietin, which transform immature T-cells into mature T-cells. It also secretes thymotaxin (thymulin), which attracts progenitor T-cells (stem cells) from the bone marrow to populate the thymus.

Besides thymus thyroid, pituitary and suprarenal glands also influence T-cell maturation. Thyroxin stimulates the cortical epithelioreticular cells to increase thymotaxin production; adrenocorticoids decrease T-cell numbers in the cortex; and somatotropin promotes the development of T-cell in the thymic cortex.

## D. Spleen

It is about the size of a clenched fist and it is the largest lymphatic organ in the body and only lymphatic organ which is the immunologic filter for the blood. It has no afferent lymphatic vessels and no lymph sinuses. It is enclosed by a well-developed capsule made up of dense connective tissue containing elastic fibers and bundles of collagen fibers. Some smooth muscle fibers may be present in the capsule. On the medial surface of the spleen, capsule form an indentation, known as hilum of the spleen through which blood vessels and nerves enter or leave the spleen. Except at the hilum, the outer surface of the capsule is covered by a mesothelium (peritoneum). Thick strands of connective tissue, known as trabeculae extend from the inner surface of the capsule and form a branching and anastomosing network. The spleen is supported throughout by a fine sponge work of reticular fibers and associated reticular cells. The reticulum blends into the trabeculae, vessels and capsule. The substance of the spleen is known as splenic pulp (Fig. 11.10A, B). The cut surface of a fresh spleen shows grey areas surrounded by red areas; the former is called white pulp and the

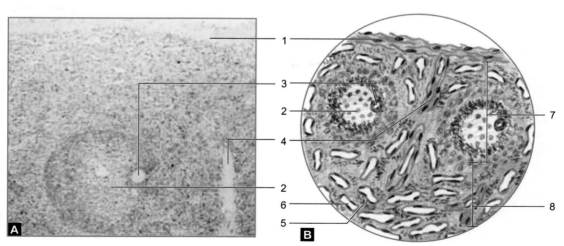

**Fig. 11.10:** Spleen, (A) micrograph, (B) sketch having white pulp (7) with an eccentric arteriole (3) in Malpighian corpuscles (2). Red pulp (8) is having cords of Billroth (5) and venous sinuses (6). Capsule (1) and trabeculae (4)

latter is called red pulp. From birth to early adulthood, the white pulp forms the greater volume of the spleen, but with increasing age, it regresses, the number of splenic nodules decreases and the red pulp becomes increasingly prominent.

a. **White pulp:** It forms the periarterial lymphatic sheaths (PALS) around the arteries, which leave the trabeculae to enter the pulp. Small lymphocytes (mostly T-cells) make up the bulk of the cells in the PALS. Frequently, enclosed within the PALS are lymphatic nodules, which are composed of B cells and these nodules may display the germinal centers. These nodules are called splenic nodules or Malpighian corpuscles (Fig. 11.11).

At the periphery of the lymphatic sheath a marginal zone is present, which separates the white pulp from the red pulp. It is composed of plasma cells, T and B lymphocytes, macrophages and dendritic cells (APCs). In addition to the cells, this zone also contains numerous sinusoids, known as marginal sinuses. Efferent lymphatic vessels originate in the white pulp and through these vessels lymphocytes go out of the spleen.

b. **Red pulp:** It is formed by large venous sinusoids. In between the sinusoids red pulp takes a shape of branching cord, known as splenic cords or cords of Billroth. The cords are composed of a loose network of reticular fibers, which is filled with a large number of cells, including all blood cells. Macrophages are particularly numerous in the area surrounding the sinusoids. The sinusoids have a wide lumen (20–40 µm in diameter) and endothelial cells of the sinusoids are elongated and fusiform. These are known as Stave or littoral or rod cells (Fig. 11.12).

There are many gaps (2–3 µm wide) in between the cells through which blood can pass in and out of the sinuses. Outside the endothelium, the wall is supported by a basement membrane which is not continuous but forms widely spaced, thick bars that encircle the sinusoid. The bars are joined by thinner strands of the same material and are continuous with the reticular fibers of the splenic cords. Red pulp is mainly concerned with the destruction of age erythrocytes and is the emergency source of erythrocytes, granulocytes and platelets, which can be instantly delivered into the circulation whenever needed.

c. **Blood circulation in the spleen:** The branches of the splenic artery enter at the hilum. These branches are then carried into the interior of the spleen within the

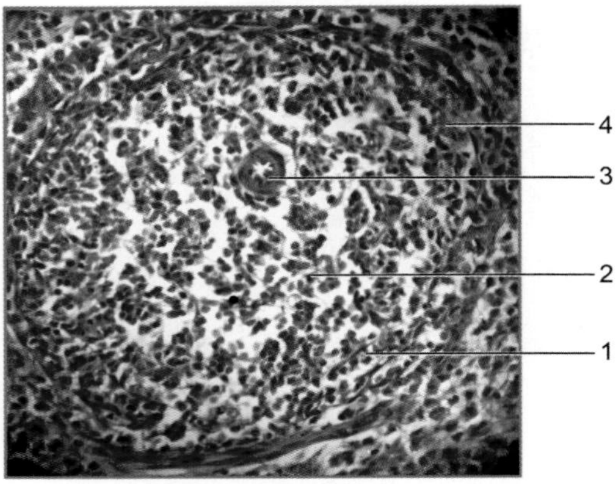

**Fig. 11.11:** Malpighian corpuscle (1) present in the white pulp. Germinal center (2), efferent arteriole (3), and corona (4)

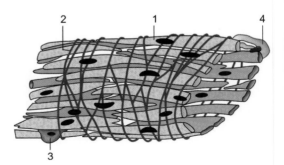

**Fig. 11.12:** Schematic diagram of a sinusoid in the red pulp of the spleen. Its narrow stave like endothelial cells (1) are held together by bars of basement membrane (2). Blood cell (3) and macrophage (4)

trabeculae. These trabecular arteries continue to branch repeatedly and when these are reduced to about 0.2 mm in diameter, these arteries leave the trabeculae. These are known as central arterioles. The tunica adventitia of these arterioles becomes loosely organized and they become surrounded by a sheath of lymphocytes, the periarterial lymphatic sheath (PALS). At various points along the course of the vessels, the lymphatic sheath is increased in amount to form splenic nodules. Where this sheath expands to form nodules, the central arteriole is displaced to one side and assumes an eccentric position in the nodule and only rarely does the vessel retain a central position in the nodular lymphatic tissue. Central arteriole gives numerous capillaries which provide supply to PALS and then continue into the marginal zone. Thus the marginal zone is the first site where blood comes in contact with the splenic parenchyma. In continuity, of course, of central arteriole, they lose their lymphatic investment and enter the red pulp, where they subdivide into several straight branches called penicilli. Some of the penicilli show a thickening in their walls

and known as sheathed arterioles. The sheath is formed by macrophages and knows as ellipsoid or Schweigger-Seidel sheath. The arterioles then branch again to form terminal capillaries. Each set of arterioles within the splenic pulp is a functional end artery. According to the open circulation theory, the terminal capillaries open in the splenic cords, then blood from here enters in the venous sinusoids (Fig. 11.13). According to closed circulation theory, the capillaries directly pour blood in the venous sinusoids. According to the compromised theory of splenic circulation, both types of circulation are present in the spleen. Splenic sinusoids then drain into the pulp veins. The pulp veins, then enter in the trabeculae as trabecular veins. The trabecular veins, then unite and leave at the hilum as the splenic vein.

d. **Functions of spleen**

  i. It is an important hemopoietic organ, generating both lymphocytes and monocytes. Lymphocytes are formed in both types of pulps, but chiefly in the white pulp. Then they pass the red pulp, and so into the sinusoids and the splenic vein. Monocytes differentiate from

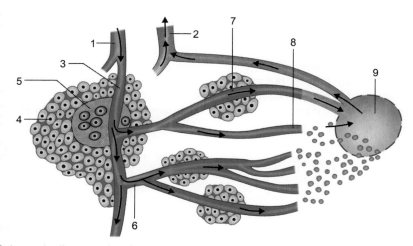

**Fig. 11.13:** Schematic diagram showing open and closed circulation in the spleen. Trabecular artery (1), trabecular vein (2), central artery (3), splenic nodule (4), PALS (5), penicilli (6), ellipsoid (7), terminal capillaries (8) and splenic sinuses (9)

hemocytoblasts in the red pulp and splenic sinuses.

ii. As the spleen is located in the way of blood circulation, the spleen is able to filter, phagocytose and mount immunological responses against blood-borne antigens. The spleen contains all the components (B and T lymphocytes, APCs and phagocytic cells) necessary for this function.

iii. Erythrocytes have an average life span of around 120 days, after which they are destroyed, by the macrophages in the splenic cords. A reduction in their flexibility and changes in their membrane seems to be the signals for their destruction. Degenerating erythrocytes are also removed from the bone marrow.

iv. Macrophages in the spleen also break down the hemoglobin of worn out erythrocytes. Iron from hemoglobin is recycled in the bone marrow, while haem is degraded and excreted into bile by liver cells.

v. The spleen serves as an important reservoir of blood in some species.

vi. The spleen is not essential to life, if it is removed then the body made readjustment through the compensatory growth of lymphoid tissue elsewhere.

For comparison among lymph node, spleen, thymus and palatine tonsil, *see* Table 22 given in Appendix I.

**Organ transplantation:** It is the moving of an organ from one body to another, for the purpose of replacing the recipient's damaged or failing organ with a working one from the donor. Organs that can be transplanted are the heart, kidneys, liver, lungs, pancreas, penis, and intestines.

**Graft rejection:** Rejection of transplanted organs is the main barrier of transplantation today. It occurs as a result of humoral and cell-mediated responses by the recipient to specific antigens present in the donor tissue. These antigens are known as major histocompatibility complex (MHC) molecules. In humans, this group of molecules is referred to human leukocyte antigen (HLA) complex molecules. The recognition of these foreign MHC antigens initiates rejection, which occurs in two stages. During the first stage, known as sensitization, lymphocytes are alerted and respond to the foreign MHC molecules. Rapid proliferation occurs in this stage. In the second 'effector' stage, the graft is destroyed by several cellular and molecular mechanisms.

**Autoimmune diseases:** These are diseases caused by the body producing an inappropriate immune response against its own tissues. Sometimes the immune system will cease to recognize one or more of the body's normal constituents as "self" and will create autoantibodies (antibodies that attack its own cells, tissues, and/or organs). This causes inflammation, damage and leads to autoimmune disorders, e.g. Graves' disease, and Hashimoto's disease.

The cause of autoimmune diseases is unknown, but it appears that there is an inherited predisposition to develop autoimmune disease in many cases. In a few types of autoimmune disease (such as rheumatic fever), a bacteria or virus triggers an immune response, and the antibodies or T-cells attack normal cells because they have some part of their structure that resembles a part of the structure of the infecting microorganism.

## Summary

| S. No. | Parameter | Lymph node | Spleen | Thymus | Palatine tonsil |
|---|---|---|---|---|---|
| 1. | Outer covering | Capsule | Capsule | Capsule | Stratified squamous nonkeratinized epithelium |
| 2. | Trabeculae or Septa | Thin trabeculae present | Abundant thick trabeculae with blood vessels | Incomplete septa are present | Both are absent |

(Contd.)

(*Contd.*)

| S. No. | Parameter | Lymph node | Spleen | Thymus | Palatine tonsil |
|--------|-----------|------------|--------|--------|-----------------|
| 3. | Cortex and medulla | Present | Absent | Present | Absent |
| 4. | Lymphatic nodules | Present | Present | Absent | Present |
| 5. | White and red pulp | Absent | Present | Absent | Absent |
| 6. | Cords and sinuses | Present | Present | Absent | Absent |
| 7. | Lymphatic vessels | Afferent and efferent | Few efferent only | Few efferent only | Efferent only |
| 8. | Unique structures | Subcapsular sinus | Malpighian corpuscle | Hassall's corpuscle | Tonsillar crypts |

## Self Assessment

1. Which of the following organs does not have outer cortex and inner medullary region?
   a. Lymph node    b. Thymus
   c. Spleen        d. Kidney

2. The lymphatic nodules are not seen in:
   a. Lymph node    b. Thymus
   c. Spleen        d. Palatine tonsil

3. Splenic sinuses are lined with:
   a. Fenestrated endothelium
   b. Continuous endothelium
   c. Cuboidal epithelium
   d. Discontinuous endothelium

4. Which one of the following is an antigen presenting cell?
   a. Langerhans cell    b. Mast cell
   c. Fibroblast         d. Erythrocyte

5. Hassall's corpuscle is seen in:
   a. Tonsil        b. Thymus
   c. Spleen        d. Lymph node

6. Which type of epithelium lines the crypts of palatine tonsil?
   a. Stratified squamous nonkeratinized
   b. Stratified squamous keratinized
   c. Pseudostratified
   d. Simple columnar

7. Which of the following lymphoid organs has both afferent and efferent lymphatics?
   a. Thymus        b. Spleen
   c. Lymph node    d. Tonsil

8. Malpighian corpuscles are seen in:
   a. Spleen        b. Thymus
   c. Tonsil        d. Lymph node

9. Which of the following lymphoid organs is having lobules?
   a. Lymph node    b. Thymus
   c. Spleen        d. Tonsil

10. Red pulp is present in:
    a. Lymph node    b. Thymus
    c. Spleen        d. Tonsil

## Answers

1. c,    2. b,    3. d,    4. a,    5. b,    6. a,    7. c,    8. a,    9. b,
10. c

# 12

# Integumentary System

The integumentary system consists of the skin and its derivatives, such as hairs, nails, sebaceous and sweat glands. Structurally, the skin consists of two layers; which differ in function, histological appearance and their embryological origin. The outer layer or epidermis is formed by an epithelium and is of ectodermal origin. The other one, the dermis, consists of connective tissue and develops from the mesoderm. Beneath these two layers a subcutaneous layer of loose connective tissue or hypodermis is present. The skin covers the entire outer surface of the body, becoming continuous with the mucous membranes of the digestive system, the respiratory system and the urogenital systems. Additionally, the skin of the eyelids becomes continuous with the conjunctiva lining the anterior portion of the orbit. Skin also lines the external acoustic meatus and covers the external surface of the tympanic membrane.

The skin constitutes about 16–20% of the total body weight. The skin protects the organism from drying out and invasion by microorganisms; it helps to regulate the temperature of the body; it absorbs ultraviolet (UV) radiation, which is necessary for synthesis of vitamin D; it is sensitve to touch, pressure, pain and temperature. Skin is also self-repairing after injury and it is essential to life.

## EPIDERMIS

It is relatively impermeable outermost tough layer. It is totally avascular and is nourished by diffusion. It consists of mainly keratinized stratified squamous epithelium and also contains the melanocytes, the Langerhans cells and the Merkel's cells. This layer itself is made up of five sublayers that work together to continuously rebuild the surface of the skin.

## A. Stratum Basale (Stratum Germinativum)

It is closest to the dermis and consists of a single layer of columnar or cuboidal cells resting on a thin basement membrane. The cells are attached to one another by desmosomes and to the underlying basement membrane by hemidesmosomes. Basal cells are the stem cells, which continuously divide and form new cells, known as keratinocytes. These cells push the older ones upwards, where they are eventually shed off. This renewal of the epidermis takes about 3 to 4 weeks. All cells contain intermediate keratin filaments and as the cells move upwards filaments increase in number.

## B. Stratum Spinosum

This thickest layer is located just above the basal layer and has many layers of keratinocytes. Keratinocytes present in this layer are larger than those in the stratum basale and have many spines or cytoplasmic processes, so this layer is known as stratum spinosum. The processes are attached to the processes of adjacent cells by desmosomes. During preparation of slides because of fixatives cells shrinks except at the desmosomes giving the cells a spiny appearance, so known as prickle cells.

The stratum basale and spinosum are together referred as the Malpighian layer.

## C. Stratum Granulosum

This layer is 1–3 cells thick and the cytoplasm of keratinocytes in this layer contains basophilic keratohyalin granules. The granules are not located in membrane-bound organelles, but forms "free" accumulations in the cytoplasm. These granules consist of protein filaggrin. The aggregation of keratin filaments with the filaggrin protein of keratohyalin granules forms keratin present within the cells of the stratum corneum. The keratin thus formed is the soft keratin of the skin. Along with this, the cytoplasm also contains the lipid containing lamellar granules. The cells release the lipids that fill the entire interstitial space, which is important for the function of the epidermis as a barrier towards the external environment.

## D. Stratum Lucidum

This layer is translucent and consists of tightly packed three to five layers of flattened cells. As the nuclei have already begun to degenerate in the outer part of the stratum granulosum, this layer does not contain any nuclei. This layer is strongly eosinophilic and contains densely packed keratin filaments.

## E. Stratum Corneum (Horny Layer)

It is the topmost layer and made up of 10–30 thin layers of continuously shedding, dead keratinocytes. The space between the cells is filled with lipids, which works as a cement to bind the cells together into a continuous membrane. The cells sloughed off continuously as new cells take its place, but this shedding process slows down with age.

Four cell types are found in the epidermis:

a. **Keratinocytes:** These cells are the predominant cells present in the epidermis. These are formed by stem cells of the stratum basale. Keratinocytes present in the stratum basale contain numerous intermediate filaments known as tonofilaments or keratin filaments. As these cells enter and move up into the stratum spinosum, the tonofilaments collect to form bundles of fibrils, known as tonofibrils. When these cells reach the stratum granulosum, filaggrin protein of keratohyaline granules promotes the aggregation of keratin filaments into keratin and thus forms the cornified cells of stratum corneum. The formation of cornified cells from granular cells, even involves the breakdown of nucleus and other organelles. The keratin formed by this process is known as soft keratin as compared to the hard keratin of hairs and nails.

b. **Melanocytes:** These cells are present in the epidermis and its appendages, in oral epithelium, some mucous membranes, the uveal tract (choroid coat) of the eyeball, parts of the middle and internal ear and in the pial and the arachnoid meninges at the base of the brain. In the epidermis, these cells are present in the stratum basale and at the junction of the epidermis to the dermis. Melanocytes are derived from neural crest cells. These cells are round to columnar cells whose long, slender processes containing melanin extend outward between keratinocytes.

The ability of melanocytes to synthesize melanin depends on the production of the enzyme tyrosinase, which converts tyrosine [through an intermediate known as 3, 4-dihydroxyphenylalanine (DOPA)] into a melanin precursor. Tyrosinase is synthesized by the rER and transfer through the Golgi apparatus to membrane vesicles known as premelanosomes. Melanin is synthesized in these vesicles, which then become melanosomes (melanin granules). The melanin granules thus formed are transferred to keratinocytes through phagocytosis by a process known as cytocrine secretion. Melanin gives skin its tan or brown color and helps in protecting the deeper layers of the skin from the harmful effects of the sun. Sun exposure causes melanocytes to increase production of melanin in order to protect the skin from damaging ultraviolet rays. In whitish persons melanin is degraded by lysosomes, while in black persons this pigment is more stable.

c. **Langerhans cells:** These cells are star shaped with numerous dendritic processes and found mainly in the stratum spinosum. Langerhans cells are antigen-presenting cells and originate in the bone marrow. These cells are smaller than keratinocytes and have a dark staining nucleus with the relatively clear cytoplasm. These cells contain characteristic paddle-shaped Birbeck (vermiform) granules, one end of which frequently distends in a vesicle, so the cells resemble a tennis racket. The exact function of these granules is not known. Langerhans cells have surface markers common to most B-cells, some T-cells, macrophages and monocytes.

d. **Merkel's cells:** These tactile cells are found in small numbers near the stratum basale and appear to be more numerous in places with special sensitivity, such as the fingertips. Merkel's cells are of neuroectodermal origin. These cells contain membrane-bound vesicles (dense core granules) in their cytoplasm and form synaptic junctions with myelinated sensory nerve twigs in the upper part of the dermis. Their communications with local neurons suggest that they have a neurosensory function.

## DERMIS (CORIUM)

It consists of dense, fibrous connective tissue whose main component is collagen. The surface of the dermis is very irregular and has many projections (dermal papillae or ridges) that interdigitate with projections (epidermal pegs or ridges) of the epidermis. Collectively, these ridges are known as the rete apparatus. These structures are more common in skin, which is subjected to frequent pressure. Dermis mainly regulates temperature and supply the epidermis with nutrient-saturated blood. Much of the body's water supply is stored within the dermis.

The texture of collagen fibers serves as the basis for recognizing two sublayers of the dermis.

### A. The Papillary Layer

This layer is made by loose connective tissue. The fibroblasts and other connective tissue cells are present in this layer; most abundant being mast cells and macrophages. It fills the hollows in the deep surface (dermal papillae) of the epidermis. Collagen fibers are thin as compared to the collagen fibers in the reticular layer. The dermal papillae contain tactile corpuscles of Meissner and small blood vessels.

In the palms, fingers, soles and toes, the influence of the papillae projecting into the epidermis forms contours in the skin's surface; these are called friction ridges. These ridges help the hand or foot to grasp by increasing friction. These ridges first appear at 13 weeks of intrauterine life in the tips of the fingers and later in the palm and sole. The patterns assumed by ridges and intervening sulci are known as dermatoglyphics. These are unique for each individual, appearing as loops, arches, whorls, or combinations of these forms. These configurations are used for personal identification (fingerprints or footprints) and probably determined by multiple genes.

### B. The Reticular Layer

This layer is made by dense irregular connective tissue and mainly consists of thick bundles of type I collagen fibers. An interwoven network of elastic fibers lies in between the bundles appearing especially abundant near sweat and sebaceous glands. Proteoglycans rich in dermatan sulfate, fill the interstices of the reticular layer. Cells are sparser in this layer than in the papillary layer. Cells present in this layer are fibroblasts, mast cells, lymphocytes, macrophages and frequently fat cells in the deeper aspects of the reticular layer. This layer strengthens the skin, and also provide elasticity. Hair follicles, smooth muscle (arrector pili), sweat glands, sebaceous glands and Pacinian corpuscles are present in this layer.

The collagen fibers mainly run parallel to the surface of the skin. Because of the direction of the fibers, lines of skin tension, i.e. Langer's lines are formed. This is of some surgical importance since incisions parallel to these lines will form fewer scars and even heal faster. Groups of smooth muscle fibers are located in the deeper regions of the reticular layer at particular sites such as the skin of the penis and scrotum and the areola around the nipples; contractions of these muscle groups wrinkle the skin in these regions.

The dermis has a rich network of blood and lymph vessels. The arteries form two plexuses. The one located between papillary and reticular layer is called papillary plexus; and the other between dermis and hypodermis is called cutaneous plexus. Similarly, veins form three plexuses, two are found on the same plane as arterial plexus and the third one is disposed in the middle of the dermis.

Sensory organs present in the dermis are:

a. **Tactile corpuscles of Meissner:** These are mechanoreceptors specialized to respond to slight deformations of the epidermis. These are found in the dermal papillae. Each one has an encapsulated sensory ending with a Pinecone-shaped structure. Their long axis is perpendicular to the skin's surface (Fig. 12.1A, B). The nerves are not easily observed in H&E stain preparations. These receptors are most common in areas of the skin that are especially sensitive to tactile stimulation, e.g. lips, external genitalia, nipple and are also distributed in the digital pulps and the palms.

b. **Lamellar corpuscles:** These are mechanoreceptors which are sensitive to pressure, vibration and acceleration of movement. These are especially observed in hypodermis and are also called Pacinian corpuscles. Like Meissner's corpuscles, lamellar corpuscle also has an encapsulated sensory ending; this sensory ending is a baroreceptor which has a unique onion-

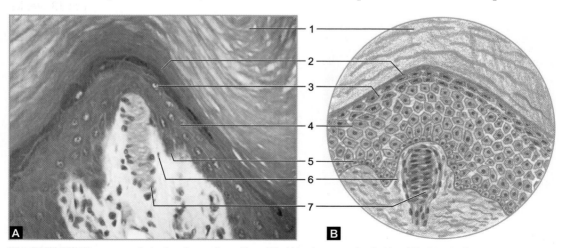

**Fig. 12.1:** Tactile corpuscle in the dermal papillae (6), (A) micrograph of skin, (B) sketch. Stratum corneum (1), stratum lucidum (2), stratum granulosum (3), stratum spinosum (4), stratum basale (5) and tactile corpuscle (7)

shaped structure (Fig. 12.2A, B). Each corpuscle is having a central myelinated axon, which is surrounded by concentric lamellae of compact collagen fibers. At periphery fibers become dense to form a capsule.

## SUBCUTANEOUS TISSUE (HYPODERMIS)

The connective tissue of the dermis grades into hypodermis, without a sharp transition or distinct boundary. Over most of the body, it is characterized by adipocytes. In some sites such as in dimples it is fibrous and binds the dermis to underlying structures. This layer is the superficial fascia of gross anatomical dissection. Individuals who are fatty or who live in cold climates contain a large amount of fat deposited in the hypodermis (superficial fascia), known as panniculus adiposus. This layer acts as a shock absorber and thermal insulator. In the penis, scrotum and eyelids, this layer is devoid of fat.

## TYPES OF SKIN

The skin is of two types: Thin skin (Fig. 12.3A, B) and thick skin (Fig. 12.4A, B). Thin skin covers

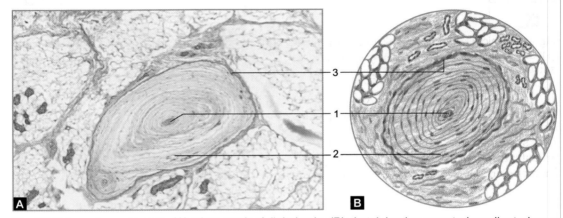

**Fig. 12.2:** Lamellar corpuscle, (A) micrograph of digital pulp, (B) sketch having a central myelinated axon (1) surrounded by concentric lamellae (2) of collagen fibers enclosed in a capsule (3)

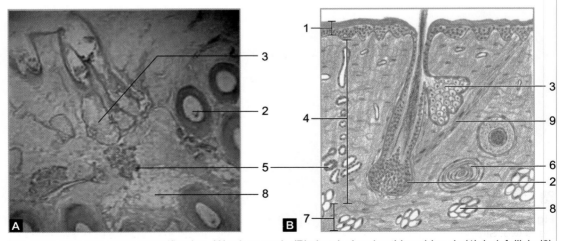

**Fig. 12.3:** Thin skin at low magnification, (A) micrograph, (B) sketch showing thin epidermis (1), hair follicle (2), sebaceous gland (3), sweat gland (5), lamellar corpuscle (6), dermis (4), hypodermis (7), adipose tissue (8) and arrector pili muscle (9)

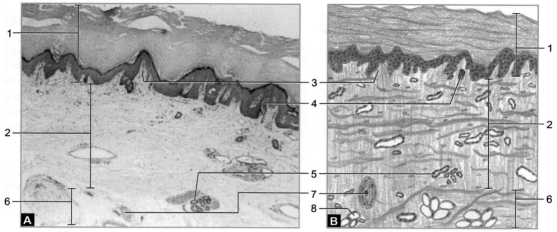

**Fig. 12.4:** Thick skin of digital pulp at low magnification, (A) micrograph, (B) sketch illustrating thick epidermis (1), sweat glands (5) are present deep in the dermis (2). Dermal papillae (3) contain tactile corpuscle (4) and capillaries. Lamellar corpuscle (7) and adipose tissue (8) are present in the hypodermis (6)

the whole body except palm and sole, while thick skin is present in palm and sole. In the thin skin, stratum corneum and spinosum are thin and stratum lucidum is absent (Fig. 12.5A, B). In thick skin, all layers of epidermis are present.

Hairs are present in the thin skin and they are absent in the thick skin.

For comparison between thin skin and thick skin, *see* Table 23 given in Appendix I.

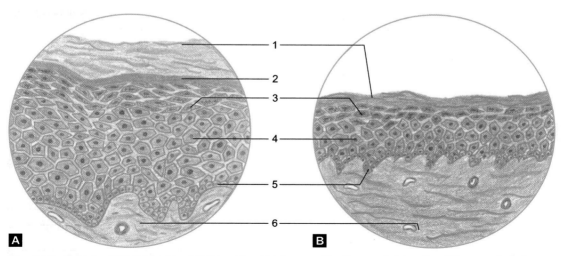

**Fig. 12.5:** Sketch of (A) thick skin, (B) thin skin at high magnification explaining the difference in between these two. Stratum corneum (1) and stratum spinosum (4) are comparatively thick in thick skin. Stratum lucidum (2) is present only in thick skin. Stratum granulosum (3), stratum basale (5) and dermis (6) are also seen

## SKIN DERIVATIVES

Organs such as hair, sweat glands and sebaceous glands that develop from the embryonic epidermis are labelled as skin derivatives or appendages of the skin.

### A. Nails

These are hard plates of tightly packed keratinized cells, and form a protective covering over the dorsal surface of each distal phalanx. Nail body is the visible portion of the nail that rests onto the nail bed (Fig. 12.6). It has a free distal edge and the stratum corneum present beneath the edge is called the hyponychium. The nail bed is highly vascular and made up only by the germinative zone (stratum basale and stratum spinosum). The matrix beneath the nail bed is very thin and does not contribute to the growth of the nail; thus known as sterile matrix. The undersurface of the nail is firmly attached to the cells in the sterile matrix, which thus prevents invasion by microbes.

The proximal hidden portion of the nail is nail root; it is embedded in a fold of skin (proximal nail fold). The germinative zone is thicker near the root and forms the germinal matrix. Cells in the matrix proliferate and form the nail substance; however, the superficial layers of the nail are formed by proximal nail fold. Distal to the proximal nail fold a crescent white area is known as lunule. The lateral margin of the nail is also overlapped by a fold of skin (lateral nail fold). The stratum corneum of the deep surface of the proximal nail pushed forward over the nail for a short distance, known as eponychium (cuticle).

### B. Hairs

These are elastic keratinized threads and consist of a free shaft (scapus) and a root embedded in the skin. The root is anchored in

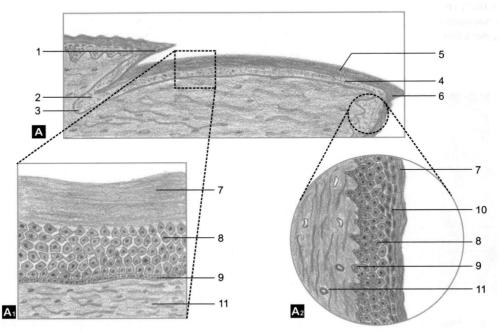

**Fig. 12.6:** (A) Nail (LS) at low magnification, (A₁) nail bed and nail body, (A₂) thin skin. Eponychium (1), nail root (2), germinal matrix (3), nail bed (4), nail body (5), hyponychium (6), stratum corneum (7), stratum spinosum (8), stratum basale (9), stratum granulosum (10) and dermis (11)

a tubular invagination of the epidermis, called as the hair follicle, which extends down into the dermis and usually, a short distance into the hypodermis. At its deepest end the follicle expands into a hair bulb, which is indented at the basal end by a connective tissue papilla. Hair papilla contains a rich plexus of blood vessels and nerves. Associated with the follicle are sebaceous glands and a bundle of smooth muscle (arrector pili). Cells in the bulb are mitotically active. Their progeny differentiates into the cell types which form the hair and the cells of root sheath.

The hair starts developing from epidermal downgrowth into the dermis in the 3rd month of intrauterine life. At 5–6 months of intrauterine life, whole body is covered with fine wool like languo (primary) hairs. These hairs are shed at birth and replaced by pale downy hairs; known as vellus (secondary hairs). Vellus are retained in most of the regions of the body except scalp, face, eyebrows, axilla and pubis, where they are replaced by coarse dark hairs known as terminal hairs (influenced by sex hormones). Hairs are absent in palms, soles, lips, glans penis, clitoris, labia minora and umbilicus.

a. **Hair shaft:** Epidermal cells of the shaft are arranged in three concentric layers (Fig. 12.7A, B):

  i. *Medulla:* It forms the central axis and consists of 2–3 layers of shrunken, cornified, cuboidal cells separated by air spaces. It is absent in thin, fine hairs (languo) and may be absent in some hairs of the scalp or extend only part way along the shaft.

  ii. *Cortex:* It contains several layers of cornified cells. The cells contain pigments in dark hairs and air bubbles in white hairs. It forms the main bulk of the hairs.

  iii. *Cuticle:* It is the superficial layer and made up by single layer of heavily keratinized cells.

b. **Hair follicle:** It is a compound sheath consisting of an external dermal root sheath and an internal epidermal root sheath. In the hair bulb these sheaths blends in a mass of primitive cells, called matrix.

  i. *Dermal root sheath:* It is composed of three layers. Outer layer is poorly defined and contains longitudinally

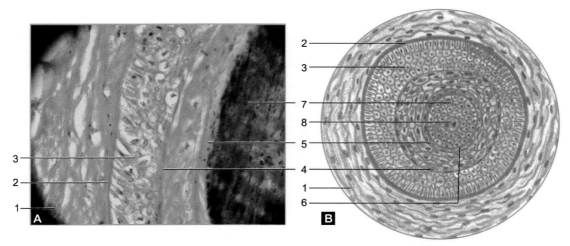

**Fig. 12.7:** Hair TS, (A) micrograph, (B) sketch demonstrating central axis of medulla (8) surrounded by cornified cells of cortex (7). Huxley's layer (5) having eosinophilic trichohyaline granules are also present in the hair. Cuticle (6), epidermal root sheath (3), dermal sheath (1), glassy membrane (2), Henle's layer (4) is also seen

running bundle of collagen fibers. Middle layer is thick, cellular and consists of circularly arranged fine connective tissue fibers. The inner layer is homogenous, the glassy membrane; consists of reticular fibers and amorphous ground substance (Fig. 12.8A, B).

ii. *Epidermal root sheath:* It is composed of an outer sheath and an inner sheath. Outer sheath contains a single row of tall cells and an inner stratum of polygonal cells. Inner sheath does not extend above the point of entry of the duct of sebaceous gland. This is further divisible into:

- Outer or Henle's layer: It is a single layer of cuboidal cells with flattened nuclei.
- Huxley's layer: It consists of several layers of elongated cells, whose cytoplasm contains eosinophilic trichohyaline granules.
- Cuticle of root sheath: It lies against the cuticle of the hair. It consists of a single layer of transparent, horny scales, the free edges of which

interdigitate with the scales of the hair cuticle.

## C. Arrector Pili Muscle

The arrector pili muscle is a tiny muscle connected at one end to the hair follicle and at the other end to the papillary layer of the dermis. It comprises a collection of smooth muscle cells, collagen fibers and non-myelinated axons of adrenergic nerves. It pulls the hair shaft outwards and presses the sebaceous glands to expel its secretion on the hair root. When it contracts it causes the hair to stand erect and a "goosebump" forms on the skin and sebaceous glands pour their secretion into the lumen of the hair follicle. Arrector pili muscles are absent from the hair present on the face and axilla and in the pubic hair and from eyelashes and eyebrows and hair around the nostrils and external auditory meatus. The hair, sebaceous gland and the arrector pili muscle together form a pilosebaceous unit (Fig. 12.3A, B).

## D. Glands of the Skin

Glands of the skin include sweat and sebaceous glands.

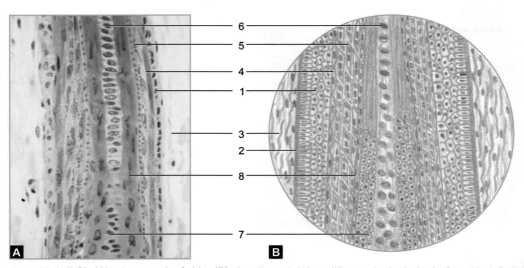

**Fig. 12.8:** Hair (LS), (A) micrograph of skin, (B) sketch explaining all layers in the hair shaft and hair follicle. Epidermal root sheath (1), glassy membrane (2), dermal sheath (3), Henle's layer (4), Huxley's layer (5), medulla (6), cortex (7) and cuticle (8)

a. **Sweat (Sudoriferous) glands:** These are widely distributed in the skin, except the nail bed, the margins of the lips, glans penis and eardrum. Sweat glands are differentiated into two types by their secretory mechanism, they also differ in their detailed histological appearance and in the composition of the sweat they secrete.

i. *Merocrine or eccrine glands*: These are simple coiled tubular glands and found over the entire body. The secretory portion of the gland lies deep in the dermis, while their duct directly opens on the skin surface. The secretory portion is having larger cells in comparison to the duct. The secretory epithelium is cuboidal or low columnar. Two types of cells are found in the secretory epithelium: Dark cells and light (clear) cells (Fig. 12.9A, B). Dark cells line the lumen of the gland and contain many mucinogen rich secretory granules. Light cells are pyramidal cells and underlie the dark cells. These cells are rich in mitochondria and glycogen and contain intercellular canaliculi that extend to the lumen of the gland. These cells secrete a watery, electrolyte-rich material. As the cells have slightly different shapes, so, the epithelium may appear pseudostratified. A layer of myoepithelial cells is found between the secretory cells of the epithelium and the basement membrane. Contraction of these cells is responsible for the rapid excretion of sweat from the duct. The excretory ducts are lined by stratified cuboidal epithelium. When the duct reaches the epidermis the ductal cells end and keratinocytes envelop the duct on its way to the sweat pore. These glands produce sweat, which is a watery mixture of salts, antibodies and metabolic wastes. Sweat helps in regulation of body temperature. Eccrine sweat glands are innervated by cholinergic (parasympathetic) nerves.

ii. *Apocrine glands*: These are present in the axillary, pubic and perianal regions. Apocrine sweat glands are much larger than merocrine sweat glands. The glands are embedded in the subcutaneous tissue and their duct empties the sweat into the upper part of the hair follicle (Fig. 12.10A, B). These glands secrete a milky sweat that encourages the growth

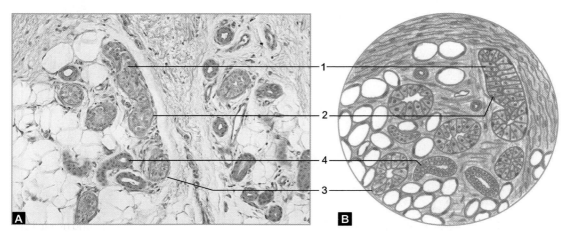

**Fig. 12.9:** Eccrine sweat gland, (A) micrograph, (B) sketch showing low columnar secretory epithelium (1) with myoepithelial cells (2) lying in between secretory epithelial cells and basement membrane (3). Excretory duct (4) lined by stratified cuboidal epithelium can also be seen in the figure

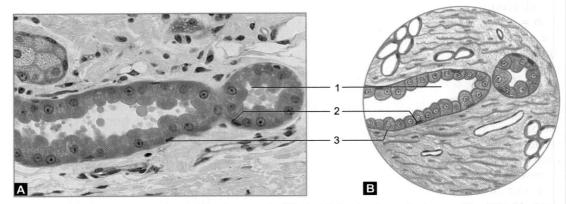

**Fig. 12.10:** Apocrine sweat gland, (A) micrograph, (B) sketch having irregular lumen (1) with secretions. Myoepithelial cells (2) are resting on the basement membrane (3)

of the bacteria responsible for body odour. Their secretion is more viscous than that of the eccrine glands.

The secretory activity of apocrine glands starts at puberty and may be analogous to the sexual scent glands of other animals. These glands are innervated by adrenergic (sympathetic) nerves. Although the term apocrine implies that a portion of the cytoplasm becomes part of the secretion, but electron micrographs have shown that these glands secrete via merocrine secretion.

b. **Sebaceous (oil) glands:** These are pear-shaped, simple branched areolar, holocrine

glands. These glands empty their secretory products into the upper parts of the hair follicles (Fig. 12.11A, B) and can be found everywhere on the body except for the palms and the soles. These glands are also found in some of the areas where no hairs are present such as in the lips, oral surfaces of the cheeks and external genitalia. At the base of the gland cells are formed by mitosis and then pushed toward the surface. Along the way, the cells become packed with lipid and then die. The secretion consists of a breakdown-products of the cells themselves.

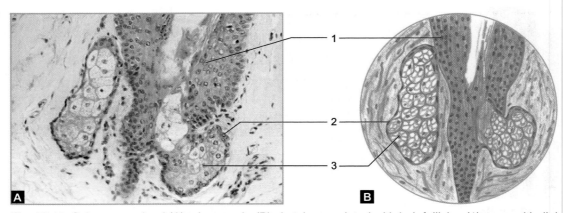

**Fig. 12.11:** Sebaceous gland (A) micrograph, (B) sketch associated with hair follicles (1), myoepithelial cells (2) surround the gland (3)

Sebaceous glands secrete the sebum (seb = oil), i.e. an oily product, which keeps the skin soft and it contains a bactericidal agent that inhibits the growth of certain bacteria (Fig. 12.12A, B). Sebum is usually secreted into a hair follicle but in a few regions of the body like lips, glans penis, areola of the nipples, labia minora, the mucous surface of the prepuce and tarsal glands of eyelids, these sebaceous glands directly pour their secretion onto the skin surface. These glands are largest in areas where the hair is very small, e.g. nose and external acoustic meatus. These glands are most abundant on the face, forehead and scalp. These glands are under the influence of sex hormones and their activity is greatly increased after puberty.

**Albinism:** This is a kind of inborn error of metabolism. This occurs due to deficiency of melanin, which results from lack of enzyme tyrosinase. Tyrosinase is necessary for the biosynthesis of melanin from its precursor, tyrosine. Albinos have blond hair, a poor vision, and severe photophobia. Chronic sun exposure may lead to precancerous lesions and even skin cancers (squamous and basal cell cancers).

**Melanoma:** It is a malignant tumor of melanocytes which are found predominantly in skin but also in the bowel, and the eye. It is one of the rare types of skin cancer but causes the majority of skin cancer related deaths. It is usually associated with excessive exposure to the sun. Dividing rapidly, malignantly transformed melanocytes penetrate the basement membrane, enter the dermis, and invade the blood and lymphatic vessels to gain wide distribution throughout the body.

**Acne:** At puberty, under the influence of sex hormones, sebaceous gland grows in size and increases their production of sebum. If the normal secretion of sebum is obstructed, then it may result in acne. Severe acne is inflammatory, but acne can also manifest in non-inflammatory forms. Acne lesions are commonly referred to as pimples, blemishes, spots, zits, or acne. Acne is most common during adolescence, affecting more than 85% of teenagers, and frequently continues into adulthood. The cause in adolescence is generally an increase in male sex hormones, which occurs in people of all genders during puberty.

## Summary

1. Skin is having 2 layers—epidermis and dermis. Epidermis is derived from ectoderm and the dermis is derived from mesoderm.

2. Epidermis: It is made up of 5 sublayers:

   • Stratum basale: Single layer of columnar or cuboidal cells (keratinocytes)

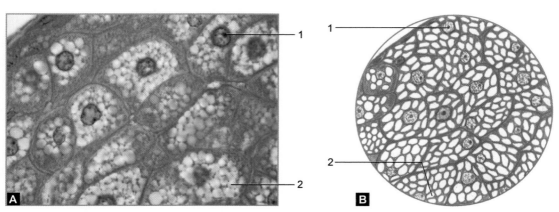

**Fig. 12.12:** Sebaceous gland (A) micrograph, (B) sketch at high magnification having similarity with multilocular adipose tissue. Nucleus (1), lipid droplets (2)

- Stratum spinosum: Many layers of keratinocytes are present. Keratinocytes have many spines.
- Stratum granulosum: 1–3 cells thick and keratinocytes contain basophilic keratohyaline granules.
- Stratum lucidum: 3–5 layers of flattened eosinophilic cells filled with keratin filaments.
- Stratum corneum: 10–30 thin layers of dead keratinocytes.

3. Dermis: It is made up of 2 sublayers.
   - The papillary layer: Loose connective tissue forms dermal papillae.
   - The reticular layer: Dense irregular connective tissue.

| 4. Parameter | Thin skin | Thick skin |
|---|---|---|
| Epidermal layers | Stratum spinosum and corneum are thin. Stratum lucidum is absent | Stratum spinosum and corneum are thick. Stratum lucidum is present |
| Epidermal thickness | ~0.1 mm | 1 mm or more |
| Epidermal ridges | Absent | Present |
| Hairs | Present | Absent |
| Sweat glands | Few | Many |
| Sensory receptors | Less | More |
| Distribution | Whole body except palm and sole | Present only in palm and sole |

5. Sweat glands: 2 types
   - Merocrine: Simple coiled tubular gland and found over the entire body.
   - Apocrine: Simple coiled tubular gland present in axillary, pubic and perianal regions.

6. Sebaceous gland: Pear-shaped simple branched alveolar holocrine gland and secrete sebum.

## Self Assessment

1. Which type of gland is sebaceous gland?
   a. Holocrine
   b. Apocrine
   c. Merocrine
   d. Endocrine

2. Which of the following function is performed by Merkel cells?
   a. Phagocytosis
   b. Detection of shape during touch
   c. Detection of sound
   d. Detection of vibrations

3. The dermis is characterized by:
   a. Vascularity
   b. Avascularity
   c. Lack of collagen fibers
   d. None of the above

4. Which of the following is not an appendage of the skin?
   a. Hair
   b. Nail
   c. Mammary gland
   d. Sebaceous gland

5. Melanocytes are present in which layer of epidermis?
   a. Stratum basale
   b. Stratum lucidum
   c. Stratum spinosum
   d. Stratum corneum

6. Which type of muscle is arrectorum pilorum?
   a. Skeletal
   b. Striated
   c. Smooth
   d. Cardiac

7. Thick skin is characterized by the presence of:
   a. Thin epidermis
   b. Hair follicle
   c. Thick stratum corneum
   d. Sebaceous gland

8. Thin skin is characterized by:
   a. Thin epidermis
   b. Hair follicle
   c. Sebaceous gland
   d. All of the above

9. Apocrine sweat gland is present in:
   a. Axilla
   b. Scalp
   c. Eyebrows
   d. Eyelashes

10. Which corpuscle has a sliced onion appearance?
   a. Pacinian
   b. Ruffini
   c. Meissner's
   d. None of the above

## Answers

1. a,    2. b,    3. a,    4. c,    5. c,    6. c,    7. c,    8. d,    9. a,
10. a

# 13

# Respiratory System

Respiratory system includes the lungs and a system of tubes that link the site of gas exchange with the external environment. The respiratory system also participates in regulation of immune responses to inhaled particles. Generally, it is divided into two main parts: Upper respiratory tract (above the vocal cords) and lower respiratory tract (below the vocal cords). However, customary it is divided into two parts: A conducting part, which consists of the nasal cavity, nasopharynx, larynx, trachea, bronchi, bronchioles and terminal bronchioles; and a respiratory portion, consisting of respiratory bronchioles, alveolar ducts and alveoli.

Patency of conducting part is maintained by bones, cartilage and fibrous tissue. Conducting part provides a passage through which air can travel to and from the lungs; along with this it also clean, moisten and warm the inspired air before it enters into the lungs. The walls of the conducting part are thicker to prevent diffusion of gas into the adjacent lung parenchyma. The air passing through the olfactory mucosa carries the stimuli for detection of odors and the air passing through the larynx is used to produce speech. Respiratory part exchanged oxygen in the inspired air from the carbon dioxide present in the blood.

## CONDUCTING PART

### A. Nasal Cavity

The nasal cavity consists of two structures: The external vestibule and the internal nasal fossa.

a. **Vestibule:** The anterior dilated portion of the nasal cavity is known as the vestibule (the first ~1.5 cm of the conductive portion following the nostrils). It is lined with a keratinized stratified squamous epithelium (epidermis) and contains vibrissae (thick, short hairs), which entrap large particles from the inspired air. The sebaceous glands are also associated with these hairs and their secretions also help in entrapment of large particles. The dermis of the vestibule is anchored by numerous collagen bundles to the perichondrium of the hyaline cartilage, which forms the supporting skeleton of the ala. Posteriorly, where the vestibule ends, epithelium undergoes a transition; from stratified squamous keratinized it becomes pseudostratified columnar ciliated epithelium with goblet cells. The sebaceous glands are absent at this site.

b. **Nasal fossa:** Nasal cavity is divided into two fossae by a median cartilaginous and bony septum. Medial wall of each fossa is smooth, but the lateral wall has an irregular contour due to the presence of three bony shelves like projections; known as superior, middle and inferior conchae (turbinates).

The middle and inferior conchae are covered with respiratory (pseudostratified columnar ciliated) epithelium, while the superior concha is covered with a specialized olfactory epithelium. Within the lamina propria of the conchae are seromucous glands, large venous plexuses and abundant lymphoid components. Venous plexuses are more in number in the lamina propria of inferior concha and known as swell bodies (cavernous bodies). These plexuses are also called erectile bodies, as the tissue containing these plexuses is capable of considerable engorgement, but it differs from the erectile tissue present in the penis due to the absence of smooth muscle containing septa. Space beneath each concha is known as meatus, which receives the opening of nasolacrimal duct and paranasal air sinuses.

Conchae increase the surface area for the inspired air and create turbulent airflow to allow more efficient conditioning of inspired air. Seromucous glands secrete mucus and watery secretion to coat and moisten the epithelium. Cilia beat synchronously to move mucus and trapped particulate matter towards the digestive tract. Vascular plexuses warm, cools and moisten the inspired air. Antibodies produced by plasma cells of lymphoid components protect the nasal mucosa against inhaled antigens as well as against microbial invasion.

c. **Olfactory mucosa:** This is present in the roof of the nasal cavity, either side of the nasal septum and superior nasal concha. This is lined by pseudostratified columnar epithelium, but this is considerably thicker than the respiratory epithelium. Three types of cells are present in this epithelium: Olfactory cells, sustentacular cells and basal cells.

i. *Olfactory cells*: These cells are present in between the supporting and the basal cells. Their apical surface extends as thin, slender (dendrite), which ends at the surface as small, round structures, called the olfactory vesicles. Radiating from each olfactory vesicles are 6 to 8 long, nonmotile olfactory cilia, which lack dynein arms necessary for motility. Nucleus lies near the basal lamina and it is spherical in shape. Axon arises from the basal region of the cell and it is unmyelinated. It penetrates the basement membrane to joins similar axons and form bundles of nerve fibers. The nerve fibers then pass through the cribriform plate in the roof of the nasal cavity to synapse with secondary neurons in the olfactory bulb. Thus the olfactory cells are modified bipolar neurons with a dendrite that reaches up to the surface and an axon that extends down into the lamina propria. The olfactory cells have a short life span of about 1 month and if these cells are injured, these are replaced by new cells produced from the division of basal cells. Besides some neurons of the enteric nervous system, olfactory neurons are the only neurons that can be replaced even during postnatal life.

ii. *Sustentacular cells:* These are tall columnar cells similar to the neuroglial cells, whose apical aspects have a striated border composed of microvilli. Their oval nuclei are present in the apical third of the cell (superficial to the olfactory cell nuclei). The apical cytoplasm of these cells contains secretory granules with a yellowish-brown (lipofuscin) pigment whose color is characteristic of the olfactory mucosa. Adhering junctions are present between the sustentacular and olfactory cells. These cells provide physical support, nourishment and electrical insulation for the olfactory cells.

iii. *Basal cells*: These are short columnar cells present at the base of the epithelium between the sustentacular and olfactory cells. These cells have microvilli on their apical surface. In the cytoplasm, vesicles and well-developed Golgi apparatus are present. The basal surface of these cells makes synaptic contact with nerve fibers that pass through the basement membrane. These nerve fibers are the terminal branches of trigeminal (Vth cranial) nerve that carries general sensation instead of olfactory sensations. These cells may be involved in absorption and secretion. These cells are capable of differentiation into the sustentacular and olfactory cells.

In the lamina propria of the olfactory mucosa serous branched tubuloacinar olfactory glands (Bowman's glands) are also present (Fig. 13.1A, B). These glands also contain lipofuscin granules. These glands produce a thin, watery secretion that is released onto the olfactory epithelial surface via narrow ducts. Odorous substances dissolved in this watery secretion are detected by the olfactory cilia. The secretion also flushes the epithelial surface, preparing the receptors to receive new odorous stimuli. Along with the watery secretion the glands also release IgA, lactoferrin and lysozyme.

d. **Paranasal sinuses:** These sinuses are air-filled closed cavities present in the bones of the walls of the nasal cavity. They are extensions from the respiratory segment of the nasal cavity and are named after their locations in the skull bones, i.e. frontal, maxillary, ethmoid and sphenoid bones. The sinuses open in the lateral wall of the nasal cavity via small openings. The sinuses are lined with a thin respiratory epithelium with a few goblet cells. The thin lamina propria resembles that of the nasal cavity and contains only a few seromucous glands and finally merges with the underlying periosteum. The paranasal sinuses communicate with the nasal cavity through small openings. The mucus produced in these cavities sweeps into the nasal passages as a result of the activity of its ciliated epithelial cells.

## B. Nasopharynx

It is the posterior continuation of the nasal cavities and becomes continuous with the oropharynx at the level of the soft palate. It is lined by pseudostratified columnar ciliated epithelium, but patches of squamous epithelium are present with increasing age, particularly near the lower end and most markedly in smokers. Lamina propria contains mucous and serous glands. Aggregation of lymphatic nodules in the lamina propria of the

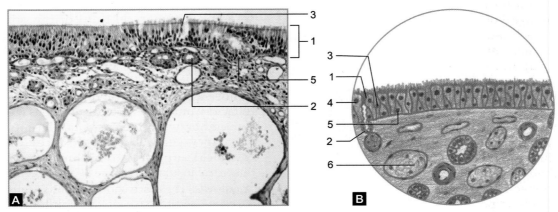

**Fig. 13.1:** Olfactory mucosa, (A) micrograph, (B) sketch, having olfactory cells (3), sustentacular cells (4) and basal cells (5) in the olfactory epithelium (1). Lamina propria contains Bowman's gland (2) and olfactory nerve (6)

posterior aspect of nasopharynx forms the pharyngeal tonsil.

## C. Larynx

It is an irregular tube that connects the pharynx to the trachea and it is 4 cm in length and approximately 4 cm in diameter. Besides form a conducting passage of the inhaled air, the larynx also serves as the organ for the production of sounds. The wall of the larynx consists of a mucosa, a poorly defined submucosa, a series of irregularly shaped cartilages connected by dense fibroelastic tissue and a group of intrinsic and extrinsic skeletal muscles which act upon the cartilages.

The cartilages are hyaline (the unpaired thyroid and cricoid cartilages and the inferior aspect of the paired arytenoids) as well as elastic (the unpaired epiglottis, the paired corniculate and cuneiform cartilages, and the tips of the arytenoids). The thyroid and cricoid cartilages provide support to the larynx, whereas the epiglottis forms a cover over the opening of the larynx. Calcification in the thyroid and cricoid cartilages begins in males during the second decade of life and at a somewhat later period in females. During respiration, the epiglottis is in the vertical position and thus permits the flow of air. While, during swallowing of food or fluid, it is in a horizontal position and closes the laryngeal opening.

Each lateral wall of the larynx has two prominent folds—vestibular fold (false vocal cord) and vocal fold (true vocal cord). A space is present in between the two folds, known as ventricle, which is lined by ciliated pseudostratified columnar epithelium. Vestibular folds are superior in position and covered by typical respiratory (pseudostratified columnar ciliated) epithelium. They are immovable and their lamina propria is formed by loose connective tissue containing seromucous glands, adipocytes and lymphoid components. Vocal folds consist of skeletal muscle (vocalis muscle) and vocal ligament (formed by a band of elastic fibers). Although vocal folds do not come in contact with the swallowed food, yet they are covered by stratified squamous non-keratinized epithelium. Stratified epithelium is more resistant to continuous stress caused by the contact of free margins of the vocal cords with each other during speech. Vocal ligament is located at the edge of the fold and keep the rim of the fold rigid. Vocalis muscle alters the shape of the vocal fold and aids in phonation. Inferior to the vocal folds, the lining epithelium changes to respiratory epithelium, which lines air passages down through the trachea and intrapulmonary bronchi. The cilia of the larynx beat toward the pharynx, transport the mucus and trapped particulate matter toward the mouth to be expectorated or swallowed.

## D. Epiglottis

It is the superior portion of the larynx that project upwards from the anterior wall of the larynx and has both a lingual (anterior) and a laryngeal (posterior) surface. On the anterior surface, where the epiglottis comes into contact with the base of the tongue during swallowing, the epithelium is stratified squamous nonkeratinized. The epithelium covering the apex and approximately upper half part of the posterior surface comes into contact with whatever is being swallowed and is therefore also subjected to wear and tear, so lined by stratified squamous non-keratinized epithelium. However, the epithelium covering the rest of the posterior surface (lower half) constitutes a part of the lining of the respiratory tract and therefore lined by pseudostratified columnar ciliated epithelium with goblet cells (Fig. 13.2A, B). Occasionally, taste buds are also present in the epithelium. A central elastic cartilage forms the framework of the epiglottis. The underlying lamina propria merges with the perichondrium of the elastic cartilage. Lamina propria contains serous, mucous, or mixed (seromucous) glands and solitary lymphatic nodules.

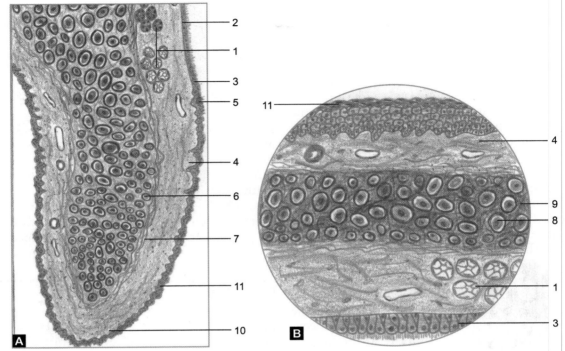

**Fig. 13.2:** LS of epiglottis, (A) low magnification, (B) high magnification. Lingual mucosa (10) is lined by stratified squamous nonkeratinized epithelium (11) covers the anterior surface, apex and half of the posterior surface. Laryngeal mucosa (2) is lined by pseudostratified columnar ciliated epithelium (3). In the lamina propria (4) lies mixed glands (1). The core is formed by elastic cartilage (6). Taste bud (5), perichondrium (7), chondrocytes (8) and elastic fibers (9)

### E. Trachea

It is a rigid hollow tubular structure through which air passes in hence, it is also known as wind pipe. It is 12 cm in length and 2 cm in diameter and begins at the cricoid cartilage of the larynx. It extends down through the lower part of the neck and superior mediastinum of the thorax, where it divides into two primary bronchi, one to each lung. The wall of the trachea is supported by 10–12 horseshoe-shaped cartilage rings (C-rings).

The wall of the trachea contains three layers (Fig. 13.3 A to C):

a. **Mucosa:** It is lined by ciliated pseudo-stratified columnar epithelium containing five types of cells. All of these cells come into contact with the thick basement membrane, but all of them do not reach the lumen.

Just beneath the basement membrane thin lamina propria is present, which is composed of a loose, fibroelastic connective tissue. It contains lymphatic nodules, lymphocytes and neutrophils as well as mixed seromucous glands, whose ducts open to the epithelial surface. The number of these glands decreases in lower parts of the trachea. A dense layer of elastic fibers; the elastic lamina, separates the lamina propria from the underlying submucosa.

The cells in the lining epithelium are:

i. *Ciliated columnar cells*: These tall, slender cells constitute the most abundant type. Each cell has about 300 long, actively

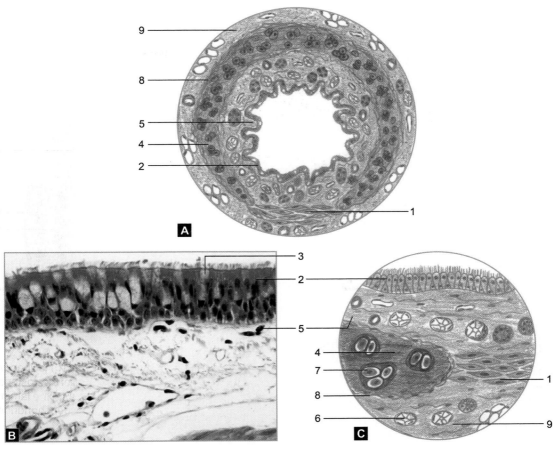

**Fig. 13.3:** Trachea, (A) sketch at low magnification, (B) micrograph and (C) sketch at high magnification, lined by pseudostratified columnar ciliated epithelium (2) with goblet cells (3). Hyaline cartilage (4) is present in "C" shaped and ends of which is joined by trachealis muscle (1). Lamina propria (5), tracheal glands (6), cell nest (7), perichondrium (8) and adventitia (9)

motile cilia on its apical surface. Cilia are anchored in the basal bodies and move inhaled particulate matter trapped in the mucus toward the nasopharynx (upwards), thus protecting the delicate lung tissue from damage (mucociliary escalator). The cells have a large Golgi apparatus, a small amount of rough endoplasmic reticulum, a few lysosomes and residual bodies. Numerous mitochondria are present near the basal bodies and provide ATP required for ciliary beating.

ii. *Goblet cells*: These cells produce mucinogen, which when secreted into an aqueous environment become hydrated and known as mucin. Mucin traps inhaled particles.

iii. *Undifferentiated short (Basal) cells*: These cells are few in number and their apical surfaces do not reach the lumen. These cells have the ability to divide and to differentiate into other cell types.

iv. *Brush cells*: These columnar cells are few in number. These cells contain varying numbers of small mucus granules and many tall microvilli. Microvilli are uniformly arranged, that is why these cells are known as brush cells. Their function is unknown, but the basal surface of the cells is in synaptic contact with an afferent nerve ending. Some investigators suggest that these cells may have a sensory role; while other investigators believe that these cells may represent an inactive stage of the goblet cell.

v. *Diffuse neuroendocrine cells*: These cells are also known as small granule cells, APUD (amine precursor uptake and decarboxylation) cells, Kulchitsky cells, Feyrter cells, P cells or entero-endocrine cells. These cells mainly lie singly in the trachea and are sparsely dispersed among other cell types. These cells contain many small granules concentrated in their basal cytoplasm, which are catecholamine-like materials and control the secretory activity of goblet cells. Some cells are present in groups in association with naked sensory nerve endings, forming pulmonary neuroepithelial bodies, which may have functioned in reflexes regulating the airway or vascular calibre. These cells can be seen with special staining techniques such as silver staining, which reacts with the granules.

b. **Submucosa:** It is composed of dense irregular fibroelastic connective tissue containing numerous seromucous glands. The ducts of these glands pass through the elastic lamina and the lamina propria to open on the epithelial surface. Lymphoid components and some adipocytes are also present in the submucosa.

c. **The adventitia:** It is composed of C-shaped hyaline cartilage rings, which is open posteriorly. The open ends of cartilage are connected by fibroelastic ligament and a band of smooth (trachealis) muscle. The fibroelastic ligament prevents over distention of the lumen and because of the presence of muscle on the posterior surface, the esophagus can dilate easily. The successive rings are separated by interspaces bridged by fibroelastic connective tissue, which provides flexibility to the trachea and as well as allows its elongation during inspiration. The cartilaginous rings mechanically hold the airway open.

Contraction of the trachealis muscle reduces the diameter of the tracheal lumen, resulting in increased velocity of expired air, which assists in the dislodging of foreign material from the larynx by coughing. Tracheal cartilage may become calcified in the elderly. The first tracheal cartilage is broadest and it is connected to the inferior border of cricoid cartilage by cricotracheal ligament. The last cartilage is thickened centrally and its lower border (carina) is a triangular hook-shaped process which curves down and backwards between the bronchi. It forms an incomplete ring on each side and encloses the beginning of a principal bronchus.

## F. Lungs

The lungs are covered by the serous membrane, known as pleura. It consists of two layers: Parietal and visceral, which are continuous in the region of the hilum of the lung. Both membranes are composed of mesothelial cells resting on a dense fibroelastic connective tissue. The connective tissue contains collagen as well as elastic fibers. The elastic fibers of the visceral pleura extend into the parenchyma of the lung and divide the right lung into 3 (upper, middle, and lower) lobes and left lung into 2 (upper and lower) lobes. In between the parietal and the visceral layers pleural cavity is present. This cavity contains a film of liquid (pleural fluid) that acts as a lubricant, so facilitates the smooth sliding of one surface over the other during respiratory movements. The trachea divides into two primary bronchi: Right and left. The right primary bronchus is wider, straighter and significantly shorter than the left primary bronchus. Right bronchus divides before entering the lung into upper and lower lobar (secondary) bronchi, with the right middle lobar bronchus arising from the latter within the lung. Normally, the left bronchus divides into upper and lower lobar (secondary) bronchi within the lung tissue. Then each secondary bronchus divides into tertiary bronchi, which supply bronchopulmonary segments; within each segment, further branching occurs and after some nine to twelve generations of branching, the size of the tube reduced to 1 mm in diameter. Such a duct is now known as bronchiole, then it further divides and form four to seven terminal bronchiole; each of which then divides into two respiratory bronchiole. These respiratory bronchioles then divide and continue into the alveolar ducts (Fig. 13.4 A, B).

a. **Bronchi:** The primary bronchi are similar in structure to the trachea except that primary bronchi are smaller in diameter and their walls are thinner. Each primary bronchus is accompanied by the pulmonary arteries, veins and lymphatic vessels.

The structure of intrapulmonary (present within the lung) bronchi slightly differs from extrapulmonary (outside the lung) bronchi. Intrapulmonary bronchi are rounded in outline and do not show a posterior flattening like trachea and extra-pulmonary bronchi. Instead of C-shaped cartilaginous rings irregular plates of hyaline cartilage are present. In the mucosa of extrapulmonary bronchi muscle layer is absent; but in intrapulmonary bronchi bundles of smooth muscle form a complete circumferential layer (Fig. 13.5). This layer of smooth muscle is controlled by the sympathetic and parasympathetic nervous systems. Sympathetic fibers cause relaxation; while, parasympathetic fibers cause con-traction of this smooth muscle layer

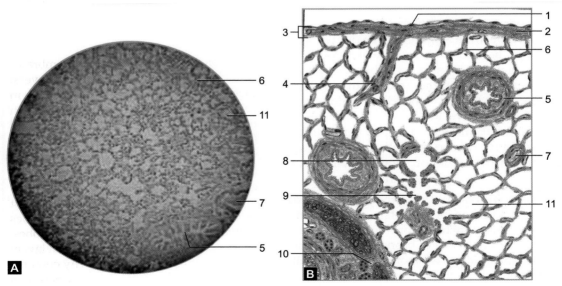

**Fig. 13.4:** Lung (A) micrograph, (B) sketch. Mesothelium (1), connective tissue (2), visceral pleura (3), connective tissue septa (4), terminal bronchiole (5), interalveolar septum (6), pulmonary artery (7), respiratory bronchiole (8), alveolar duct (9), intrapulmonary bronchus (10) and alveolar sac (11)

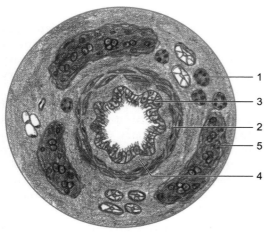

**Fig. 13.5:** Intrapulmonary bronchus, with plates of hyaline cartilage (5) and lined by pseudostratified columnar ciliated epithelium (3). Bronchial glands (1), smooth muscle layer (2) and lamina propria (4)

(reduced diameter of the lumen of the bronchi), thus the smooth muscle control the diameter of the lumen. In histological section, bronchial mucosa appears folded because of contraction of this muscle layer after death.

With successive divisions of the bronchi, they become smaller in diameter and even the amount of cartilage decreases. But the smooth muscle layer becomes more conspicuous as the amount of cartilage decreases. Height of the cells even decreases; with successive divisions it becomes simple columnar ciliated from pseudostratified columnar ciliated epithelium. At the sites of the divisions of bronchi lymphatic nodules are particularly numerous.

b. **Bronchioles:** With further divisions of bronchi when its diameter reaches 1 mm, it is now known as bronchioles. The lining epithelium in larger bronchioles is simple columnar ciliated with some goblet cells; with further divisions into smaller bronchioles, the goblet cells disappear and the cells now become low columnar or cuboidal (many with cilia). In between the ciliated cells,

there are a few nonciliated cells, called Clara cells. Clara cells are columnar cells having short microvilli and apical secretory granules. These cells secrete a glycoprotein surfactant-like material which protects the bronchiolar lining from inhaled particles. These cells secrete a surface-active agent, a lipoprotein that covers the bronchial epithelium and break down the luminal stickiness of mucus produced in the larger bronchioles for more efficient respiration. The lipoprotein, also reduces the surface tension to reduce the tendency of the alveoli of collapse. In addition, Clara cells also secrete a Clara cell secretory protein (CC16). Clara cells also act as progenitor cells in the regeneration of damaged bronchiolar epithelium. In larger bronchioles ciliated cells are more in number as compared to the Clara cells. However, as bronchioles become smaller, the relative proportion of the Clara cells increase.

Seromucous glands and lymph nodes are absent in the lamina propria. The lamina propria is formed by fibroelastic connective tissue surrounded by a loose meshwork of smooth muscle fibers. Elastic fibers radiate from this tissue and connect it to the elastic fibers ramifying from other branches of the bronchial tree. Although the walls of bronchioles and their branches have no cartilage, yet they show no tendency to collapse during inhalation. Because when the lung expands in volume, the elastic fibers, apply tension on the bronchiolar walls; by pulling it uniformly in all directions and thus help to maintain the patency of the bronchioles.

When the bronchioles have a diameter of less than 0.5 mm, they are known as terminal bronchioles. In the lining epithelium, Clara cells are more in number than the cuboidal (with few cilia) cells. The narrow lamina propria consists of fibroelastic connective tissue and is surrounded by one or two layers of smooth muscle fibers (Fig. 13.6 A, B).

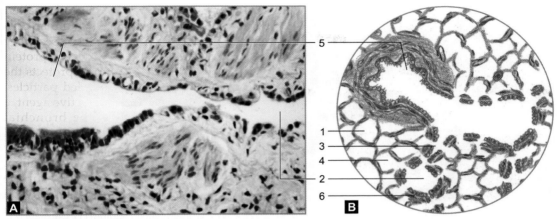

**Fig.13.6 A, B:** Terminal and respiratory bronchiole, (A) micrograph, (B) sketch. Respiratory bronchiole (2) is supported by a thin collagen layer (6) with some smooth muscle and elastic fibers. Alveoli (1), alveolar duct (3), alveolar sac (4) and terminal bronchiole (5)

## RESPIRATORY PART

### A. Respiratory Bronchiole

The respiratory passage begins from respiratory bronchioles. They are lined by cuboidal epithelium with Clara cells. Goblet cells are absent. The epithelium is supported by a thin collagenous layer in which smooth muscle and some elastic fibers are found. Each respiratory bronchiole ends by dividing into 2 or 3 alveolar ducts. Wall of these bronchioles is interrupted by thin-walled outpocketings, known as alveoli. These alveoli increase in number and come to lie close together with branching of the respiratory bronchiole (Fig. 13.6 A, B).

### B. Alveolar Ducts

These are cone-shaped thin wall tubes lined by simple squamous epithelium. This epithelium is supported by a small amount of fibroelastic tissue. These ducts open in the atrium, which give rise to the alveolar sacs. Sacs are composed of two or more small clusters of alveoli.

Smooth muscles present in the respiratory bronchioles and alveolar ducts regulate movements of air. Alveolar ducts, the atria and alveoli are supplied by a rich capillary network.

### C. Alveoli

Each alveolus is a small outpocketing (200 µm in diameter) and forms the primary structural and functional unit of the respiratory system, as their thin walls permit the gaseous exchange. They form the parenchyma of the lung and also give a spongy texture to the lung. An adult respiratory system contains approximately 300 million alveoli, so because of the large numbers their walls are frequently pressed against each other. A very thin connective tissue septa are present in between the alveoli; the interalveolar septa. The one side of alveoli opens into the alveolar sac and these openings are circumscribed by reticular and elastic fibers.

The interalveolar septum is rich in elastic fibers and type III collagen (reticular) fibers and also has an extensive capillary bed composed of continuous capillaries. Capillaries are thick in relation to the rest of the wall, so bulge in the alveoli and thus the greater portion of their surface is presented to the alveolar air (Fig. 13.7A, B). The interalveolar septum contains alveolar pores (pores of Kohn) between neighboring alveoli that function to equalize air pressure in adjoining alveoli and promote the collateral circulation

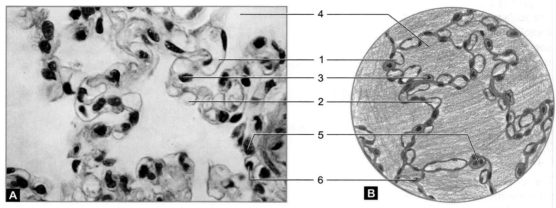

**Fig. 13.7:** Alveoli, (A) micrograph, (B) sketch. In between two alveoli (4) lie interalveolar septum (1). Capillary (2), type II pneumocyte (3), alveolar macrophage (5) and type I pneumocyte (6)

of air when a bronchiole is obstructed. Human being has up to seven pores per alveolus, ranging in size from 2 to 13 μm.

The walls of the alveoli are composed of two types of cells: Type I pneumocytes and type II pneumocytes.

a. **Type I pneumocytes (type I alveolar cells):** These are thin squamous cells and occupy 95% of the alveolar surface. Their main role is to provide a barrier of minimum thickness, which is easily permeable to gases. The cells are not able to divide and their cytoplasm contains abundant pinocytotic vesicles, which may play a role in the turnover of surfactant and the removal of small particulate matter from the outer surface. In addition to the desmosomes, all type I cells have occluding junctions that prevent the leakage of tissue fluid into the alveolar air space.

b. **Type II pneumocytes (type II alveolar cells, great alveolar cells or septal cells):** These cuboidal cells occupy only about 5% of the alveolar surface, but these cells are more numerous than type I pneumocytes and form occluding junctions with type I pneumocytes. These cells are usually found in groups of two or three along the alveolar surface at points at which the

alveolar walls unite and form angles. Their apical surface has short microvilli and a centrally placed nucleus. The cells have an abundance of rER, a well-developed Golgi apparatus and mitochondria. In histological sections, the cells exhibit a characteristic vesicular or foamy cytoplasm because of the presence of lamellar bodies, which are rich in a mixture of lipids, proteins and phospholipids; which is secreted by exocytosis to form a surface covering over alveolus and known as pulmonary surfactant. Type II pneumocytes are able to divide and can regenerate both types of pneumocytes.

**Pulmonary Surfactant** It is synthesized on the rER of type II pneumocytes and is composed of two phospholipids: Dipalmitoyl phosphatidylcholine and phosphatidylglycerol; neutral lipid; and four proteins (surfactant apoproteins) SP-A, SP-B, SP-C and SP-D. The surfactant is modified in the Golgi apparatus and then released into secretory vesicles, known as composite bodies (precursors of lamellar bodies). The surfactant is released by exocytosis into the lumen of the alveolus.

Surface tension at the alveolar surface is very high, because the alveoli are minute. This opposes expansion during inspiration and tends to collapse the alveoli in expiration. The detergent-like properties of pulmonary surfactant greatly reduces the surface tension and makes ventilation of the alveoli much more efficient. The surfactant also has some bactericidal properties. The surfactant layer is not static but is constantly being turned over. The lipoproteins are gradually removed from the surface by the pinocytotic vesicles of the squamous epithelial cells, by macrophages and by type II alveolar cells.

## D. Alveolar Macrophages (Alveolar Phagocytes)

These cells are also known as dust cells, as they remove the inhaled dust, bacteria and other particulate matter that is small enough to reach the alveoli. These cells are found in the connective tissue of the interalveolar septum and lumen of the alveolus. These are the monocytes derived from bone marrow and belong to the mononuclear phagocytic system. After becoming filled with debris these cells migrate to the bronchioles. From there, these cells are transported via ciliary action to the pharynx, where these are swallowed or expectorated. These cells may also exit by migrating into the pulmonary interstitium and leaving via lymphatic vessels. Their cytoplasm appears granular because they contain phagocytosed particles. In smokers, the particles have a characteristic appearance and are called tar bodies.

## E. The Blood–Air Barrier

This barrier is formed by the structures through which gaseous exchange occurs between air in the alveoli and blood in the capillary. Oxygen passes from the alveolus into the capillary and carbon dioxide passes from the capillary blood into the alveolus. The thin regions of the barrier are 0.2 µm or less in thickness and consist of the following layers:

a. A thin layer of surfactant and type I pneumocytes
b. Fused basal lamina of type I pneumocytes and capillary endothelial cells
c. Endothelial cells of the continuous capillary

Thick regions of the barrier measure about 0.5 µm in thickness and have an interstitial area in between the two basal lamina (basal lamina of type I pneumocytes and basal lamina of endothelial cells of the capillary), which are not fused. Most of the gaseous exchange may occur through the thin regions of the blood–air barrier.

For comparison between various parts of respiratory system, *see* Table 24 given in Appendix I.

## F. Pulmonary Blood Supply

The lung has both pulmonary and bronchial circulations.

a. **Pulmonary circulation:** The pulmonary arteries leave the right ventricle and carry deoxygenated blood to the lungs. Branches of these vessels accompany the bronchial tree and are surrounded by adventitia of the bronchi and bronchioles. At the level of the alveolar duct, the branches of this artery form a capillary bed composed strictly of continuous capillaries in the interalveolar septum. The blood in the capillary bed becomes oxygenated and then collected by pulmonary venous capillaries that drain into veins of increasing diameter. These tributaries of the pulmonary vein carry oxygenated blood and travel in the interlobular septum of the lung. Thus, the veins follow a path that is different from that of the arteries, until they reach the apex of the lobule, where they accompany the bronchial tree to the hilum of the lung to deliver oxygenated blood to the left atrium of the heart.

b. **Bronchial circulation:** Bronchial arteries are branches of the thoracic aorta; provide nutrients to the bronchial tree, interlobular septa and pleura of the lungs. They follow the branching pattern of the bronchial tree and form anastomoses with the pulmonary vessels near capillary beds. Bronchial veins drain only the connective tissue of the hilum of the lungs. The rest of the blood reaching the lungs through bronchial arteries leaves the lungs via the pulmonary veins.

## G. Pulmonary Lymphatic Vessels

The lung has dual-lymphatic drainage; a superficial system of vessels drains the surface of the lung and lies in the visceral pleura. A deep network of vessels follows the bronchi and the pulmonary vessels and also found in the interlobular septum. Lymphatic vessels are not found in the terminal portions of the bronchial tree or beyond the alveolar ducts. Both the systems have numerous inter-connections and finally drain into the hilar (bronchopulmonary) lymph nodes at the root of each lung. Efferent lymphatic vessels from these lymph nodes deliver their lymph to the thoracic duct or the right lymphatic duct.

## H. Pulmonary Nerve Supply

Both parasympathetic and sympathetic efferent fibers innervate the lungs. Most of the nerves are found in the connective tissues surrounding the larger airways. Parasympathetic stimulation causes contraction of bronchial smooth muscle causing bronchoconstriction; while sympathetic stimulation causes relaxation of bronchial smooth muscle and thus bron-chodilation.

**Bronchial asthma:** It is a disease caused by increased responsiveness of the tracheobronchial tree to various stimuli. A patient suffering from asthma has a tendency to bronchospasm, which leads to obstruction of airways, and air trapping. The bronchospasm (airway obstruction) may be due to smooth muscle spasm in the wall of smaller bronchi and bronchioles, increased mucus secretion, and swelling of mucosa.

**Hyaline membrane disease (HMD) or respiratory distress syndrome (RDS):** It is one of the most common problems of premature babies. The course of illness with hyaline membrane disease depends on the size and gestational age of the baby. HMD occurs when there is not enough surfactant in the lungs. Thus, tiny alveoli collapse with each breath. The respiratory bronchioles and alveolar ducts are dilated and contain edema fluid. A fibrin-rich eosinophilic material called hyaline membrane lines the alveolar ducts. Synthesis of surfactant can be induced by administration of glucocorticoids.

**Heart failure cells:** These cells are haemosiderin containing macrophages present in the alveoli. The main causes are left heart failure and chronic pulmonary edema. In left heart failure, the left ventricle cannot keep pace with the incoming blood from the pulmonary veins. The resulting backup causes increased pressure on the alveolar capillaries, and red blood cells leak out. Alveolar macrophages ingest the red blood cells, and become engorged with brownish haemosiderin. In pulmonary edema, alveolar septa get thick and fibrous, again increasing pressure on alveolar capillaries and resulting in leakage of red blood cells which undergo phagocytosis by alveolar macrophages.

## Summary

| Parameter | Vestibule | Nasal fossa | Olfactory mucosa | Paranasal sinuses | Nasopharynx | Larynx | Trachea and primary bronchi | Intrapulmonary bronchus | Terminal bronchiole | Respiratory bronchiole | Alveoli |
|---|---|---|---|---|---|---|---|---|---|---|---|
| Epithelium | Stratified squamous keratinized | Pseudostratified columnar ciliated | Pseudostratified columnar ciliated | Pseudostratified columnar ciliated (thinner) | Pseudostratified columnar ciliated | Pseudostratified columnar ciliated and stratified squamous non-keratinized | Pseudostratified columnar ciliated | Pseudostratified columnar ciliated | Simple cuboidal (with a few cilia), and more number of Clara cells | Simple cuboidal and Clara cells | Simple squamous |
| Goblet cells | Absent | Present | Absent | Present | Present | Present | Present | Present | Absent | Absent | Absent |
| Ciliated cells | Absent | Present | Absent | Present | Present | Present | Present | Present | Present | Absent | Absent |
| Glands | Sebaceous and sweat glands | Seromucous glands | Bowman's glands | Seromucous glands | Mucous and serous glands | Mucous and seromucous glands | Mucous and seromucous glands | Mucous and seromucous glands | Absent | Absent | Absent |
| Skeleton | Hyaline cartilage | Bone | Bone | Bone | Muscle | Hyaline and elastic cartilage | Hyaline cartilage (C-shaped) | Hyaline cartilage (irregular plates) | Absent | Absent | Absent |

## Self Assessment

1. In the larynx, stratified squamous epithelium is seen over:
   a. Vestibular folds
   b. Vocal folds
   c. Lower half of posterior surface of epiglottis
   d. Ventricle

2. Which of the following is the smallest active functional unit (including conduction and air exchange) of the lung?
   a. An alveolus
   b. A respiratory bronchiolar unit
   c. A bronchopulmonary segment
   d. Segmental bronchi

3. Which of the following lung cells is known as congestive heart failure cells?
   a. Type I pneumocytes
   b. Type II pneumocytes
   c. Macrophages
   d. Erythrocytes

4. Which of the following is a part of the blood–air barrier in the lungs?
   a. Fused basal lamina of epithelial and endothelial cells
   b. Alveolar pores of Kohn
   c. Alveolar macrophages
   d. Type II pneumocytes

5. Ciliated epithelial cells are not present in:
   a. Olfactory mucosa
   b. Trachea
   c. Bronchiole
   d. Alveoli

6. Alveoli are mainly lined by which epithelium?
   a. Simple columnar
   b. Simple cuboidal
   c. Simple squamous
   d. Pseudostratified

7. Bowman's glands are present in:
   a. Olfactory mucosa
   b. Bronchiole
   c. Trachea
   d. Esophagus

8. Cartilage present in the bronchial tree is:
   a. Hyaline          b. Elastic
   c. Fibrocartilage   d. None of the above

9. Surfactant is produced by which cells?
   a. Type I pneumocytes
   b. Type II pneumocytes
   c. Alveolar macrophages
   d. Heart failure cells

10. Bronchiole is characterized by:
    a. Presence of cartilage
    b. Presence of glands
    c. Absence of Clara cells
    d. Absence of cartilage

## Answers

1. b,    2. b,    3. c,    4. a,    5. d,    6. c,    7. a,    8. a,    9. b,
10. d

# 14

# Digestive System

The digestive system consists of a long, muscular tubular structure, which extends from the mouth to the anus. Glands, such as salivary glands, liver and the pancreas, are also part of this system. Although these glands are located outside the tube, but they pass their secretion into the tube by the duct system. The main function of the digestive system is to break down the food mechanically and chemically (digestion) for absorption of the nutrients and the waste is thrown out through the anus. The digestive system also separates the ingested food and water from intake of air.

## ORAL TISSUES

The oral tissues include the lips, palate, teeth and associated structures, as well as the tongue and the major salivary glands. Mostly, these structures are covered by stratified squamous epithelium whose ridges interdigitate with subjacent connective tissue ridges. The epithelial and connective tissue ridges are collectively known as the rete apparatus.

## A. Lip

The core of the lip is composed of skeletal muscle (orbicularis oris) embedded in the fibroelastic connective tissue. Its external surface is covered by thin skin and internally its surface is covered by mucous membrane.

The mucous membrane is lined by a thick stratified squamous nonkeratinized epithelium, with mucous glands in its lamina propria. The submucosa contains many small mucous and mucoserous salivary (labial) glands, the secretion of which passes to the surface via short ducts and provides lubrication. Fibers of orbicularis oris muscle are arranged in such a way that they represent the formation of folds and thus reduce the chances of biting of mucous membrane during mastication (Fig. 14.1).

The external and internal surfaces meet at the free border of the lip, known as red margin or vermilion border, which is covered by modified skin having keratohylin granules. It is very translucent because of the presence of thick stratum lucidum. Dermis is having high papillae with a rich vascular plexus, so the margin appears red. There is no hair, sweat or sebaceous glands in this margin.

## B. Palate

It is divided into an anterior hard palate (with a shelf like bony core) and a posterior soft palate (with a skeletal muscle core). The palate separates the nasal cavity from the oral cavity, so it has a nasal surface and an oral surface. On the nasal surface hard as well as the soft palate is lined by pseudostratified ciliated columnar epithelium (respiratory epithelium).

The oral surface of the hard palate is lined by stratified squamous parakeratinized to

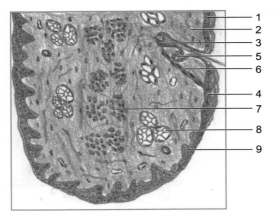

**Fig. 14.1:** Lip (LS) at low magnification showing thin skin (4) covering the external surface. Dermis (2) with hair follicle (3), sebaceous gland (5) and arrectorum pilli muscle (6) is present beneath the epidermis (1). The core of lip containing orbicularis oris muscle (7) can be seen in the figure. Internal surface is covered by stratified squamous non-keratinized epithelium (9). Mucus secreting labial glands (8) are present in the connective tissue

stratified squamous keratinized epithelium. Submucosa is present in the hard palate except in the area adjacent to the gums and in the midline. In anterior one-third submucosa contains adipose tissue, while in posterior two-thirds it contains mucous salivary glands. Parakeratinized epithelium is similar to keratinized epithelium except its superficial cells contain highly condensed (pyknotic) nuclei, which remain until the cell is exfoliated. The oral surface of the soft palate is lined by stratified squamous nonkeratinized epithelium. Mucous salivary glands are present in its submucosa.

## C. Tongue

It is a muscular organ covered by the stratified squamous epithelium. It has a root, an apex, a curved dorsal surface and a ventral surface. By the root tongue is attached to the hyoid bone and mandible. The apex is the anterior most part, touching the incisor teeth.

The dorsal surface of the tongue is divided into anterior two-thirds (oral surface) and posterior one-third (pharyngeal surface) by a V-shaped sulcus, known as sulcus terminalis (Fig. 14.2).

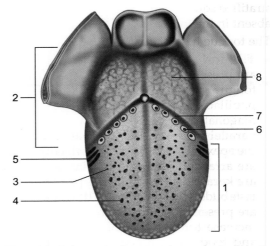

**Fig. 14.2:** Schematic diagram of tongue showing its dorsal surface. Anterior two-thirds (1), posterior one-third (2), filiform papillae (3), fungiform papillae (4), foliate papillae (5), circumvallate papillae 6), sulcus terminalis (7) and lingual tonsils (8)

The surface of the posterior one-third is irregular because of the presence of lymphatic nodules (lingual tonsil). The anterior two-thirds surface is covered by a number of small eminences formed by epithelium and a core of connective tissue (lamina propria) known as papillae. The papillae are useful in the manipulation of food as well as in the sense of taste. 5–20 tall secondary papillae projects from the papillae. The core of the tongue consists of bundles of skeletal muscle fibers arranged in vertical, transverse and longitudinal planes. This arrangement of muscle fibers allows enormous flexibility and precision in the movements of the tongue, which are essential to human speech as well as its role in digestion and swallowing. Lamina propria is formed by dense fibrous connective tissue with numerous elastic fibers.

It firmly binds the epithelium to the skeletal muscle core and also separates the bundles of skeletal muscle fibers.

The ventral surface of the tongue is smooth and thin in comparison to the dorsal surface. This surface is lined by nonkeratinized stratified squamous epithelium. Submucosa is absent in the tongue (Fig. 14.3 A, B).

The tongue has four types of papillae.

a. **Filiform papillae:** These conical papillae are present over the entire surface of the tongue, so these are the most numerous papillae. These papillae are arranged in diagonal rows that extend anterolaterally, parallel with sulcus terminalis, except at the apex of the tongue, where these papillae are arranged transversely. These papillae are keratinized on their tips and have no taste buds (Fig. 14.4 A, B). Secondary papillae are present on all surfaces. These papillae increase the friction between the tongue and food and facilitate the movement of particles by the tongue within the oral cavity.

b. **Fungiform papillae:** These papillae are relatively a few in number and are dispersed among the filiform papillae. These are more numerous near the tip of the tongue. These papillae resemble a mushroom of the common edible variety. These are covered by stratified squamous nonkeratinized epithelium, with 1–5 taste buds associated with them on their free surface (Fig. 14.4 A, B). Secondary papillae are present on all surfaces. The connective tissue core of these papillae is richly vascularized, giving it a red appearance. Serous glands are present in association with these papillae.

c. **Foliate papillae:** These papillae are covered with nonkeratinized stratified squamous epithelium. These are leaf-shaped and present at the posterolateral margin. These have numerous taste buds on their side. Secondary papillae are present on all surfaces. Infants may have 4–8 well-developed papillae, but in adults these papillae are rudimentary. In lagomorphs (rabbits) these papillae are the main site of aggregation of

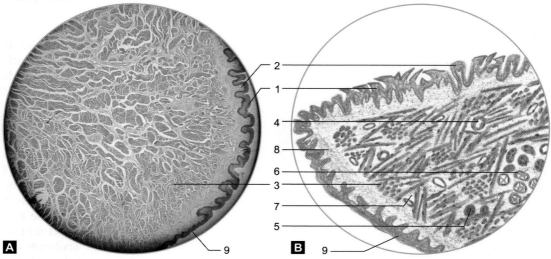

**Fig. 14.3:** LS of the anterior part of the tongue, (A) micrograph, (B) sketch showing filiform (1) and fungiform (2) papillae. The core of the tongue consists of skeletal muscle fibers (3) running in various directions. Ventral surface of tongue is smooth and lined by nonkeratinized stratified squamous epithelium (9). Serous acini (5), mucous acini (6), intralobular duct (4), connective tissue (7) and lamina propria (8) are also seen in the figure

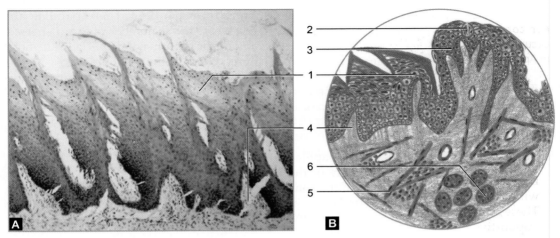

**Fig. 14.4:** Tongue: Filiform and fungiform papillae, (A) micrograph and (B) sketch. The figure shows the dorsal surface of the tongue having filiform papillae (1) with keratinized tips and fungiform (3) papillae with taste buds (2) on the free surface. Lamina propria (4), skeletal muscle fibers (5) and serous acini (6) are also seen

taste buds. Serous glands are present in association with these papillae.

d. **Circumvallate papillae:** These papillae are dome shaped, largest in size and arranged in a row just anterior to the sulcus terminalis. These papillae are 8–12 in number and contain numerous taste buds arranged around the sides of the papilla. These papillae do not

project above the surface. These papillae are surrounded by a deep circular sulcus or trench or moat (Fig. 14.5 A, B). Trench is flushed for reception of new tastes by the secretion of serous glands (von Ebner), which is present beneath the papillae and their duct open at the bottom of the trench. Secondary papillae are present only on its top surface.

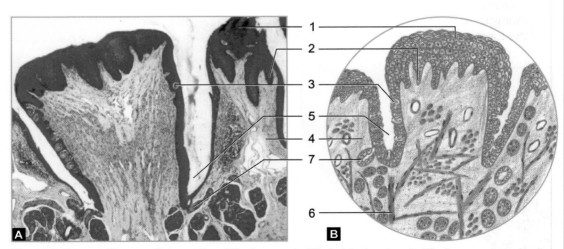

**Fig. 14.5:** Tongue: Circumvallate papillae, (A) micrograph, (B) sketch showing stratified squamous epithelium (1) covering papillae. Underlying lamina propria (4) exhibits numerous secondary papillae (2) and contain von Ebner's gland (7). Taste buds (3) are present on the lateral surface of papillae. A deep trench (5) surrounds the base of each papilla. The core of the tongue consists of skeletal muscle fibers (6) running in various directions

For comparison among filiform, fungiform, circumvallate and foliate papilla, *see* Table 25 given in Appendix I.

e. **Taste buds:** These buds are mainly present in relation to the papillae and also present occasionally in the oral cavity such as the soft palate and the epiglottis. These are barrel-shaped bodies, which are embedded in the whole thickness of the epithelium. Each bud has a small cavity that communicates with the exterior through the taste pores. These are composed of three types of cells: Supportive or sustentacular cells, taste or gustatory cells and basal cells (Fig. 14.6 A, B). Sustentacular cells are less numerous and lie at the periphery. In between the sustentacular cells lie neuroepithelial taste cells. Both types of cells are elongated and have long apical microvilli (taste hairs), which projects in the taste pore. The endings of afferent nerves end in relation to taste cells.

Basal cells lie at the periphery near the basal lamina and are stem cells for the other two cell types. The four basic taste sensations are: Sweet, salty, bitter and sour. Each can be perceived maximum at some region of the tongue. In general, taste buds at the tip of the tongue detect sweet stimuli, those at the margin detect salty stimuli and those over the dorsum detect sour stimuli. Taste buds on the circumvallate papillae detect bitter stimuli. But there is no difference in the structure of these taste buds according to taste sensations.

## D. Teeth and Associated Structures

In adult humans, the 32 permanent teeth are arranged in two bilaterally symmetric arches in the maxillary and mandibular bones. There are 8 teeth in each quadrant: 2 incisors, 1 canine, 2 premolars and 3 molars. In humans two sets of teeth develop and the first set (the baby, milk, primary or deciduous set) has 20 teeth. All primary teeth are replaced with permanent counterparts, except for molars, which are replaced by permanent premolars. In each tooth a visible crown projects above the gum or gingiva with roots buried in the alveolus of maxilla or mandible. Incisors, canines and premolars have one root each, except for the first premolar of the maxilla, which has two roots. Molars have three and rarely, four roots. The crown is covered by enamel, while the roots are covered by cementum. These two coverings meet at the neck (cervix) of the tooth. Each tooth contains a calcified material (dentin), which surrounds

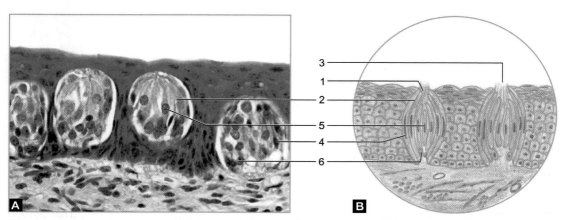

**Fig. 14.6:** Tongue: Taste buds at higher magnification, (A) micrograph, (B) sketch. Three types of cells are present in taste buds (2), supportive (4), taste (5) and basal (6) cells. Buds open on the surface by a taste pore (3). Supportive and taste cells have long apical microvilli (1)

a connective tissue-filled pulp cavity. This cavity extends up to the root canal (apex of the root), where an apical foramen permits the entrance and exit of blood vessels, lymphatics and nerves of the pulp cavity. The periodontal ligament holds the tooth in its socket or alveolus (Fig. 14.7).

a. **Dentin:** It is the second hardest tissue in the body and forms the bulk of a tooth. It provides main strength to enamel and it is the first mineralized component of the tooth to be deposited. It is composed of a calcified organic matrix similar to that of bone. The inorganic component constitutes a somewhat larger proportion of the matrix of dentin than that of bone and exists mainly in the form of hydroxyapatite crystals. It is produced by odontoblast cells, which are tall columnar cells and lies at the periphery of the pulp, i.e. on the inner aspect of dentin. Long, thin processes of odontoblast cells known as dentinal tubules occupy the tunnel like spaces within the dentin. As odontoblasts remain functional, so the formation of dentin continues through adult life. Thus dentin has the capacity for self-repair.

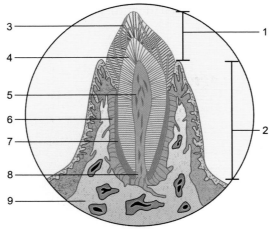

**Fig. 14.7:** LS of tooth showing crown (1), root (2), enamel (3), dentin (4), pulp cavity (5), periodontal ligament (6), cementum (7), apical foramen (8) and alveolar bone (9)

b. **Enamel:** It is a translucent substance and its color is due to the color of underlying dentin. It is the hardest and most dense tissue of the body. It forms a protective covering of the teeth, rendering them suitable for mastication. It contains 96% inorganic material (hydroxyapatite) and only a small amount (4%) of organic substance and water. Structurally, it is composed of enamel rods or prisms and interprismatic substance.

Enamel rods are elongated columns, which extends over the entire thickness of enamel from the dentinoenamel junction to the surface of enamel. Enamel is produced during tooth development before eruption, by ameloblast cells. These cells die before the tooth erupts into the oral cavity, so enamel persists throughout life as acellular tissue and body cannot repair it.

c. **Dental pulp:** It is a jelly-like ground substance. It consists of connective tissue resembling embryonic mesenchyme and intercellular material composed of fine collagen fibers. Usually, a single arteriole and two venules enter the pulp cavity through the root canal and form a capillary plexus beneath and within the layer of odontoblasts.

d. **Associated structures:** The structures responsible for maintaining the teeth in the bone are:

i. *Cementum:* It is a thin layer of bone-like material, but the haversian system is absent. It contains coarse bundles of type I collagen fibers in a calcified matrix. It is thicker in the apical region of the root, where osteocytes like cells (cementocytes) are present. Like osteocytes, cementocytes are also enclosed in lacunae that communicate through the canaliculi that extend toward the vascular periodontal ligament. Cementum is continuously elaborated after tooth eruption, compensating for the decrease in tooth length, resulting from abrasion of the enamel.

ii. *Periodontal ligament:* It is a special type of dense irregular collagenous (type I collagen) connective tissue. The ends of these collagen fibers are embedded in the alveolus and cementum as Sharpey's fibers, which permit the periodontal ligament to suspend the tooth in its socket.

iii. *Gingiva:* It is the mucosal tissue firmly bound to the periosteum of the maxillary and mandibular bones. It is composed of stratified squamous nonkeratinized epithelium, bound to the tooth enamel by means of a cuticle that resembles a thick basal lamina. As the gingiva is exposed to strong frictional forces, its stratified squamous epithelium is either fully keratinized (orthokeratinized) or partially keratinized (parakeratinized).

e. **Development of tooth:** Tooth bud is an aggregation of cells that eventually forms a tooth. These cells are derived from the ectoderm of first branchial arch and the ectomesenchyme of the neural crest. At about 6 weeks of gestation, this ectoderm proliferates and forms a horseshoe-shaped band known as the dental lamina. A little later, at 10 regions of lamina, ectodermal cells multiply more rapidly and form a little knobs in the underlying mesenchyme **(Bud stage)** (Fig. 14.8).

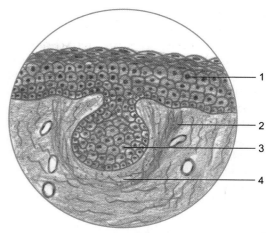

**Fig. 14.8:** Developing tooth: Bud stage. Tooth bud (3) is derived from oral ectoderm (1). Underlying condensed mesenchyme (4) starts forming dental sac (2)

Each knob represents the beginning of enamel organ of tooth bud. Enamel organ consists of outer low columnar cells and central polygonal cells. As the cells proliferate, each enamel organ increases in size and as it develops takes the shape of the cap **(Cap stage)** (Fig.14.9A, B). Cells at the convexity of the cap are cuboidal (outer enamel epithelium) and at the concavity are tall columnar (inner enamel

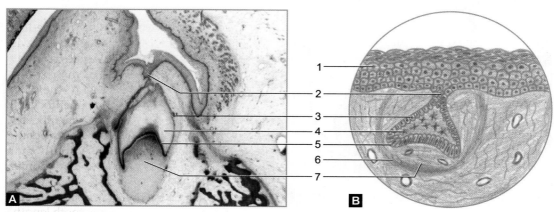

**Fig.14.9:** Developing tooth: Cap stage (A) micrograph, (B) sketch. Cuboidal cells of tooth bud at convexity form outer enamel epithelium (3) and tall columnar cells in concavity form inner enamel epithelium (5), stellate reticulum (4) is the network form of star-shaped cells. Oral ectoderm (1), dental lamina (2), dental sac (6) and the dental papilla (7) are also well marked

epithelium). At the site of the depression of the cap, the ectomesenchymal cells proliferate and condense to form the dental papilla. Ectomesenchymal cells form the dental sac or dental follicle, which surround the enamel organ and the dental papilla.

Central polygonal cells begin to separate due to the water being drawn from surrounding dental papilla, so the cells become star-shaped. These cells form a network, called stellate reticulum. Peripheral cells of the dental papilla adjacent to the inner enamel epithelium enlarge and later differentiate into odontoblasts. Depression occupy by the dental papilla become deeper until the enamel organ takes shape like a bell **(Bell stage)** (Fig. 14.10 A, B).

In the bell stage crown shape is determined. The junction between outer and inner enamel epithelium is called cervical loop. The inner enamel epithelial cells differentiate into ameloblasts. Stratum intermedium is formed by a few layers of squamous cells, which lie in between the inner enamel epithelium and the stellate reticulum. Stellate reticulum expands further and before the beginning of enamel formation it collapses, so that the distance between centrally situated ameloblasts

is reduced. Smooth surface of outer enamel epithelium is laid in folds containing capillary loops. Odontoblasts secrete predentin, which get mineralized and form dentin. After the first layer of dentin formation ameloblasts form the enamel. The dental follicle gives rise to three important entities: Cementoblasts, osteoblasts and fibroblasts. Cementoblasts form the cementum of a tooth. Osteoblasts give rise to the alveolar bone around the roots of teeth. Fibroblasts develop into periodontal ligaments. Mesenchymal cells within the dental papilla are responsible for formation of dental pulp.

## GASTROINTESTINAL TRACT (GIT)

GIT or alimentary canal extends from the esophagus to the anal canal. In this, esophagus and anal canal are only for the transport, while stomach to the rectum is the proper digestive tract.

### A. General Organization

The entire GIT presents some common structural characteristics. It is a hollow tube made up of a lumen of variable diameter, surrounded by a wall made up mainly of 4 layers or tunics: The mucosa, submucosa, muscularis externa

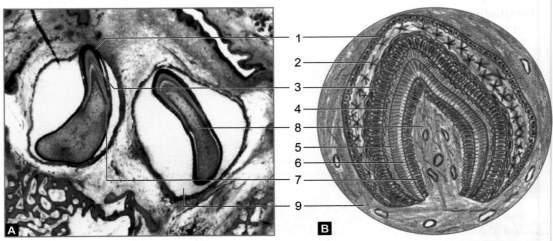

**Fig.14.10:** Developing tooth: Bell stage, (A) micrograph, (B) sketch. Inner enamel epithelial cells differentiate into ameloblast (3), which forms the enamel (4). Odontoblasts (7) secrete predentin (6), which then form dentin (5). Outer enamel epithelium (1), stellate reticulum (2), mesenchyme of dental papilla (8) and dental sac (9) are also well developed

and serosa. The structures of these layers are:

a. **The mucosa:** It comprises an epithelial lining resting on a basement membrane; a lamina propria; and the muscularis mucosae or muscularis interna. Type of epithelium depends upon the function. Sites of the GIT, which are exposed to friction comparatively have a thick epithelium, e.g. esophagus. The main functions of the epithelial lining are to provide a selectively permeable barrier, to facilitate the transport and digestion of food, to help the absorption of the products and to produce hormones that affect the activity of the digestive system. Cells in the epithelial layer also produce mucus for lubrication and protection.

Supporting lamina propria is located just below the epithelium. It is made up of either loose areolar or reticular connective tissue. It usually possesses digestive glands along with plenty of capillaries, macrophages and lymphatic tissue. Lymphatic tissue can range from solitary lymphocytes to large lymphoid nodules. Some of lymphoid cells actively produce antibodies (mainly IgA).

The muscularis mucosae usually consist of a thin inner circular layer and outer longitudinal layer of smooth muscle fibers. Contraction of these muscles produces movement of the mucosa independent of other movements of the digestive tract. Contractions are generated and coordinated by nerve plexuses (Meissner's), which are composed mainly of nerve cell aggregates that form small parasympathetic ganglia. The number of these ganglia varies along the GIT; they are more numerous in the regions of greatest motility.

b. **Submucosa:** It is composed of dense connective tissue with larger blood vessels. These vessels provide supply to the mucosa, muscularis externa and serosa. In some organs there are compound glands in the submucosa. It also contains a submucosal (Meissner's) nerve plexus. Mucosa and submucosa make folds which projects into the lumen. These folds increase the surface area for absorption and greatly vary in size.

c. **Muscularis externa:** It consists of two thick layers of smooth muscle fibers: An inner circular and an outer longitudinal. Esophagus is the exception as its wall also contains skeletal muscle fibers. The muscles in this layer mix and propel the food in the GIT. The myenteric (Auerbach's) nerve plexus is located in between the two muscle layers and controls the motor activity of smooth muscle fibers (Fig. 14.11A, B). At some sites

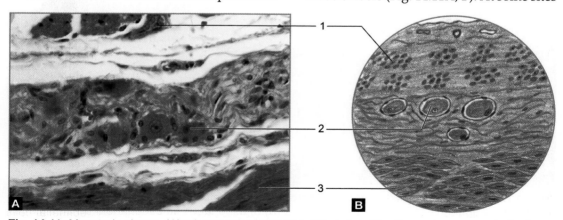

**Fig. 14.11:** Myenteric plexus, (A) micrograph of intestine, (B) sketch. The figure shows myenteric plexus (2) in between the inner circular (3) and outer longitudinal (1) layers of smooth muscle fibers of the muscularis externa

the circular muscle layer gets thickened and form sphincters.

d. **Serosa:** It consists of loose connective tissue. Often its connective tissue blends with that of the surrounding tissues and then it is known as adventitia; however, in many regions it is covered by peritoneum (simple squamous epithelial cells) and there it is known as serosa. Through this layer vessels and nerves pass to the deeper layers of the wall.

## B. Esophagus

It is a relatively straight, muscular tube, which is continuous above with the pharynx at the inferior border of the cricoid cartilage and below it opens into the stomach. It transports the bolus of food to the stomach. Its lumen is irregular due to the presence of deep longitudinal folds and grooves. Its wall shows the four layers as described previously:

a. **Mucosa:** The mucous membrane shows several longitudinal folds and in the distended tube the folds disappear. Esophagus has to withstand a certain amount of abrasion by rough textured food, so it is lined with stratified squamous nonkeratinized epithelium. At the lower end, it shows an abrupt transition to the simple columnar epithelium of the stomach. Only the basal cells of the esophagus continue into the stomach. The connective tissue of lamina propria forms processes, which project in the epithelium. These processes are permanent and not affected by the distension of the esophagus. In the lamina propria of the region near the pharynx and near its junction with the stomach groups of mucus secreting glands (esophageal cardiac glands) are present (Fig. 14.12A, B).

Esophageal cardiac glands are compound tubuloalveolar glands of mucous type and secrete neutral mucus, which protects esophageal wall from regurgitated gastric content. In the lamina propria lymphatic infiltration is present only around the orifices of the mucous glands. The muscularis mucosa varies in thickness and having only longitudinally running smooth muscle fibers. Fibers are thick in the proximal part of the esophagus and may be function as an aid in swallowing.

b. **Submucosa:** Dense irregular connective tissue of submucosa is very elastic allowing

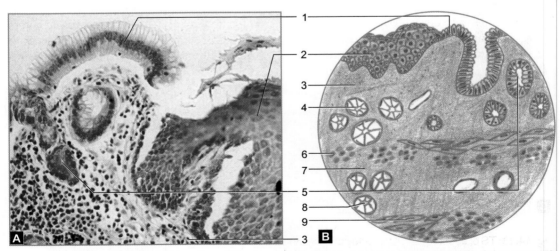

**Fig. 14.12:** Gastroesophageal junction, (A) micrograph, (B) sketch showing cardia (1) of the stomach along with esophagus (2). In the lamina propria (3) of esophagus lie esophageal cardiac glands (4). Muscularis mucosae (6) of esophagus have an only longitudinal layer of smooth muscle fibers, in comparison, stomach have inner circular and outer longitudinal layer of muscle fibers. Cardiac glands (5), submucosa (7), proper esophageal gland (8) and muscularis externa (9)

the esophagus for expansion when food is present. It also contains small groups of compound, tubulo-alveolar mucus secreting glands (esophageal glands). The mucus secreted by these glands is slightly acidic in nature and lubricate the mucosa. Esophageal glands are more in number in the upper half of esophagus.

c. **Muscularis externa:** It consists of inner circular and outer longitudinal layers. The fibers at the upper one-third of the esophagus are skeletal, a continuation of the muscles of the pharynx. In the lower one-third fibers are smooth muscle fibers. Both skeletal as well as smooth types of fibers are present in the middle one-third (Fig. 14.13 A to D).

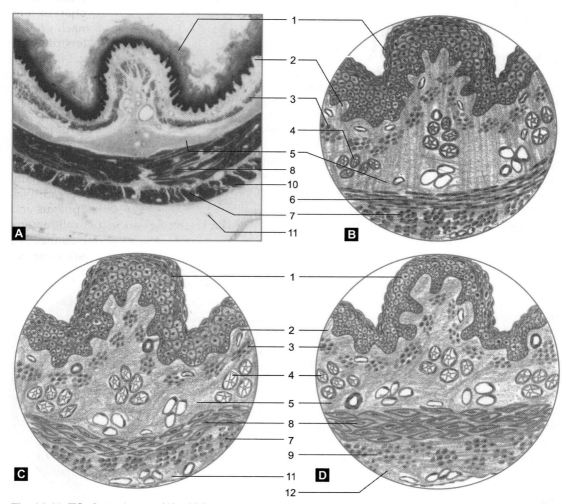

**Fig. 14.13:** TS of esophagus, (A) middle part—micrograph, (B) upper part—sketch, (C) middle part—sketch, (D) lower part—sketch. Stratified squamous nonkeratinized epithelium (1), lamina propria (2), muscularis mucosae (3), esophageal glands (4), submucosa (5), inner circular layer of skeletal muscle fibers (6), outer longitudinal layer of skeletal muscle fibers (7), inner circular layer of smooth muscle fibers (8), outer longitudinal layer of smooth muscle fibers (9), muscularis externa (10), adventitia (11) and serosa (12). Note the change in arrangement of muscle fiber in various parts of esophagus

Myenteric plexus present in this layer produces peristaltic activity.

> The striated muscle present in the upper part is innervated by somatic motor neurons of the vagus nerve (from nucleus ambiguous). The smooth muscle of the lower part of the esophagus is innervated by visceral motor neurons of the vagus nerve (from dorsal motor nucleus). These motor neurons make synapse with postganglionic neurons whose cell bodies are located in the esophagus.

d. **Serosa or adventitia:** Only a small piece that lies below the diaphragm is lined by serosa; the rest of the esophagus is fixed and covered by adventitia.

## C. Stomach

It is a dilated segment of the GI tract, which connects the esophagus to the intestine. It receives the bolus of the food from esophagus, which undergoes mechanical and chemical breakdown in the stomach, to form chyme. Solid foodstuffs are broken up by a strong muscular churning action, while a chemical breakdown is produced by gastric juices secreted by the gastric glands and bolus of the food changes into a semiliquid material, known as chyme. Once chyme formation is completed, the pyloric sphincter relaxes and allows the chyme to pass into the small intestine for further digestion and absorption. Stomach is also a storage depot for food and it can retain food for two hours or more.

Grossly, it has four parts: Cardia, fundus, body, and pylorus (Fig. 14.14). The cardia surrounds the esophageal orifice; the fundus lies above the level of a horizontal line drawn through the esophageal orifice; the body is the middle portion of the stomach; and the pylorus is the lower funnel-shaped part, lying near the junction of the stomach and duodenum.

Microscopically, the fundus and the body are identical. In the empty stomach, the mucosa and submucosa is thrown into longitudinal folds called rugae, and in full stomach the rugae are much reduced in size

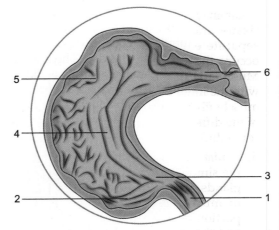

**Fig. 14.14:** Schematic diagram of the stomach showing its parts: Cardia (3), fundus (2), body (4) and pyloric (6). Esophagus (1), gastric rugae (5)

due to distension. The rugae do not change the surface area; rather, their function is to accommodate expansion of the stomach during its filling. The layers in the stomach are:

a. **Mucosa:** The lining epithelium is columnar and it invaginates to a varying extent into the lamina propria, forming gastric pits or foveolae. Several simple branched, tubular gastric glands (cardiac, fundic and pyloric) feature of each region of the stomach opens in one gastric pit. The apical parts of surface epithelial cells are filled with mucinogen granules, so these cells look empty (mucinogen granules are removed during tissue processing). At base cells looks basophilic, because of the presence of small amount of rough endoplasmic reticulum. These cells are renewed approximately every 3–5 days.

The mucus secreted by these cells is known as visible mucus, because of its insolubility and cloudy appearance. It forms a thick coat over the epithelial surface and protects it from acidic pH and hydrolytic enzymes contain in the gastric juice. The bicarbonate ions trapped in this mucus layer form a relatively alkaline pH at the surface, despite the acidic pH of the lumen.

Lamina propria consists of loose connective tissue and difficult to recognize as a separate entity because it is split up to occupy the spaces between pits and glands. Muscularis mucosae is having two layers with the inner circular layer sending a few muscle fibers towards the lumen. Mucosa of the different parts of the stomach shows some different characteristics, these are:

i. *Cardia:* The gastric pits are shallow, and the simple or branched tubular cardiac glands occupy the rest of the thickness of mucosa (Fig.14.15). The terminal portion of these glands is often coiled and the glands are having a relatively large lumen. In comparison to other parts even the mucosa is thin. The cells produce mucus and lysozyme, a bactericidal enzyme. A few parietal cells may be present.

ii. *Fundus and body:* The gastric pits are not deep and they extend into the one-fourth of the thickness of the mucosa. The remaining mucosa is occupied by simple branched tubular fundic glands, which lie at right angle to the mucosal surface. Each gland has three different parts: Isthmus, neck and base. The distribution of cells in these glands is not uniform. Isthmus lies close to the gastric pit and contains differentiating mucous cells, undifferentiated cells, and parietal cells; neck contains undifferentiated cells, mucous neck cells, a few entero-endocrine cells and parietal cells; base contains parietal cells, enteroendocrine cells and chief cells (Fig. 14.16A, B). The isthmus is the site for replication of cells.

- Undifferentiated cells: These are low columnar cells with oval nuclei near the bases of the glands. These are present in the isthmus and neck region, but few in number. Cells are having a high rate of mitosis, some of them move upwards to replace the damaged cells, while the rest of the

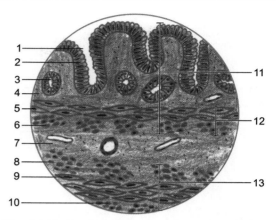

**Fig. 14.15:** Cardia of the stomach showing gastric pits (1). Simple columnar epithelium (2), gastric glands (3), lamina propria (4), inner circular layer (5), outer longitudinal layer (6), submucosa (7), inner oblique layer (8), middle circular layer (9), outer longitudinal layer (10), mucosa (11), muscularis mucosae (12) and muscularis externa (13)

cells move downwards to maintain the cell population of fundus.

- Mucous neck cells: These cells are found dispersed between the parietal cells. Cells are irregular in shape, with their nuclei at the base. These are much shorter than the surface mucous cells and contain less mucinogen granules in the apical parts. The mucus is soluble mucus, which protects other glandular cells from the action of proteases and HCl. The life span of these cells is approximately 6 days. Release of mucinogen granules is stimulated by the vagus nerve, so secretion from mucous neck cells does not occur in the resting stomach.

- Parietal (oxyntic) cells: These are mainly present in the upper half of the gastric glands and scarce at the base. These are ovoid or polyhedral cells with a large central nucleus that contain distinct eosinophilic cytoplasm (Fig. 14.17A, B). The cells

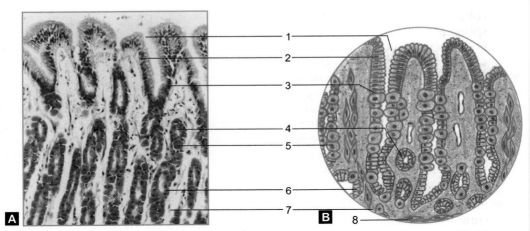

**Fig.14.16:** Fundic gland with gastric pits (1) extending into one-fourth of the mucosa. (A) micrograph, (B) sketch. Surface epithelial cells (2), mucus neck cell (3), gastric gland (4), parietal cell (5), chief cell (6), lamina propria (7) and muscularis mucosae (8)

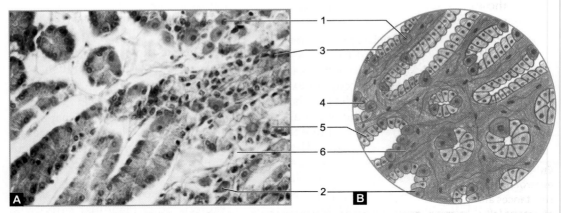

**Fig. 14.17:** Cells of the fundic glands at high magnification. (A) Micrograph, (B) sketch. Parietal cells (1) are large polyhedral cells with eosinophilic cytoplasm (2). Chief cells (3) are cuboidal cells with basophilic cytoplasm (4). Gastric gland (5) and lamina propria (6) are also seen

have no protein secretion function, so a little RNA is present in the cytoplasm.

The parietal cells secrete HCl and intrinsic factor, needed for absorption of vitamin $B_{12}$. Vitamin $B_{12}$ is important for the maturation of red blood cells in the bone marrow and lack of this vitamin results in pernicious anaemia. HCl keeps the pH of gastric juice low to activate gastric enzymes. HCl also

destroys most of the bacteria entering the stomach along with food. The parietal cells often bulge outwards (in lamina propria) creating a beaded appearance. These cells have the longest life span of approximately 150–180 days.

• Chief (peptic or zymogen) cells: These are found mostly near the base of the gastric glands. These are cuboidal or columnar cells with basally placed spherical nucleus and basal cytoplasm is basophilic filled with many ribosomes. Apical cytoplasm is eosinophilic due to the presence of secretory granules, which contain pepsinogen. It is converted to pepsin in the acidic medium of the stomach. Pepsin breaks down proteins to small peptides. Chief cells also secrete a weak lipase. The life of these cells is approximately 60–80 days.

- Enteroendocrine, APUD (amine precursor uptake and decarboxylation) [Argentaffin or Argyrophilic or Enterochromaffin or DNES or Kultschitsky] cells: These are found mainly near the bases of the glands. Several types of these cells are present; some of them secrete serotonin, gastrin, glucagon, and somatostatin. These cells lie in between the chief cells and the basement membrane, so do not reach up to the lumen. Unlike the other types of secretory cells, these cells release their products into the lamina propria. The life span of these cells is approximately 60–80 days.

**Enteroendocrine cells** These cells are known as enteroendocrine cells as they secrete hormone-like substances and these are located in the epithelium of enteric (alimentary) canal. These cells are known as APUD cells as some of them can take up the precursors of amines and decarboxylate them. These cells are known as argentaffin or argyrophilic cells as they take silver stains. These cells are known as enterochromaffin cells as they can be stained by chromium salts. These cells are known as DNES cells as these are the members of the diffuse neuroendocrine system of cells. G cells are present in the pyloric part of the stomach and secrete gastrin, which stimulates secretion of HCl by parietal cells. D cells are present in the upper and lower parts of the stomach and secrete somatostatin, which inhibits the release of gastrin and thus indirectly inhibits HCl secretion. EC cells are scattered throughout the gastric mucosa and secrete serotonin, which influences motility of gastrointestinal tract. A cells are present in the upper part of the stomach and secrete glucagon, which stimulates hepatic glycogenolysis.

iii. *Pylorus:* The gastric pits are deep and occupy two-thirds of the thickness of the mucosa. The rest of the mucosa is occupied by branched tubular pyloric glands (Fig.14.18). The terminal part is often coiled. A few parietal and enteroendocrine cells may be present. Pyloric glands secrete the gastrin hormone.

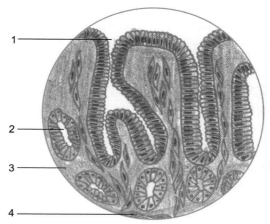

**Fig. 14.18:** Pylorus of stomach having deeper gastric pits (1) occupying two-thirds of the thickness of the mucosa. Gastric gland (2), lamina propria (3) and muscularis mucosae (4)

b. **Submucosa:** It is composed of dense connective tissue with blood and lymphatic vessels; it is infiltrated by lymphoid cells, macrophages and mast cells.

c. **Muscularis externa:** This is formed from three layers of smooth muscle fibers: Inner oblique, middle circular and outer longitudinal layer. These layers are responsible for mixing of gastric contents and emptying of the stomach. At the pyloric region, the middle circular layer thickened to form the pyloric sphincter (Fig. 14.19A, B).

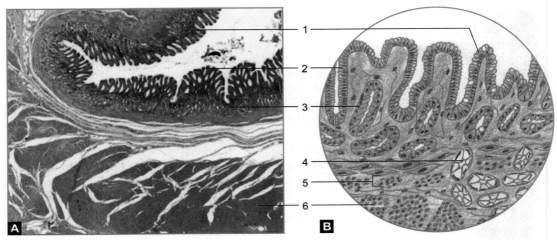

**Fig.14.19:** Duodeno-pylorus junction, (A) micrograph, (B) sketch. Pyloric sphincter (6) is formed by a thickened inner circular layer of the muscularis externa. Submucosa of the duodenum contains Brunner's gland (4). Intestinal epithelium (1), epithelium of stomach (2), pyloric glands (3) and muscularis mucosae (5). Note the presence of goblet cells in the duodenal/intestinal epithelium

> For comparison between cardia, fundus and pylorus of stomach *see* Table 26 given in Appendix I.

d. **Serosa:** It is thin and covered by mesothelium.

## D. Small Intestine

It is the part of the GIT where the major part of digestion and absorption takes place. Chyme from the stomach enters in the duodenum and exocrine secretion of the pancreas and liver is even delivered into the duodenum. These secretions along with the secretion from small intestine continue the digestion process. Anatomically and histologically, it has three parts: Duodenum, jejunum and ileum. Layers in the wall of the small intestine are:

a. **Mucous membrane:** The lining of the small intestine shows a series of permanent circular or spiral folds, plicae circulares (Kerckring's valve), consisting of mucosa and a core of submucosa. These folds are present in the distal half of the duodenum, the entire jejunum (most developed), and proximal half of the ileum. These folds disappear in the distal half of the ileum. The plicae increase the surface area of the mucosa two to threefold and slow down the passage of the contents.

The surface area is further increase by the presence of finger-like projections of the mucosa, the villi (tenfold). Each villus is covered by epithelium and has a core of lamina propria (Fig. 14.20A, B).

> For comparison between pylorus and duodenum, *see* Table 27 given in Appendix I.

In duodenum villi are broad, tall and leaf-shaped, in jejunum they have clubbed end and in ileum they become shorter and appear finger like. Proceeding from duodenum towards ileum villi decreases in number also. Between the villi are small openings of simple tubular glands called intestinal glands (crypt of Lieberkühn). In the upper half of the intestinal glands lie tall columnar absorptive cells. Cells in the basal half of the gland are mostly undifferentiated, enteroendocrine and Paneth cells, and only a few goblet cells. Absorptive cells are absent in the basal half.

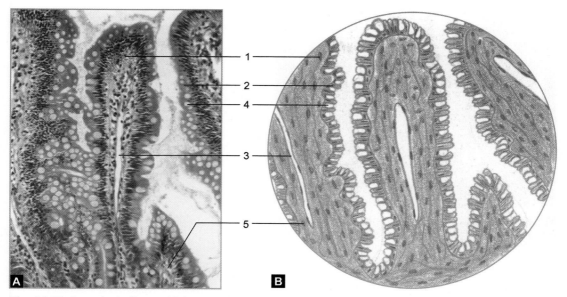

**Fig. 14.20:** Intestinal villus at high magnification, (A) micrograph, (B) sketch, showing simple columnar epithelium (2) with goblet cells (4). Central lacteal (3) is visible in villi (1). Lamina propria (5) is also seen

i. *Columnar (absorptive cells or enterocytes):* These tall columnar cells rest upon a basal lamina. Each cell has a striated border formed by closely packed, parallel microvilli. The microvilli increases the surface area of the mucosa about 20-fold and their external surface is coated with filamentous glycoproteins, known as glycocalyx. The glycocalyx is resistant to protease attack and thought to protect the underlying epithelium against pancreatic enzymes in the intestinal lumen. It also serves to absorb a number of pancreatic enzymes. Epithelial cells are joined to each other and to adjacent goblet cells by junctional complexes, which form a barrier in between the contents of lumen and epithelial cells. These cells absorb sugars and amino acids from the gut lumen; these substances pass through the cells of the blood capillaries in the lamina propria.

ii. *Goblet cells:* These are interspersed between the columnar cells and their number increases from the duodenum to the ileum. These are more numerous in the upper half of the intestinal glands. The cells are flask-shaped and have a slender, dark staining base that contains the flattened nucleus. The apex of cells contains mucus secreting granules. These cells produce acid glycoproteins whose main function are to protect and lubricate the lining of the intestine. These cells also play a role in the immune defense of the membrane. The goblet cells endocytose IgA secreted by B lymphocytes present in the underlying lamina propria and then discharge them to the surface of the mucosa.

iii. *Paneth cells:* These pyramidal cells are found at the bases of the crypts. In GIT these cells are most numerous in the small intestine and appendix. These cells have a comparatively long life span of 20 days. Basal cytoplasm of these cells is basophilic due to the presence of rough endoplasmic reticulum and apical is eosinophilic due to the presence of large eosinophilic granules (Fig. 14.21A, B).

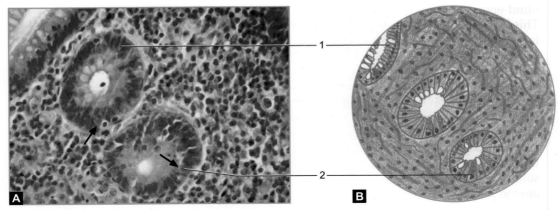

**Fig.14.21:** Paneth cells, (A) micrograph, (B) sketch. The figure is showing sections of intestinal glands (1) with Paneth cells (2, arrow) having eosinophilic granules

These granules accumulate during fasting and disappear during digestion and contain defensins (antimicrobial peptides) as well as lysozyme (digest the capsules of bacteria). These chemicals represent the bodies "first-line" of defense against microbes that enter through the digestive tract. Thus, the Paneth cells play an important role in regulating the normal bacterial flora of the small intestine. These cells also produce "tumor necrosis factor-α".

iv. *Enteroendocrine cells:* These cells are found both in the crypt and on the villi. In GIT these cells are most numerous in duodenum and appendix. These cells contain membrane bound vesicles filled with neuroactive substances and secrete hormones such as secretin, somatostatin, enteroglucagon and serotonin; one hormone per type of cell. These hormones are discharged either into the neighborhood, which they influence (paracrine secretion), or they are directly discharged into the blood capillaries and act on distant organs (endocrine secretion).

> **Enteroendocrine cells** D cells secrete somatostatin, which inhibit endocrine, exocrine and neurotransmitter secretion and are present in the duodenum. EC cells

prevalent throughout the intestines and secrete serotonin, motilin and substance P. These hormones increases gut motility. G cells are present in the duodenum and secrete gastrin, which stimulates secretion of HCl by parietal cells. I cells are present in the small intestine and secrete cholecystokinin which influences pancreatic secretion and gallbladder emptying. K cells are present in the small intestine and secrete gastric inhibitory peptide (GIP) which inhibit secretion of gastric acid and stimulate release of insulin. L cells are present in the small intestine as well as in the colon, and secrete glucagon like peptide-1(GLP-1), which stimulates insulin secretion and inhibits glucagon secretion. S cells are present in the small intestine and secrete secretin which modifies pancreatic and biliary water and ion secretion.

v. *Undifferentiated stem cells:* These columnar cells lie at the bases of crypts and are the source of other cells both in the crypts and on the villi. The rate of cell division is high in these cells.

b. **Lamina propria:** It is a loose areolar tissue with lymphoid tendencies and it also contains meshwork of reticular fibers. Reticular cells, lymphocytes and macrophages are present in this meshwork. A single smooth muscle cells oriented lengthwise in the cores of villi are closely related to blind-ended lymphatic capillaries (lacteal). This lacteal is responsible for absorption of fatty acids and glycerol. In addition to scattered lymphocytes, a large number of solitary follicles (more numerous distally) are present. The amount of lymphoid tissue increases from duodenum to ileum. In the ileum follicles aggregates into large masses of lymphatic tissue, called Peyer's patches or aggregated nodules, which extend through the muscularis mucosae into the submucosa. Peyer's patches are maximum around puberty and are antimesenteric in site.

**M (Microfold) cells** These are specialized epithelial cells overlying the lymphatic follicles of Peyer's patches and other large lymphatic nodules. They are derived from undifferentiated cells of the crypts of Lieberkühn. Instead of microvilli microfolds are present on their apical surface. M cells can endocytose antigens and transport them to the underlying macrophages and lymphoid cells.

c. **Muscularis mucosae:** It contains inner circular and outer longitudinal layers of smooth muscle fibers. In the ileum where Peyer's patches are large, it is thin or even absent. Muscle fibers of inner circular layer enter in the villi and extend as far as the basement membrane of mucous membrane. During digestion, these muscle fibers contract rhythmically and shorten the villi. Contraction of muscle fibers even causes milking of the lacteals.

d. **Submucosa:** It is composed of dense connective tissue with blood and lymph vessels. In the duodenum, it contains clusters of branched, tubuloalveolar, mucous glands; known as duodenal glands (Brunner's gland) (Fig. 14.22A, B). These glands are abundant and crowded in upper duodenum, in the lower two-thirds they become smaller and less in number; they disappear entirely before the duodenum comes to an end. The duct of these glands

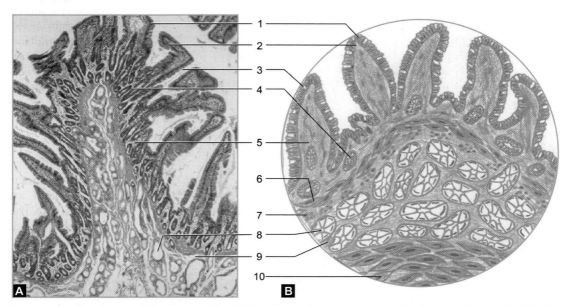

**Fig. 14.22:** Duodenum, (A) micrograph, (B) sketch, having mucus secreting Brunner's gland (8) in the submucosa (9). Simple columnar epithelium (1), villi (2), goblet cell (3), intestinal gland (4), lamina propria (5), an inner circular layer of muscularis mucosae (6), outer longitudinal layer of muscularis mucosae (7) and an inner circular layer of muscularis externa (10)

pierces the muscularis mucosae and opens in the crypts of Lieberkühn. These glands secrete an alkaline mucus and urogastrone (human epidermal growth factor). Urogastrone is a polypeptide hormone that increases epithelial cell division and inhibits gastric HCl production. Mucus

protects the duodenal mucosa against the effect of the acid gastric juice. In the jejunum (Fig. 14.23A, B) and ileum (Fig. 14.24A, B) submucosa is similar to the rest of the GIT.

e. **Muscularis externa:** It is made up of an inner circular layer and an outer longitudinal layer of smooth muscle fibers. Two types

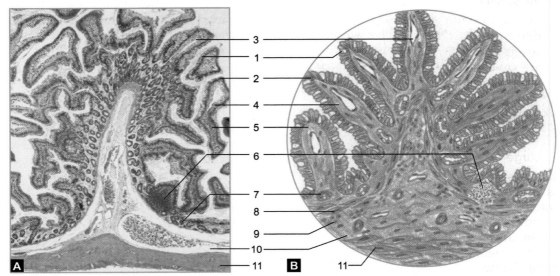

**Fig. 14.23:** Jejunum, (A) micrograph, (B) sketch. Solitary lymphatic follicle (6) can be seen in the lamina propria (5). Goblet cell (1), simple columnar epithelium (2), lacteal (3), villi (4), intestinal gland (7), inner circular layer of muscularis mucosae (8), outer longitudinal layer of muscularis mucosae (9), submucosa (10), inner circular layer of muscularis externa (11)

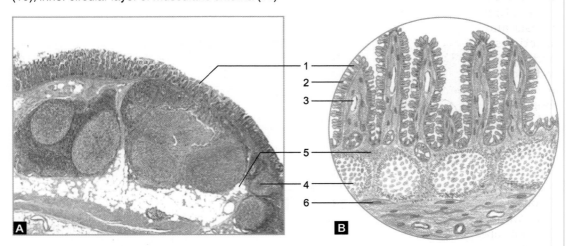

**Fig. 14.24:** Ileum, (A) micrograph, (B) sketch. Peyer's patches (4) are present in the lamina propria (5). Muscularis mucosae (6) is incomplete. Simple columnar epithelium (1), goblet cells (2) and lacteal (3) are also present

of muscular contractions occur in the small intestine: Local and peristaltic contractions. Local contractions, which mainly involved circular muscle layer; circulate the chyme and mixes it with digestive enzymes. Peristaltic contractions, mainly involved longitudinal muscle layer; moves the intestinal contents distally.

f. **Serosa:** Except second and third parts of the duodenum and terminal parts of ileum it covers all of the small intestine. These parts are covered by adventitia and therefore remain fixed to the abdominal wall.

For comparison between duodenum, jejunum and ileum, *see* Table 28 given in Appendix I.

## E. Large Intestine

It consists of colon, rectum and anal canal. It is much larger in caliber than the small intestine except the appendix, which is very narrow. Villi are present in the fetal life, but absent in postnatal life. The crypts are longer, more numerous and closer together than the small intestine. The number of goblet cells gradually increases along the length of the large intestine. No digestive enzymes are produced by the cells of the large intestine. It houses bacteria that produce vitamin $B_{12}$ and vitamin K; the former is necessary for hemopoiesis and the latter for coagulation. It functions mainly in the absorption of electrolytes, fluids and gases. Dead bacteria and indigestible remnants of the ingested material are compacted into faeces. It produces abundant mucus, which lubricates its lining and facilitates the passage and the elimination of faeces.

a. **Colon:** It is situated in between the terminal part of the ileum and rectum. It is composed of the caecum, ascending colon, transverse colon, descending colon and sigmoid colon.
  i. *Mucosa:* The plicae circulares and villi are absent, so the surface is smooth. Crypts of Lieberkühn are present. The lining epithelium is columnar with striated border and numerous goblet cells. Paneth cells are absent in the adult, but can be seen in the children. Thick lamina propria is occupied by crypts and contains diffuse lymphatic tissue and sometimes lymphatic nodules. Muscularis mucosae contain inner circular and outer longitudinal layers of smooth muscle fibers.
  ii. *Submucosa:* It is composed of fibroelastic connective tissue.
  iii. *Muscularis externa:* The inner circular layer is thin and outer longitudinal layer is gathered into three bands, known as taenia coli (Fig. 14.25A, B). In between the taenia thin longitudinal layer is present. Taenia puckers or sacculate the wall of the colon; forming haustrations. Two types of muscular contractions occur in the large intestine: Local and peristaltic contractions. Peristaltic contractions propel the contents distally.
  iv. *Serosa:* The posterior surface of ascending and descending colon is covered by adventitia; the rest of the colon is covered by serosa. Small pouches of serosa filled with fat are present, known as appendices epiploicae. They are more numerous on the sigmoid and transverse colon.

b. **Rectum:** The rectum is structurally similar to the colon except:
  i. The surface epithelium and crypts contain abundant goblet cells. Crypts are deeper here, but are a few in number (Fig. 14.26A, B).
  ii. Taenia coli are absent, so the outer longitudinal muscle coat is continuous.
  iii. Serosa is present at the sides and in front of upper part; only front of the middle part and the rest of the rectum is covered by adventitia.
  iv. Appendices epiploicae are not present.

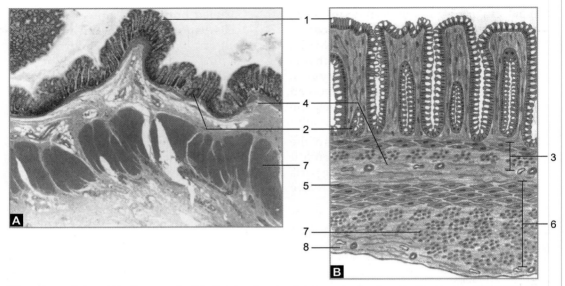

**Fig. 14.25:** Colon, (A) micrograph, (B) sketch, showing thickened outer longitudinal layer of the muscularis externa (6) forming taenia coli (7). Simple columnar epithelium with plenty of goblet cells (1), intestinal glands (2), muscularis mucosae (3), submucosa (4), inner circular layer (5) and serosa (8)

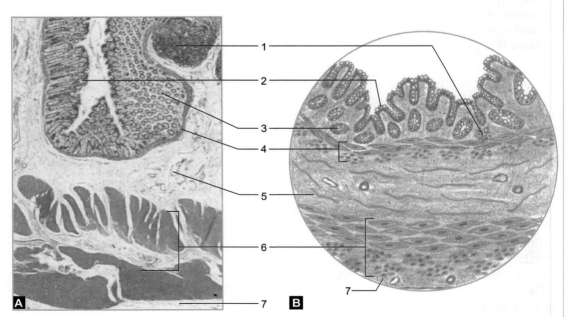

**Fig. 14.26:** Rectum, (A) micrograph, (B) sketch, lined by simple columnar epithelium with abundant goblet cells (2). Lymphatic nodule (1), intestinal gland (3), muscularis mucosae (4), submucosa (5), muscularis externa (6) and adventitia (7)

c. **Anal canal:** The lining epithelium of the upper part of the canal is columnar. In the upper part 6–10 vertical mucosal folds (Morgagni's columns) are present. Dentate line lies at the level of the bases of the columns, where tiny flaps and pockets are present, known as anal valves and sinuses. Apocrine sweat glands (anal glands) open in each anal sinus. In the middle part of the canal epithelium is stratified squamous nonkeratinized and columns are absent. This middle part is called a transitional zone or pectin. The lower part of anal canal is lined by true skin, which contains sebaceous and apocrine glands. Lamina propria is composed of fibroelastic connective tissue and contains sebaceous glands, circumanal glands, hair follicles and large veins. Submucosa contains prominent venous sinuses. It is surrounded by inner circular and outer longitudinal layers of smooth muscle fibers. The circular layer of smooth muscle thickens terminally as the internal anal sphincter. More superficially the nearby skeletal muscle forms the external anal sphincter. Adventitia is the outermost layer (Fig. 14.27A, B).

For comparison between small and large intestines *see* Table 29 given in Appendix I.

d. **Appendix:** It is a small, slender, blind diverticulum of the caecum. The lumen is small and usually of irregular outline. Lumen often contains cellular debris and may be completely occluded. Villi are absent and only a few intestinal glands are present. The lining epithelium is simple columnar with striated border and also contains a few goblet cells, a few Paneth cells and many enteroendocrine cells. The lamina propria is occupied by many large and small lymphatic nodules that may extend up to the submucosa (Fig. 14.28A, B). The muscularis mucosa is incomplete. Muscularis externa is thin, but contain usual two layers. The serosa forms the outermost layer covering it completely.

## GLANDS OF GI TRACT

Associated with the GIT are eight major glands: The three paired salivary glands, pancreas and liver.

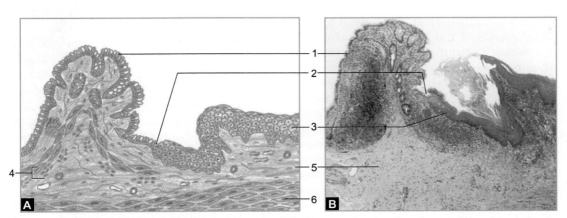

**Fig. 14.27:** Recto—anal junction, (A) sketch, (B) micrograph, showing the transition (2) of simple columnar epithelium (1) of rectum in stratified squamous nonkeratinized epithelium (3) of the anus. Muscularis mucosae (4) is absent in anal canal. Submucosa (5) and inner circular layer of muscularis externa (6)

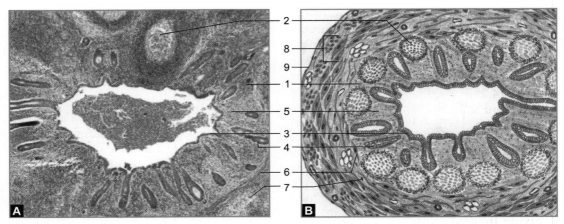

**Fig. 14.28:** Vermiform appendix, (A) micrograph, (B) sketch, showing lymphatic nodules with germinal center (2) in the lamina propria (5). Muscularis mucosae (6) is incomplete. Diffuse lymphatic tissue (1), simple columnar epithelium with goblet cells (3), intestinal glands (4), submucosa (7), inner circular layer and outer longitudinal layer of muscularis externa (8) and serosa (9)

## A. Salivary Glands

The salivary glands are accessory glands of digestion and pour their secretion (saliva) into the oral cavity. Saliva lubricates and cleanses the oral cavity through its water and glycoprotein content. The three major salivary glands are: Parotid, submandibular and sublingual. Besides these major salivary glands, numerous minor accessory glands are also present in oral mucosa. Some minor salivary glands are lingual glands of tongue, labial glands of the lips and buccal glands of cheeks. The minor salivary glands continuously secrete the saliva, whereas the major salivary glands secrete saliva in response to parasympathetic stimulation. Major salivary glands are compound tubuloalveolar glands. The alveolar cells can be either of serous type or mucous or a mixture of both types. Some of the mucous cells may have a cap of serous cells; they are called serous demilunes or crescents of Giannuzzi or crescents of Heidenhain. Small canaliculi from the serous demilunes pass between the mucus secreting cells to open into the lumen. Recent studies indicate that the presence of demilune is an artifact of fixation (use of formalin). Due to fixation serous cells swell and they burst out of their position. After sectioning, the cells resembled the common demilune shape. When samples were preserved by quick-freezing in liquid nitrogen and then fixed with osmium tetroxide in acetone, demilunes were not present.

**Saliva:** Salivary glands produce about 1 liter of saliva per day. Saliva mainly contains water; it also contains ions, mucus, enzymes and antibodies. Saliva performs various functions, such as:

1. It moistens the oral mucosa and chewed food.
2. It lubricates the bolus so that it can easily swallow.
3. Salivary amylase, produced by the serous acini is present in the saliva which initiates the breakdown of starch into smaller carbohydrates.
4. Lysozyme, produced by the serous acini hydrolyzes the capsules of bacteria and thus controls the bacterial flora of the oral cavity.
5. Saliva contains various proteins, glycoproteins and electrolytes.
6. IgA is produced by the plasma cells in the connective tissue surrounding the secretory acini of the salivary glands. Acini secrete a protein component that forms a complex with IgA, which helps to provide defense against oral bacteria.

a. **Parotid gland:** This is the largest salivary gland. It has a well-defined capsule. Septa divide the gland into lobes and lobules. Alveoli are almost entirely serous in nature but occasionally mucous alveoli are present (Fig. 14.29A, B). In the parotid gland abundant scattered fat cells are present. Myoepithelial (basket) cells are present. These cells are highly branched and help to expel the watery secretion from the lumen of the alveoli.

b. **Submandibular gland:** This is a mixed type of gland. It has a well-defined capsule. Septa divide the gland into lobes and lobules. The gland has more serous alveoli in comparison of mucous alveoli (Fig. 14.30A, B). At some places serous demilunes are also present. Myoepithelial cells are present and these cells are spindle-shaped.

c. **Sublingual gland:** This is also a mixed type of gland. It has no definitive capsule. Septa divide the gland into lobes and lobules. The gland is made up predominantly of mucous alveoli (Fig. 14.31A, B). Pure serous alveoli are rarely present, but the demilunes are present in some places.

d. **Duct system of salivary glands:** Alveolar cells secrete their product directly into intercalated ducts, which are lined by low cuboidal cells. Intercalated ducts of serous and mixed glands secrete $HCO_3^-$ and absorb $Cl^-$ from secretions of acini. From the intercalated duct the secretion passes in larger striated ducts that are lined with a simple columnar epithelium. These epithelial cells are packed with basal infoldings between which lie numerous mitochondria. This peculiar feature gives rise to the striated appearance of these cells. Striated duct add $K^+$ and $HCO_3^-$ to the saliva and absorb sodium from it to make the saliva hypotonic. From the striated duct secretion passes in excretory ducts, which initially are lined by columnar cells and terminate as tubes lined by stratified squamous epithelium continuous with the same epithelium covering the oral cavity. Excretory ducts are believed to be involved in electrolyte transport. The duct system is most conspicuous in the parotid gland and least conspicuous in the sublingual gland. In submandibular gland, the striated ducts are longer and appear more prominent in histological sections than the other salivary glands. The intercalated ducts of the sublingual gland are composed primarily of mucous cells in the form of the tubules

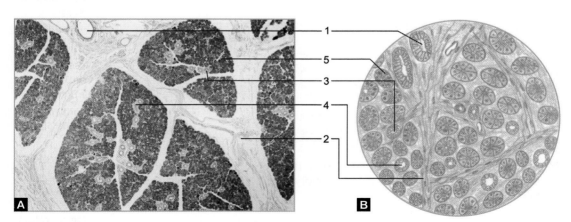

**Fig. 14.29:** Parotid gland, (A) micrograph, (B) sketch, made up of serous acini (5). Connective tissue septa (2) divide it into many lobules. A duct system of parotid includes intercalated duct (4), striated duct (3) and intralobular excretory duct (1)

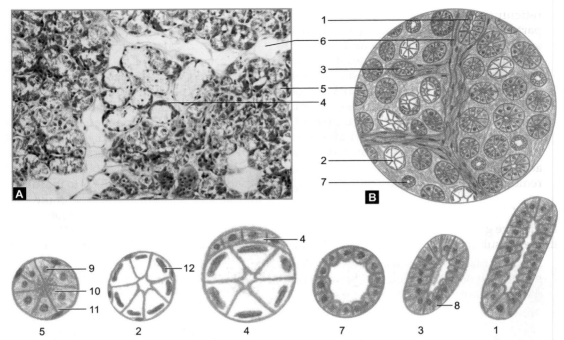

**Fig. 14.30:** Submandibular gland, (A) micrograph, (B) sketch, made up mainly by serous acini (5) with a few mucous acini (2) and serous demilune (4). Interlobular excretory duct (1), striated duct (3), connective tissue septa (6), intercalated duct (7), basal striation (8), round nucleus (9), apical zymogen granules (10), basal basophilic cytoplasm (11) and flat nucleus (12)

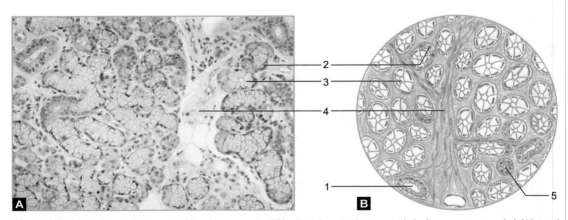

**Fig. 14.31:** Sublingual gland, (A) micrograph, (B) sketch, made up mainly by mucous acini (3) and a few serous demilunes (2). Interlobular excretory duct (1), connective tissue septa (4) and intercalated duct (5)

and link to very short secretory ducts. The final excretory segment is similar in all three glands.

e. **Passage of secretion:** The salivary glands secrete enzymes rich saliva. They are synthesized in the rough endoplasmic reticulum, which is pushed to the basal parts of the cells by the secretions in the apical part. Because of this basal part is having a basophilic tinge. The secretions are then transported to the Golgi apparatus from where they are thrown into the apical part in the form of secretory granules. The granules are eosinophilic in the serous acini, so apical part looks pink with eosin. In contrast to that apical part of mucous acini looks empty (mucinogen granules are removed during tissue processing).

## B. Liver

It is a large gland covered by a thin connective tissue capsule (Glisson's capsule). The capsule is thick at the hilum (porta hepatis), where the portal vein and hepatic artery enter in the liver and hepatic ducts and lymphatic exits. In the cross section shape of a lobule is hexagonal and at the angles of these hexagons there are small triangular areas containing portal triads (Fig. 14.32A to D). The outline of the hexagon may be marked out by a condensation of connective tissue in some animals, e.g. liver of pigs, such an appearance is lacking in man. In the center of the lobule lies the central vein and radiating from the vein lies plates of hepatocytes. Central vein can be regarded as a venule as its walls are poorly developed. These plates are usually one cell thick and anastomose to form a 3-D network. In children

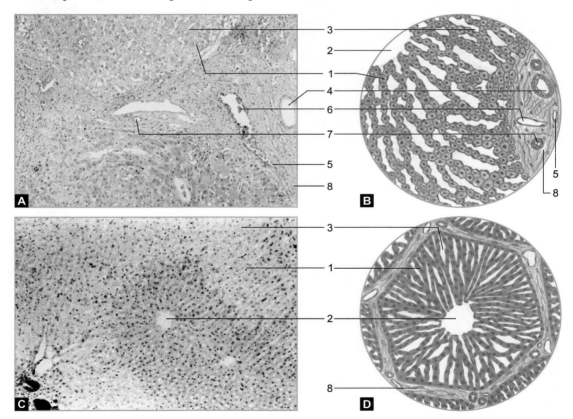

**Fig. 14.32:** Liver, (A) micrograph, (B) sketch at high magnification and (C) micrograph, (D) sketch at low magnification showing plates of hepatocytes (1). Portal triad includes branches of the hepatic artery (7), portal vein (6) and bile duct (4). Central vein (2), hepatic sinusoids (3), lymphatic vessels (5) and connective tissue septa (8)

up to 6 years hepatocytes are arranged in two-cell thick plates.

Blood from the branches of the portal vein and hepatic artery enter into the sinusoids, which lie between the plates of hepatocytes (Fig. 14.33).

Sinusoids are lined by fenestrated endothelial cells and phagocytic Kupffer cells. The

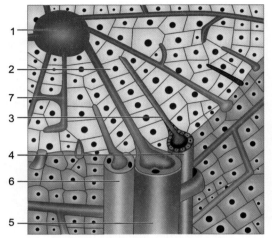

Fig. 14.33: Schematic diagram showing part of a liver lobule. Central vein (1), plates of hepatocytes (2), bile ductules (3), bile duct (4), portal vein (5), hepatic artery (6) and sinusoids (7)

fenestrations permit blood plasma to wash freely over the exposed surfaces of the hepatocytes in this space. Kupffer (stellate macrophage) cells, either lie by the side of endothelial cells (Fig. 14.34) or lie over its surface and send cytoplasmic processes between cells. The space between the endothelium and the plates is known as perisinusoidal space (space of Disse). This space contains the short microvilli of hepatocytes, reticular fibers, lipocytes (hepatic stellate or Ito cells) and occasional nonmyelinated nerve fibers. Lipocytes store vitamin A and usually secrete growth factors, cytokines and extracellular matrix proteins. Through the space of Disse exchange of material occurs between the bloodstream and hepatocytes as the hepatocyte does not lie in direct contact with the bloodstream.

Small, irregular microvilli project into the space of Disse from the hepatocyte. These microvilli increase the surface area and the rate of exchange of metabolites between hepatocytes and plasma. The structural framework of the liver is formed by a delicate network of reticular fibers embedded in the extracellular matrix. The network of reticular fibers provides supports to the hepatocytes

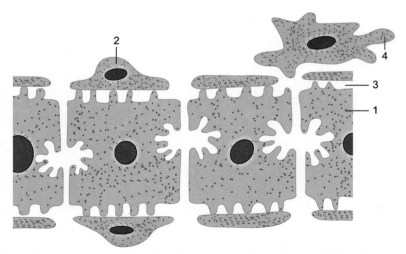

Fig. 14.34: Schematic diagram showing plate of hepatocytes (1), endothelial lining of sinusoid (2), space of Disse (3) and Kupffer cell (4)

and endothelial lining of sinusoids. At the periphery of the liver, this network of reticular fibers becomes continuous with the Glisson's capsule of the liver.

The portal triads include branches of the hepatic artery, portal vein (venule) and interlobular bile duct. The largest tube with largest lumen is the portal vein. It differs from the other veins because its lumen is open instead of being collapsed. The second largest tube is the hepatic artery. The bile duct is smaller than the above vessels and is lined by low cuboidal epithelium in contrast to the simple squamous epithelium of other tubes.

The space between the wall that surrounds the portal triad and portal triad is called the space of Mall. This space is thought to be one of the sites where lymph arises. Bile canaliculi, formed by apical surfaces of adjacent hepatocytes, form a network of tiny passages contained within each plate. Blood flows from the periphery to the center and bile flows from center towards the periphery.

a. **Functions of liver:**

i. The liver acts as an exocrine gland by producing and secreting bile.

ii. The liver produces most of the circulating plasma proteins, including albumins, globulins, lipoproteins, glycoproteins and clotting factors prothrombin and fibrinogen.

iii. The liver stores several vitamins such as vitamins A, D and K. Some of these vitamins are also modified by the liver.

iv. The liver detoxifies various drugs, metabolic waste products such as bilirubin and toxins.

v. The liver synthesizes almost all proteins required for transport and metabolism of iron and thus functions in storage and metabolism of iron.

vi. The liver maintains the normal level of blood plasma through synthesis, storage and breakdown of glycogen.

vii. The liver plays an important role in metabolism of fat and protein.

viii. The liver acts as an endocrine gland by modification of the structure and function of many hormones. Thyroxine hormone is secreted by the thyroid gland as $T_4$ and in the liver it is converted into the active form, i.e. $T_3$. The action of growth hormone is modified by GHRH (growth hormone releasing hormone) produced by the liver. In the liver insulin and glucagon hormone produced by the pancreas is degraded.

b. **Lobules in the liver:** Following three kinds of lobules are described in the liver (Fig 14.35):

i. *Classical liver lobule:* It has a vein in the center and portal triads at the edges (as mentioned above).

ii. *Portal lobule:* In this type portal triad lies in the center, while the central vein lies at the edges. Blood flows from the center to the periphery.

iii. *Liver acinus of Rappaport:* This acinus may be as large as one-sixth of the hepatic lobule and its hepatocytes receive blood from one hepatic arteriole and one portal

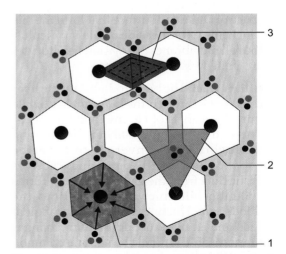

**Fig. 14.35:** Schematic diagram showing three kinds of lobules. Classical liver lobule (1), portal lobule (2), liver acinus of Rappaport (3)

venule; bile from the same hepatocytes is delivered to the accompanying bile ductule. The acinus can be divided into three zones of approximately equal size; these are known as zone 1, zone 2 and zone 3. Zone 1 is nearest to the blood supply (periportal) and zone 3 includes the terminal hepatic venule (central vein). Zone 2 is located between zones 1 and 3. There is an oxygen gradient (from high to low) is evident in between the zones 1 and 3. After a meal, glycogen will be stored first in the zone 1, later in zone 2 and finally in zone 3. The reverse is true when glucose is needed.

c. **Hepatocytes:** Each hepatocyte is a large polyhedral cell. The nucleus is large, spherical and occupies the centre of the cell. Many cells of adult liver are even binucleated. The cytoplasm contains numerous mitochondria, abundant rER and sER, well developed Golgi complex, lysosomes, peroxisomes and vacuoles containing various enzymes. The cytoplasm contains glycogen and lipid granules and also stores iron.

Numerous microvilli are present on the surface of hepatocyte towards the perisinusoidal space of Disse and surface that form the bile canaliculi. On either side of bile canaliculus, the cell membranes of adjacent hepatocytes are united by tight junctions.

d. **Biliary tract:** The bile produced by the liver cells flows through the bile canaliculi, bile ductules (canals of Hering) and bile ducts. These structures gradually merge, forming a network that converges to form the hepatic duct. The hepatic duct receives cystic duct from the gall bladder and forms common bile duct that opens into the duodenum. Ductules are lined by cuboidal cells and in bile duct epithelium changes to columnar. The hepatic, cystic and common bile duct all are lined by simple columnar epithelium with an inconspicuous layer of smooth muscle.

## C. Gall Bladder

It is a hollow, pear-shaped organ attached to the inferior surface of the liver. Its wall is composed of three layers:

a. **Mucosa:** It is having abundant folds that are particularly visible in the empty gall bladder. In between the mucosal folds, diverticula or crypts are present that form deep indentations in the mucosa. The lining epithelium is simple columnar cells with brush border of microvilli. The lamina propria is composed of a vascularized loose connective tissue with elastic fibers and collagen fibers. In the neck of the gall bladder, the lamina propria sometimes contains simple tubuloalveolar glands, which produce mucus in very small amount to lubricate the lumen of the neck. These glands are more common in the inflamed gall bladder. The muscularis mucosae and submucosa are absent.

b. **Muscularis externa:** It is composed of randomly arranged smooth muscle fibers with interlacing collagen fibers and elastic fibers (Fig. 14.36A, B). Contractions of these muscle fibers force the contents of the gall bladder out through the cystic duct.

c. **Serosa or adventitia:** Serosa is present only on the inferior surface; the rest of the gall bladder is covered by adventitia.

The gall bladder stores and concentrates the bile by actively absorbing sodium, coupled with water and anions. Bile produced by the liver reaches to gall bladder for storage via cystic duct. In response to the presence of fat into the proximal duodenum, the enteroendocrine cells of the small intestine produce cholecystokinin (CCK). CCK stimulates contractions of the smooth muscles of the gall bladder and concentrated bile is discharged into the duodenum via the common bile duct.

## D. Pancreas

The pancreas serves both exocrine and endocrine functions. These two components are very different structurally and functionally

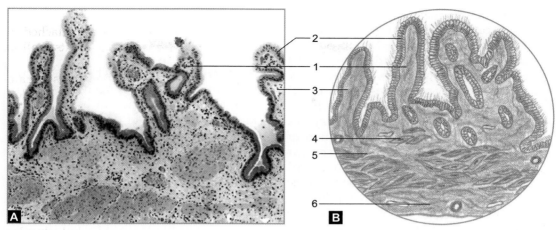

**Fig. 14.36:** Gall bladder, (A) micrograph, (B) sketch, having abundant mucosal folds (1) lined by simple columnar epithelium with microvilli (2). Lamina propria (3), smooth muscle fibers (4), elastic fibers (5) and adventitia (6)

but are intermingled within the gland. Only about 5% of the volume of the pancreas consists of endocrine cells, rest of it consists of exocrine cells. The pancreas is covered by a poorly developed sheath of loose connective tissue and from this sheath thin interlobular septa of loose connective tissue extends into the gland and divide it into ill-defined lobules.

a. **Exocrine pancreas:** It is compound tubulo-alveolar and serous gland (Fig. 14.37 A, B). It has many small lobules and each lobule is surrounded by connective tissue septa through which vessels, nerves, lymphatics and interlobular ducts run. Alveolar cells are pyramidal, arranged around a small lumen and show biphasic staining

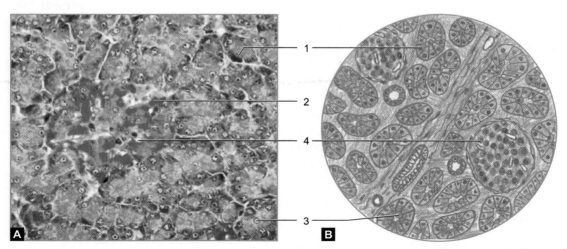

**Fig. 14.37:** Pancreas, (A) micrograph, prepared by immunohistochemical method + H and E stain, (B) sketch of H and E stain. Beta cells (2) of pancreatic islet (4) look brown due to the DAB reaction, when insulin antibody is used. Serous acini (1) of the pancreas are stained with H and E. Centroacinar cells (3) can be seen in the serous acini

properties with H and E. The basal regions of these cells are rich in rough ER and stain intensely with hematoxylin. The apical region contains zymogen granules and stains with eosin. These granules are released by exocytosis. Zymogen granules contain several digestive enzymes in an inactive form. These inactive enzymes or proenzymes are: Pancreatic amylase for digestion of carbohydrates, pancreatic lipases for digestion of lipids, ribonuclease and deoxyribonuclease for digestion of nucleic acids, and the proteolytic enzymes trypsinogen, chymotrypsinogen, procarboxypeptidase and proaminopeptidase.

Pancreatic proenzymes are produced in the acinar cells, but they become activated only upon reaching the lumen of the duodenum. The enterokinase present in glycocalyx of the intestinal mucosa converts trypsinogen to trypsin. Trypsin then converts all other proenzymes into an active form for digestion of food products in the chyme. In between the cells and the lumen centroacinar cells are interposed, which are in continuity with the intercalated or intralobular ducts. These ducts are lined with low cuboidal epithelial cells that secrete large amounts of watery fluid rich in sodium and bicarbonate ions. The bicarbonate ions serve to neutralize the acidity of the chyme that enters the duodenum from the stomach. These ducts, then lead into larger interlobular ducts, which are lined with a low columnar epithelium. Interlobular ducts empty into the main pancreatic duct, which is lined by tall columnar cells with occasional goblet cells. There are no striated ducts in the pancreas.

The secretory activity of the exocrine pancreas is mainly regulated by vagal stimulation and two hormones: Cholecystokinin-pancreozymin (CCK) and secretin. These two hormones are secreted by enteroendocrine cells of the duodenum. CCK triggers the acinar cells to secrete their proenzymes. Secretin induces the duct cells to produce large amounts of watery fluid rich in bicarbonate ions.

b. **Endocrine pancreas:** The cells of the endocrine part are arranged in round or oval-shaped areas rich in blood vessels known as the islets of Langerhans or they may be scattered throughout the exocrine parts of the pancreas. Islets are more in the tail region of the pancreas. The islets are closely applied on a capillary or sinusoid, as the secretions have to be discharged directly into the blood. There are several types of cells in the islet or other regions, each secreting a different peptide hormone. These cells cannot be distinguished by H and E stain. Different cells of the endocrine pancreas are:

   i. *Alpha cells*: 20%, and larger with eosino-philic granules. These cells are mainly found on the periphery of islets and produce the hormone glucagon, which decreases uptake of glucose; raises the blood glucose level.

   ii. *Beta cells*: 75%, and smaller with bas-ophilic granules. These cells are mostly found in the center of islets and produce insulin, which increases uptake of glucose by most cells; reduces blood's glucose level.

   iii. *Delta cells*: 5%, with large argyrophil granules; form somatostatin, which inhibits insulin and glucagon release.

   iv. *F cells/PP cells*: Present in islets and among exocrine cells, making pancreatic polypeptide (PP), acts centrally on the brainstem to influence the vagal control of GI functions and liver.

For comparison between pancreas and parotid glands, *see* Table 30 given in Appendix I.

**Pernicious anemia (Biermer's anemia, Addison's anemia, or Addison-Biermer anemia)** It is a form of megaloblastic anemia due to vitamin $B_{12}$ deficiency. Vitamin $B_{12}$ cannot be produced by the human body, and must therefore be obtained from the diet. Normally, dietary vitamin $B_{12}$ can only be absorbed by the ileum, when it is bound by the intrinsic factor produced by the parietal cells. Because of impaired absorption of vitamin $B_{12}$ due to the absence of intrinsic factor (in atrophic gastritis, and in loss of gastric parietal cells) leads to this anemia.

**Ulcer** This refers to a site of inflammation where an epithelial surface (gastric epithelium, colonic mucosa, bladder epithelium) has become necrotic and eroded; it is often associated with subepithelial acute and chronic inflammation. The peptic ulcer of the stomach or duodenum shows the typical findings.

**Gastritis** It is not a single disease, but includes several different conditions that all have inflammation of the stomach lining. Gastritis can be caused by drinking too much alcohol, prolonged use of non-steroidal anti-inflammatory drugs (NSAIDs) such as aspirin or ibuprofen, or infection with bacteria such as *Helicobacter pylori* (*H. pylori*). Sometimes gastritis develops after major surgery, traumatic injury, burns, or severe infections. Certain diseases, such as pernicious anemia, autoimmune disorders, and chronic bile reflux can cause gastritis as well.

**Hirschsprung's disease or megacolon** It is a congenital disorder of the colon that occurs due to failure of neural crest cells to form the myenteric plexus within the sigmoid colon, and rectum. This results in loss of peristalsis in the colon distal to the normal innervated colon. Patients suffering from this disease come with faecal retention and distension of the abdomen.

**Diabetes** It is caused by impaired function of beta cells of islets of Langerhans. In this condition, these cells are unable to make the required amount of insulin. Persons suffering from this disease have high levels of blood glucose. The glucose may also get excreted from urine. If the disease remains untreated; it may lead to atherosclerosis, and partial blindness.

**Cirrhosis** It is a term that refers to a group of chronic diseases of the liver in which normal liver cells are damaged and replaced by scar tissue. The distortion of the normal liver structure by the scar tissue interferes with the flow of blood through the liver. The patient gradually becomes weak and develops jaundice due to the obstruction in the flow of bile. Cirrhosis is most commonly caused by alcoholism, hepatitis B & C and fatty liver disease, but has many other possible causes.

**Regeneration of liver** The liver has a remarkable capacity to regenerate after injury and to adjust its size to match its host. Within a week after partial hepatectomy, hepatic mass is back essentially to what it was prior to surgery. In the few cases where baboon livers have been transplanted into people, they quickly grow to the size of a human liver.

Hepatocytes or fragments of liver transplanted in extrahepatic locations remain quiescent but begin to proliferate after partial hepatectomy of the host. Partial hepatectomy leads to proliferation of all populations of cells within the liver, including hepatocytes, biliary epithelial cells and endothelial cells. DNA synthesis is initiated in these cells within 10 to 12 hours after surgery and essentially ceases in about 3 days. Cellular proliferation begins in the periportal region (i.e. around the portal triads) and proceeds toward the center of lobules. Proliferating hepatocytes initially form clumps, and clumps are soon transformed into classical plates. Similarly, proliferating endothelial cells become fenestrated typical of those seen in sinusoids.

**Chalones** Any of several polypeptides that are produced by a body tissue and cause the reversible inhibition of mitosis in the cells of that tissue are known as chalones. These have recently been found in the epidermis and in some other tissues. Recently, the use of such substances in the treatment of cancer has been suggested on the basis of experiments with transplanted tumors and small pieces of such tumors *in vitro*. It seems well documented that some tumors contain chalone-like substances and that the rate of proliferation in some tumors can be influenced by the tissue-specific chalone. However, from the present knowledge of chalones, it seems unlikely that they can be used in cancer therapy.

## Summary

1.

| Parameter | Filiform papilla | Fungiform papilla | Circumvallate papilla | Foliate papilla |
|---|---|---|---|---|
| Distribution | Anterior 2/3. These are most numerous papillae | Anterior 2/3 (among filiform). These are more numerous at tip | In front of and parallel to the sulcus terminalis | Posterolateral margin (rudimentary in men, but well developed in lagomorphs) |
| Shape | Conical (with keratinization on tip) | Like a mushroom | Dome shaped (surrounded by a circular sulcus) | Leaf-shaped |
| Secondary connective tissue papillae | On all surfaces | On all surfaces | Only on its top surface | On all surfaces |
| Taste buds | Absent | Few on the free surface | On the sides | On the sides |
| Glandular association | Absent | Present (serous) | Present (serous—von Ebner's gland) | Present (serous) |

2. In each tooth a visible crown projects above the gum or gingiva with roots buried in the alveolus of maxilla or mandible.

3. Dentin is the second hardest tissue in the body and forms the bulk of a tooth.

4. Enamel is a translucent substance and it is the hardest and most dense tissue of the body. It forms a protective covering of the teeth.

5. Cementum is a thin layer of bone-like material, but the Haversian system is absent.

6. Esophagus is lined by stratified squamous nonkeratinized epithelium. In the submucosa small groups of compound, tubulo-alveolar mucus secreting glands (esophageal glands) are present.

7.

| Parameter | Cardia | Fundus | Pylorus |
|---|---|---|---|
| Gland | Very short gland, ½ is body and ½ is duct | Tubular gland. Lower ¾ is secretory and upper ¼ is conducting | Coiled pyloric glands. Lower 1/3 is secretory and upper 2/3 is conducting |
| Cells of gland | Mucous cells and a few parietal cells | Undifferentiated, mucous neck, parietal, chief, and a few argentaffin cells | Mucous cells, and fewer parietal, and argentaffin cells |
| Muscularis externa | Inner oblique, middle circular, and outer longitudinal | Inner oblique, middle circular, and outer longitudinal | Circular muscle layer thickened to form pyloric sphincter |

8.

| Parameter | Duodenum | Jejunum | Ileum |
|---|---|---|---|
| Epithelium | Columnar epithelium with striated border and a few goblet cells are seen | Columnar epithelium with striated border and goblet cells are seen | Columnar epithelium with striated border and goblet cells are more in number |
| Villi | Broad, tall, and leaf-shaped villi | Villi have clubbed end | Villi are shorter and finger shaped |
| Lymphatic tissue in lamina propria | Scattered lymphocytes are present | Scattered lymphocytes, and a large number of lymphatic follicles are present | Peyer's patches are present |
| Submucosa | Mucus secreting Brunner's glands are typical feature | Only connective tissue, blood vessels, and nerves | Peyer's patches extend in the submucosa |

9.

| Parameter | Small intestine | Large intestine |
|---|---|---|
| Villi | Villi are present | Villi are absent |
| Crypts of Lieberkühn | Crypts of Lieberkühn are fewer and less deep | Crypts of Lieberkühn are deeper and more in number |
| Goblet cells | Goblet cells are less in number | Goblet cells are more in number |
| Taenia coli | Longitudinal coat of muscularis externa is uniformly thick | Longitudinal coat of muscularis externa is thickened to form three taenia coli |
| Sacculations | No sacculations | Taenia are shorter than the length of the large intestine, so sacculations appear |
| Appendices epiploicae | No appendices epiploicae | Peritoneal pouches filled with fat are present. These are called appendices epiploicae |

10. Appendix is a small, slender, blind diverticulum of the cecum. Villi are absent and only a few intestinal glands are present. The lining epithelium is simple columnar with striated border and the lamina propria is occupied by many lymphatic nodules that may extend up to the submucosa.

11. Parotid gland is having serous acini, in submandibular gland serous acini are more than mucous acini, while in sublingual gland mucous acini are predominantly present.

12. Liver is covered by a Glisson's capsule and its structural framework is formed by a delicate network of reticular fibers embedded in the extracellular matrix.

13. In the liver, blood flows from the periphery to the center and bile from center towards the periphery.

14. The liver acts as an exocrine gland by producing bile and acts as an endocrine gland by modification of the structure and function of many hormones.

15. Gall bladder is lined by mucosa, fibromuscular muscularis externa and serosa or adventitia.

16. The pancreas serves both exocrine and endocrine functions. These two components are very different structurally and functionally but are intermingled within the gland. The cells of the endocrine part are arranged in round-to-oval shaped areas rich in blood

vessels known as the islets of Langerhans and these are more in number in the tail region of the pancreas.

## Self Assessment

1. Which of the following glands has serous demilunes?
   a. Parotid            b. Submandibular
   c. Sebaceous          d. Pancreas

2. Which of the following organs has glands in its submucosa?
   a. Gall bladder       b. Duodenum
   c. Ileum              d. Large intestine

3. The goblet cells are absent in the:
   a. Jejunum            b. Large intestine
   c. Stomach            d. Trachea

4. Which of the following organs has both skeletal and smooth muscle fibers in the muscularis externa?
   a. Colon              b. Esophagus
   c. Stomach            d. Ileum

5. The α-cells of pancreas secrete:
   a. Insulin
   b. Glucagon
   c. Somatostatin
   d. Pancreatic polypeptide

6. Which of the following statements describes the papillae of the tongue?
   a. Circumvallate papillae contain taste buds
   b. Filiform papillae contain taste buds
   c. The predominant papillae present in the tongue is fungiform
   d. Fungiform papillae are keratinized on the top surface

7. Oxyntic cells are present in which organ?
   a. Esophagus
   b. Stomach
   c. Small intestine
   d. Pancreas

8. Mucous membrane is not formed by:
   a. Epithelium
   b. Lamina propria
   c. Muscularis mucosae
   d. Muscularis externa

9. Dentin of tooth is formed by which cells?
   a. Ameloblast         b. Cementoblast
   c. Odontoblast        d. Chondroblast

10. Portal triad is formed by:
    a. Bile duct          b. Portal vein
    c. Hepatic artery     d. All of the above

## Answers

1. b,    2. b,    3. c,    4. b,    5. b,    6. a,    7. b,    8. d,    9. c,
10. d

# 15

# Urinary System

The urinary system consists of paired kidneys and ureters and the unpaired urinary bladder and urethra. This system contributes to the maintenance of homeostasis by eliminating various waste metabolic products in the form of urine. The kidneys produce urine, control acid–base balance, maintain extracellular fluid volume and regulate total body water. Kidneys also act as an endocrine organ by producing two hormones: Erythropoietin and renin. Kidneys also convert vitamin D into an active form (calcitriol), which helps the body to absorb dietary calcium into the blood. Ureter conduct urine from the kidneys to the urinary bladder, which is responsible for temporary storage of urine and then it is released in the exterior by the urethra. The two kidneys receive a large volume of circulating blood because the renal arteries are large and they are direct branches of the abdominal aorta. About 1220 ml of blood enters the two kidneys each minute, from which 125 ml of glomerular filtrate is formed per minute; 124 ml is absorbed in the organ, and only 1 ml is released into the ureter as urine.

## KIDNEYS

These bean-shaped structures are 10 cm in length, 6.5 cm in breadth and 3 cm in thickness. These are covered by a dense, irregular collagenous capsule with some elastic fibers called the renal capsule. The renal artery and nerves enter the kidney on the medial border at a concavity known as the hilum, which also serves as the point of exit for the renal vein, lymphatics and ureter. The upper expanded part of the ureter is known as renal pelvis. Pelvis is divided into 2–3 major calyces, which further divide into 8–12 minor calyces. The kidney has an outer cortex and an inner medulla (Fig. 15.1).

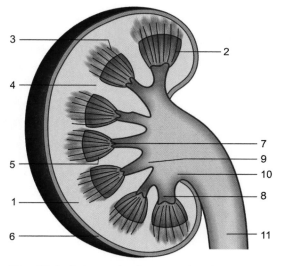

**Fig. 15.1:** Schematic diagram showing general organization of kidney. Cortex (1), medulla (2), medullary ray (3), renal column (4), medullary pyramid (5), capsule (6), renal papilla (7), minor calyx (8), major calyx (9), pelvis (10) and ureter (11)

The medulla consists of 10–18 conical structures, known as medullary pyramids. The broad base of each pyramid is directed towards the cortex and the apex (renal papilla) fits into a minor calyx. From the base of each pyramid parallel array of tubules, the medullary rays (of Ferrein) penetrate the cortex. The cortex at the margin of each pyramid extends inward between the pyramids as renal columns (columns of Bertin). The mass of cortical tissue surrounding each pyramid represents a renal lobe. Each medullary ray with the surrounding connective tissue is considered as a renal lobule.

Each kidney is composed of 1–4 million nephrons, which is the basic structural and functional unit of the kidney. A nephron and the collecting tubule into which it drains form a uriniferous (renal) tubule. The space between uriniferous tubules and blood vessels is known as the renal interstitium. It occupies a very small volume in the cortex, but increases in the medulla (Fig. 15.2).

Interstitium contains a small amount of connective tissue with fibroblasts and some collagen fibers. It is mainly present in the medulla and over there it contains interstitial cells and a highly hydrated ground substance rich in proteoglycans. Interstitial cells contain cytoplasmic lipid droplets and secrete pro-staglandin, which regulates the blood pressure.

## A. Nephron

Nephron consists of a dilated portion, the renal corpuscle: The proximal convoluted tubule (PCT), the loop of Henle and the distal convoluted tubule (DCT) (Fig. 15.3). The urine produced by the nephron is collected by collecting tubules and ducts, which conduct it to the renal pelvis. Renal corpuscles, greater parts of PCT and DCT, collecting tubules are located in the cortex in between the medullary rays, whereas loop of Henle and collecting

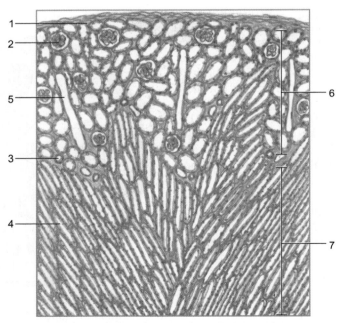

**Fig. 15.2:** Kidney at low magnification showing outer cortex (6) and inner medulla (7). Kidney is covered by a dense collagenous capsule (1). Glomerulus (2), arcuate artery (3), medullary ray (4) and interlobular artery (5) are also seen in the section

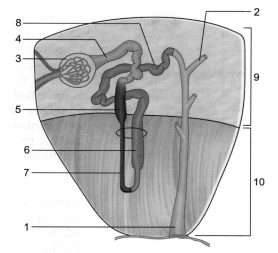

**Fig. 15.3:** Schematic diagram showing parts of a juxtamedullary nephron and its collecting duct (1) and tubule (2). Renal corpuscle (3), PCT (4), thick descending limb (5), thick ascending limb (6), thin limb (7), DCT (8), cortex (9) and medulla (10)

ducts lie in the medullary ray and in the substance of pyramid.

Nephrons produce urine, so functionally they correspond to the secretory part of other glands. The collecting ducts finally concentrate the urine and are similar to the ducts of other glands. Unlike the typical gland in which the secretory and duct portions arise from a single epithelial outgrowth, nephron and their collecting ducts arise from separate primordia and only later become connected. Nephron develops from a mass of inter-mediate mesoderm known as the metanephric blastema, whereas the collecting ducts are derivatives of the ureteric bud, an outgrowth of the mesonephric duct. Number of nephron decreases with age and a lost nephron can never be replaced.

Nephrons can be classified into cortical (subcapsular) and juxtamedullary, depending on the location of the renal corpuscle. All intergrades between these two extreme types occur. Cortical nephrons have their renal corpuscle in the superficial part of the cortex, while in the juxtamedullary

nephrons these are located near the base of the medullary pyramid. Approximately one-eighth of all nephrons are juxtamedullary nephrons. Juxtamedullary nephrons have very long Henle's loops, which extend up to the medulla. These loops consist of a long thin descending and ascending limbs. Cortical nephrons have short Henle's loops, which consists of short thin descending limbs and even thin ascending limbs are absent.

a. **Renal (Malpighian) corpuscle:** Each spherical corpuscle (diameter 200 µm) consists of a tuft of fenestrated capillaries; the glomerulus, surrounded by a double-walled epithelial capsule called Bowman's capsule. There is a narrow slit-like space (urinary or capsular space) in between the outer or parietal layer (capsular epithelium) and the inner or visceral layer (glomerular epithelium). This space receives the fluid filtered through the capillary wall and the visceral layer. Corpuscle has a vascular pole, where afferent and efferent arterioles enter and leave the glomerulus; and a urinary pole at the opposite side, where the proximal convoluted tubule begins (Fig. 15.4A, B). The parietal layer consists of simple squamous epithelium and at the urinary pole it changes to low columnar, which is a characteristic feature of the PCT. Cells of the visceral layer are close to the endothelial lining of capillaries (fenestrated but without diaphragm) and they become modified; known as podocytes. The podocytes contain actin filaments and lysosomes and they have both contractile and phagocytic functions. Each podocyte has a cell body, which gives rise to several primary processes. Each primary process gives rise to numerous small foot-like secondary processes, known as pedicles, that embraces the capillaries of the glomerulus. The pedicles of adjacent podocytes interdigitate with each other and thus completely surround the capillary loops of the glomerulus. The

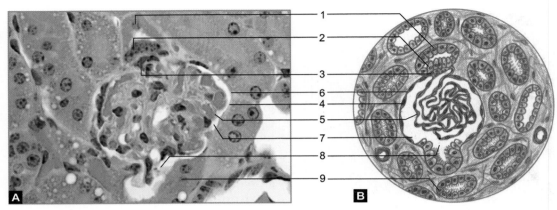

**Fig. 15.4:** Kidney: Cortex at high magnification, (A) micrograph, (B) sketch, showing capsular space (7) present in between the parietal (4) and visceral (5) layers of Bowman's capsule (6). PCT (9) and DCT (1) are clearly visible with their lining epithelium. Macula densa (2), juxtaglomerular cells (3) and urinary pole (8)

pedicles are separated from each other by narrow spaces called filtration slits, or slit pores (40 nm wide). These pores are occupied by a thin diaphragm, known as slit membrane (Fig. 15.5).

In between the endothelium of capillaries and podocytes; lies a basal lamina, which is manufactured by both cell populations. It is the thickest basal lamina in the body (300–370 nm). The basal lamina consists of three layers: A central electron-dense layer (lamina densa) and, on each side, a more electron-lucent layer (lamina rara). The two lamina rara contain fibronectin, while lamina densa is a meshwork of type IV

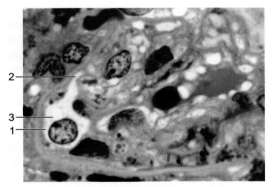

**Fig. 15.5:** Podocyte (1) with its foot processes (2) stain by iron hematoxylin. Its cytoplasm (3) appears clear

collagen and laminin in a matrix containing proteoglycan heparan sulfate. Fibronectin and laminin assist the pedicles and endothelial cells to maintain their attachment to the basal lamina.

Besides endothelial cells and podocytes, the glomerular capillaries have mesangial cells [lacis cells or cells of Goormaghtigh or polkissen (pole cushions)] adhering to their wall in places where the basal lamina forms a sheath that is shared by two or more capillaries (Fig. 15.6A, B).

These cells are stellate in shape with long cytoplasmic processes that contains numerous filaments. These cytoplasmic processes pass between the endothelial cells to reach the capillary lumen. These cells phagocytose large protein molecules and debris, which may accumulate during filtration or in certain disease states. These cells are contractile and have receptors for vasoconstrictors such as angiotensin II and thus reduce blood flow through the glomerulus. These cells also give structural support to the glomerulus. Similar to the mesengial cells, the extraglomerular mesengial cells, lie outside the glomerulus at the vascular pole and form part of the juxtaglomerular apparatus.

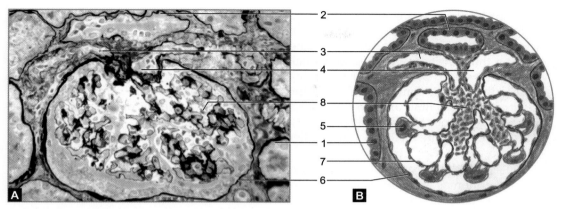

**Fig. 15.6:** Renal corpuscle-PAM + H and E stains, (A) micrograph, (B) sketch. PAM positive structures look black and these are glomerular basement membrane, glomerular capsule (6), the uriniferous tubule (1) and endothelial lining of afferent (3) and efferent (4) arteriole. Glomerular endothelial cells (7). DCT (2), podocyte (5) and mesengial cells (8) are also seen in the sections

- *The renal filtration barrier:* It is composed of the endothelium of the glomerular capillaries, the basal lamina and the filtration slits between pedicles. This barrier prevents passage of red blood cells, leukocytes, platelets and proteins of more than 70,000 d. It permits passage of water, ions and other small molecules from the bloodstream into the urinary space.

b. **Proximal convoluted tubule (PCT):** It follows a tortuous course and terminates by straightening out and passing into the nearest medullary ray, where it becomes continuous with the loop of Henle. At its commencement, there is a narrow region (neck) where a rapid transition from squamous (Bowman's capsule) to low columnar epithelium takes place. The cells of tubule are strongly eosinophilic (numerous mitochondria) with brush border and basal striations. The brush border is composed of long, closely packed microvilli with an extracellular glycocalyx, which gives them a physical and chemical protection. Basal striations are due to the extensive infolding of the basal plasma membrane, between which are numerous elongated mitochondria. The nucleus is large, spherical and centrally located. Prominent interdigitations are present along the lateral borders, which interlock adjacent cells. PCT is longer and more convoluted than DCT and forms the bulk of the cortex.

PCT is the initial and major site of reabsorption. It reabsorbs about 65% of the ultra-filtrate received from the urinary space of Bowman's capsule. In the cells of PCT, transmembrane proteins $Na^+/K^+$ ATPase are present on the lateral folds of plasma membranes. These proteins reabsorb $Na^+$ into the lateral intercellular space by active transport and in response of it $Cl^-$ is diffused. Thus NaCl accumulates in the lateral intercellular space which creates an osmotic gradient that draws water from the lumen into the intercellular compartment. In the plasma membrane water channel is present which allows the movement of water without requirement of energy from intercellular compartment to the cell. Almost 100% of the filtered glucose and amino acid is also reabsorbed by PCT. It also reabsorbs polypeptides from the lumen. It secretes organic acids, e.g. creatinine, bases and certain foreign substances into the filtrate, which has to be eliminated in the urine.

c. **Loop of Henle:** It is a U-shaped structure consisting of a thick descending limb (proximal straight tubule); a thin descending limb; a thin ascending limb; and a thick ascending limb. Structure of the thick descending limb is similar to PCT, but the cells of the thick limb are shorter, with a less well developed brush border (Fig. 15.7). Mitochondria in the thick limb are smaller than those of PCT.

Cells of thick limb are not as specialized for absorption as are those of PCT. In the outer medulla, the thick descending limb suddenly narrows and continuous as thin descending limb. The lumen of this segment is wide because the wall consists of squamous epithelial cells whose nuclei only slightly protrude in the lumen. A brush border is absent, but short, irregularly spaced microvilli are present. The epithelial cells of thin limb have simple junctional complexes with a few strands in the occluding junctions and simple infoldings of the basal cell membrane. The thin limb even closely resembles the blood capillaries. The thin ascending limb of the loop is also composed of squamous epithelial cells, but with more extensive junctional complexes than the descending limb. As the thin ascending limb approaches the transition to the thick portion, the cell borders become more irregular. The thick ascending limb closely resembles in structure to DCT; however, the height of the cells is shorter, so the lumen is wider. A few short, apical microvilli are present, but there is no brush border.

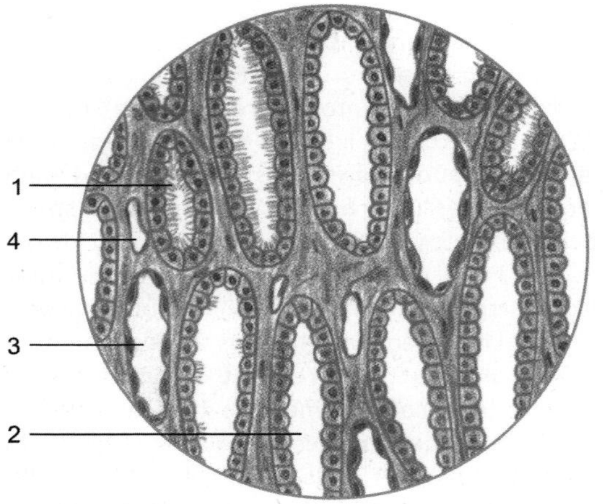

> **Loop of Henle** mainly generates a high osmotic pressure in the extracellular fluid of the renal medulla by counter-current exchange multiplier system. Thin descending limb of the loop is freely permeable to water and reabsorbs water by osmosis. It is much less permeable to solutes like NaCl and urea. Thin ascending limb is highly permeable to NaCl but impermeable to water as the salt concentration increases in interstitium. Thus hypertonicity created in the medullary interstitium by Henle's loop influences the concentration of the urine.
>
> Thick ascending limb is also impermeable to water. The apical cell allowed the movements of $Cl^-$, $Na^+$ and $K^+$ between the cell and the lumen. $Na^+$ is actively transported by $Na^+/K^+$ATPase pump, while $Cl^-$ and $K^+$ diffuse out by $Cl^-$ and $K^+$ channels.

**Fig. 15.7:** Ducts of the medullary region. Thick segment of loop of Henle (1), collecting tubule (2), thin segment of loop of Henle (3) and vasa recta (4)

d. **Distal convoluted tubule:** When the thick ascending limb penetrates the cortex, it becomes tortuous and is known as DCT. It is lined by simple cuboidal epithelium without any brush border, but basal striations are present. Cytoplasm is less eosinophilic and the lumen is larger in comparison to PCT.

Along the path in the cortex, it establishes contact with the vascular pole of the corpuscle of its parent nephron. At the point of contact, cells of the DCT are taller and narrower than adjacent tubular cells. The nuclei of these cells are closer together and more prominent, so this region appears dark under microscope and is known as macula densa.

**DCT** is the major site of salt and water control in the body. It reabsorbs sodium ions from the filtrate and actively transports them into the renal interstitium; this process is stimulated by aldosterone. It also transfers potassium, ammonium and hydrogen ions into the filtrate from the interstitium. Macula may monitor the osmolarity and volume of the fluid in the DCT and transmit this information to juxtaglomerular cells via the gap junctions existing between the two cell types.

For comparison between proximal and distal convoluted tubule, *see* Table 31 given in Appendix I.

## B. Collecting Tubules and Ducts

Urine passes from the DCT to collecting tubules that join each other to form larger straight collecting ducts; the papillary ducts of Bellini, which gradually widen as an approach to the tips of the pyramids. Collecting tubules have segments in cortex as well as in the medulla, which join to form larger tubules.

Cortical collecting tubules are located primarily within medullary rays, although a few are interspersed among the convoluted tubules in the cortex. These are lined by simple cuboidal epithelium containing two types of cells: Principal (light) cells and intercalated (dark) cells. Principal cells are cuboidal with centrally-placed round nuclei and a light staining cytoplasm. The cell boundaries of these cells are very distinct. Short, scattered microvilli are present at the apex and the basal plasma membrane has many infoldings. Intercalated cells are less in number. These cells have numerous mitochondria and more intense staining cytoplasm.

In the outer medulla, medullary collecting tubules are similar in structure to cortical collecting tubules and contain both types of cells. In the inner medulla, the collecting tubules are lined only by principal cells. Papillary ducts are large collecting tubules and they open at the area cribrosa of the renal papilla to deliver the urine into the minor calyx of the kidney. These ducts are lined by simple columnar epithelium.

**Collecting tubules** The filtrate that enters the collecting tubule is hypotonic. Light cells have abundance of ADH-regulated water channels. So, in the absence of antidiuretic hormone (ADH), the cells of the collecting tubule are completely impermeable to water. However, in the presence of ADH, they become permeable to water. So, the urine becomes concentrated (hypertonic).

## C. Juxtaglomerular Apparatus

Adjacent to the renal corpuscle, the tunica media of afferent arteriole consists of specialized smooth muscle cells containing secretory granules. These cells are known as juxtaglomerular cells (JG cells). The macula densa of DCT is located close to the region of afferent arteriole containing JG cells. The JG cells and the macula densa are collectively called juxtaglomerular apparatus. It also includes mesangial and extraglomerular mesengial cells. JG cells are the source of the erythropoietin and enzyme renin (proteolytic).

**Erythropoietin** stimulates the production of RBCs in red bone marrow. Thus it helps to regulate the concentration of erythrocytes in the blood. When rennin is released into the blood, it acts on a plasma protein known as angiotensinogen and converts it into angiotensin I. An enzyme from the endothelial cells of lung capillaries called angiotensin-converting enzyme (ACE), then converts angiotensin I to angiotensin II, which acts upon the zona glomerulosa of the adrenal cortex and stimulates it to release aldosterone. Aldosterone acts on the distal tubule and increases the absorption of sodium and chloride ions. Angiotensin II reduces the luminal diameter of blood vessels, thus constricting the efferent glomerular arterioles and elevates blood pressure within the glomerulus.

## D. Blood Supply of Kidney

Kidneys are highly vascular organs; they receive approximately 25% of the cardiac output. Approximately 90–95% of the blood passing through the kidney is in the cortex; 5–10% is in the medulla. At the hilum, the renal artery divides into a few segmental arteries, which further form interlobar arteries. The interlobar arteries are located in between the pyramids. At the base of pyramid these arteries form arcuate arteries, which form an arch over the base of the pyramid. The interlobular arteries branch off at right angles from the arcuate arteries (Fig. 15.8) and then run into the cortex perpendicular to the renal capsule. From interlobular arteries arise the afferent arterioles, which divide into primary branches that further divide into capillaries and form renal glomerulus. Glomerulus is a rete mirabile, interrupting an arteriole in its course.

> **Rete mirabile** is a capillary-like plexus inserted in the course of an arteriole or venule. It is a 'marvelous network' because an afferent arteriole (or venule) feeds blood to it and an efferent arteriole (or venule) drains it. Rete is uncommon in mammal; however, an arteriolar example is the renal glomerulus.

Blood is drained from glomerulus by efferent arterioles. Lumen of efferent arteriole is smaller than afferent since it is carrying less blood; because of this a pressure gradient is created which causes active filtration driving many components of blood in the urinary space. The efferent arterioles of cortical nephrons branch and form a peritubular capillary plexus around the convoluted tubules, whereas the efferent arterioles of the juxtamedullary nephrons give rise to long straight, thin capillary vessels, called vasa recta that pass into the medulla and loop back towards the corticomedullary junction. These looped blood vessels play an important role in maintaining the osmotic gradient of the interstitium of the medulla. These vessels join other vessels in the cortex to form stellate veins, which empty into the interlobular veins. Blood from interlobular veins flows into arcuate veins and from there to the interlobar veins. Interlobar veins converge to form the renal vein through which blood leaves the kidney.

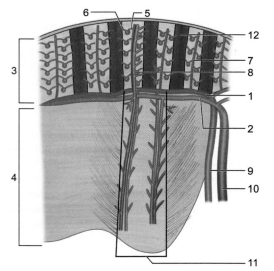

**Fig. 15.8:** Schematic diagram showing circulation of blood in the kidney. Arcuate arteries (1) and veins (2) are seen in the border between the cortex (3) and the medulla (4). Afferent arteriole (5), efferent arteriole (6), interlobular artery (7), interlobular vein (8), interlobar artery (9), interlobar vein (10), renal lobule (11) and medullary ray (12)

## URETER

The lining of the mucosa is transitional epithelium (4–5 layers thick) supported by a collagenous lamina propria. Mucosa has several longitudinal folds, giving the lumen a stellate shape in the cross-section (Fig. 15.9). There is no boundary between lamina propria and the deeper submucosa.

The muscularis externa is thick and consist of bundles of smooth muscle fibers separated by strands of connective tissue. These smooth muscle fibers are arranged in two layers: Inner longitudinal and outer circular; in addition to this, the middle and lower part of ureter has an extra, outer longitudinal coat. These three

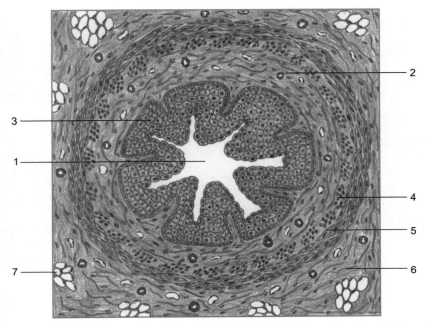

**Fig. 15.9:** TS of ureter with stellate-shaped lumen (1) and lined by transitional epithelium (3). Lamina propria (2), inner longitudinal layer (4), outer circular layer (5), adventitia (6) and fat cells (7)

layers of muscles are not well defined and difficult to be mark off from each other. The connective tissue adventitia, rich in vessels and nerves surrounds the ureter. The distal end of the ureters, the intramural portion, passes obliquely through the wall of the bladder to empty into its lumen. When the bladder fills with urine, because of oblique path of ureter, its wall are pressed together and it thus prevents backflow of urine. The circular layer of smooth muscle disappears and the contractions of the longitudinal layers help in dilatation of the lumen of the distal ureter so that urine can enter in the bladder.

## URINARY BLADDER

In the empty bladder the mucous membrane is thrown into numerous folds (rugae), which disappear when the bladder is distended. The lining of the mucosa is transitional epithelium supported by a wide collagenous lamina propria without glands (Fig. 15.10A, B).

Epithelium of empty bladder is 6–8 layers thick and superficial cells are low cuboidal or columnar and appear dome-shaped. Also, some superficial cells may be binucleated. In distended bladder, epithelium is 2–3 layers thick and superficial cells appear squamous due to stretching. Apical plasma membranes of superficial surface cells have unusually thick plaques and apical cytoplasm contains fusiform vesicles. The lateral borders of these cells are connected by desmosomes and tight junctions. All these features make the epithelium impermeable to urine. Three smooth muscle tunics, i.e. transverse, oblique and longitudinal interweave in the muscularis externa and are difficult to distinguish. Contraction of these muscle tunics, also called detrusor muscle, is responsible for emptying of the bladder. A connective tissue adventitia having blood vessels, lymphatic vessels, nerve fibers and ganglion cells surround the bladder. The part of the bladder facing the pelvic cavity (superior surface) has a serosa.

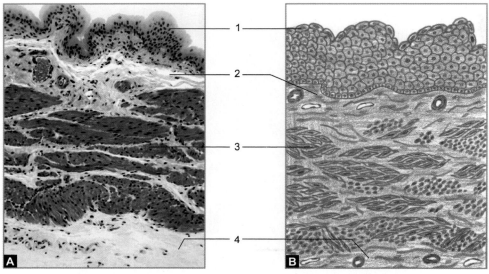

**Fig. 15.10:** Urinary bladder, (A) micrograph, (B) sketch, lined by transitional epithelium (1) and having thick muscle coat made up of smooth muscle fibers (3) running in transverse, oblique and longitudinal direction. Lamina propria (2) and adventitia (4)

## URETHRA

The urethra is a tube that carries the urine from the bladder to the exterior. In the male, sperm also passes through it during ejaculation, while in the females it is only a passage for urine.

### A. Male Urethra

It consists of 3 parts: Prostatic, membranous and spongy. Prostatic part is lined by transitional epithelium but changes to a pseudostratified columnar or stratified columnar in the rest of the urethra. The terminal dilatation (fossa navicularis) of the urethra is lined by stratified squamous epithelium. A few mucus secreting goblet cells are present. Lamina propria is present, made up of loose, fibroelastic connective tissue. The mucosa shows invaginations or recesses into which the mucous glands (Littre's gland) open. These glands are found along the entire length, but most numerous on the terminal urethra. The submucosa consists of loose connective tissue. The muscular coat consists of outer circular and inner longitudinal layers of smooth muscle

fibers and well defined only in the membranous and prostatic parts. The spongy part is surrounded only by occasional fibers. The membranous part is also surrounded by striated muscle that forms the external urethral sphincter (Fig. 15.11A, B).

### B. Female Urethra

It is structurally similar to the male urethra but it is much shorter than that. The lining epithelium is mainly stratified columnar or pseudostratified. Although in the proximal part it is lined by transitional epithelium, while in the terminal part the lining epithelium is stratified squamous nonkeratinized (Fig. 15.12).

Lamina propria, Littre's glands and submucosa are present. Lamina propria contains an extensive venous plexus, so it resembles the corpus spongiosum in the male. The muscle coat consists of an outer circular and an inner longitudinal layer of smooth muscle fibers. External urethral sphincter is surrounded by striated muscle.

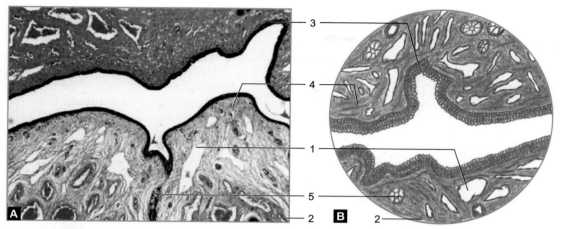

**Fig. 15.11:** Male urethra—spongy part, (A) micrograph, (B) sketch, lined with stratified columnar epithelium (3). In the lamina propria (4) lies mucus secreting Littre's gland (5). Cavernous sinus (1) and trabeculae (2)

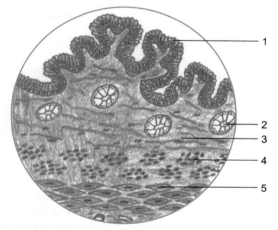

**Fig. 15.12:** Female urethra, lined by stratified columnar epithelium (1). Littre's gland (2), lamina propria (3), inner longitudinal layer (4) and outer circular layer (5)

## Summary

1. The kidney has an outer cortex and an inner medulla.

2. Each kidney is composed of 1–4 million nephrons, which is the basic structural and functional unit of the kidney.

3. Nephron consists of a dilated portion, the renal corpuscle: PCT, the loop of Henle and DCT. The urine produced by the nephron is collected by collecting tubules and ducts, which conduct it to the renal pelvis.

4. Renal corpuscles, the greater parts of PCT and DCT, collecting tubules are located in the cortex in between the medullary rays, whereas loop of Henle and collecting ducts lie in the medullary ray and in the substance of pyramid.

5. Nephrons can be classified into cortical (subcapsular) or juxtamedullary, depending on the location of the renal corpuscle.

6. Renal (Malpighian) corpuscle consists of a tuft of fenestrated capillaries; the glomerulus, surrounded by a double-walled epithelial capsule called Bowman's capsule.

7. The renal filtration barrier is composed of the endothelium of the glomerular capillaries, the basal lamina and the filtration slits between pedicles.

8. The cells of PCT are strongly eosinophilic (numerous mitochondria) with brush border and basal striations.

9. Loop of Henle is a U-shaped structure consisting of a thick descending limb (proximal straight tubule); a thin

descending limb; a thin ascending limb; and a thick ascending limb.

10. DCT is lined by simple cuboidal epithelium without any brush border, but basal striations are present. Cytoplasm is less eosinophilic and the lumen is larger in comparison to PCT.

11. The JG cells and the macula densa are collectively called juxtaglomerular apparatus. It also includes mesangial and extraglomerular mesengial cells. JG cells are the source of the erythropoietin and enzyme renin (proteolytic).

12. The lining of the mucosa in the ureter is transitional epithelium (4–5 layers thick) supported by a collagenous lamina propria. Mucosa has several longitudinal folds, giving the lumen a stellate shape in the cross-section.

13. In the empty bladder the mucous membrane is thrown into numerous folds (rugae), which disappear when the bladder is distended. The lining of the mucosa is transitional epithelium supported by a wide collagenous lamina propria without glands.

## Self Assessment

1. The number of nephron in one kidney is approximately:
   a. One million    b. Ten million
   c. Ten thousand   d. Fifty thousand

2. Glomerular capillaries are lined by:
   a. Fenestrated endothelium
   b. Continuous endothelium
   c. Simple columnar
   d. None of the above

3. In renal cortex all of the following structures are present EXCEPT:
   a. Proximal convoluted tubule
   b. Distal convoluted tubule
   c. Renal corpuscle
   d. Thick segment of loop of Henle

4. Macula densa is seen in:
   a. Afferent arteriole
   b. Efferent arteriole
   c. Proximal convoluted tubule
   d. Distal convoluted tubule

5. JG cells:
   a. Secrete rennin
   b. Produce glomerular filtrate
   c. Secrete erythropoietin
   d. Support the glomerulus

6. Aldosterone acts on:
   a. Proximal convoluted tubule
   b. Distal convoluted tubule
   c. Collecting duct
   d. Collecting tubule

7. Urinary bladder is lined by which epithelium?
   a. Stratified squamous keratinized
   b. Transitional
   c. Stratified columnar
   d. Stratified cuboidal

8. Shape of lumen of ureter is:
   a. Triangular    b. Circular
   c. Star          d. Oval

9. Urothelium is another name used for which epithelium?
   a. Transitional
   b. Stratified columnar
   c. Stratified cuboidal
   d. Pseudostratified

10. Ducts of Bellini are present in:
    a. Kidney
    b. Ureter
    c. Urinary bladder
    d. Urethra

## Answers

1. a,    2. a,    3. d,    4. d,    5. a,    6. b,    7. b,    8. c,    9. a,
10. a

# 16

# Male Reproductive System

The male reproductive system consists of a pair of testes, accessory genital glands, their ducts and penis. The accessory genital glands are the paired seminal vesicles, the single prostate gland, and the two bulbourethral glands (of Cowper).

## TESTES

These are bilateral compound tubular gonads, lying outside the body within a common musculocutaneous sac, the scrotum. The temperature of the testis is about 3–4°C lower than the normal body temperature. This lower temperature is necessary for functioning of testis, i.e. production of sperm. Besides the external location of the testes, the evaporation of sweat from the scrotal surface also contributes to maintain the lower temperature of the testes. Special arrangements of blood vessels are also helpful in maintaining lower temperature. Each testis is supplied by a testicular artery, which is surrounded by the pampiniform plexuses of veins. The cooler venous blood returning from the testis cools the arterial blood before it enters in testis through the counter-current heat exchange mechanism between arterial and venous blood.

In adult human testes are about 5 cm in length, 2.5 cm in width and weighs about 10–15 gm. Testes serve as both exocrine (production of spermatozoa) and endocrine (production of testosterone) gland. Each testis is covered on the anterior and lateral side by a simple squamous epithelium, known as visceral layer of the tunica vaginalis. On the posterior surface of the testis, this epithelium reflects onto and lines the scrotum to form the parietal layer of the tunica vaginalis. The serous cavity between the visceral and parietal layers allows the testis to move freely and reduces the chance of injury due to increased pressure on the external surface of the scrotum. Deep to the visceral layer, whole testis is covered by a white fibrous capsule made by dense connective tissue known as the tunica albuginea (Fig. 16.1).

On the posterior surface of the testis, the tunica albuginea thickens and projects inward as the mediastinum testis. Blood vessels, lymphatic vessels and genital excretory ducts pass through the mediastinum as they enter or leave the testis. Septa extending internally from the tunica albuginea incompletely divide the stroma into about 250 lobules. The tunica vasculosa is vascular, loose connective tissue layer present beneath the tunica albuginea and lines the lobules. Lobules are pyramidal in shape with their apices directed towards the mediastinum and their bases directed towards the surface of the testis. Each lobule contains 1–4 convoluted seminiferous tubules, which are 30–70 cm long with a diameter of 150–250 μm. Tubules are separated from one

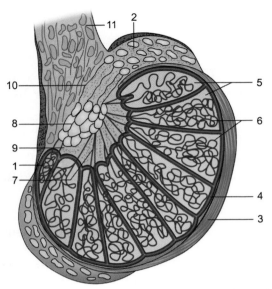

**Fig. 16.1:** Schematic diagram showing testis (1) and epididymis (2). Tunica vaginalis (3), tunica albuginea (4), lobule of testis (5), seminiferous tubules (6), tubulus rectus (7), rete testis (8), mediastinum (9), efferent ductules (10) and spermatic cord (11)

another by a connective tissue stroma, which contains blood and lymphatic vessels, nerves and interstitial (Leydig) cells (Fig. 16.2A, B).

Each seminiferous tubule is lined by a stratified epithelium, which acts as germinal epithelium consisting of 4 to 8 cell layers. These layers contain spermatogenic cells and Sertoli cells (Fig. 16.3A, B). Epithelium rests on a fine basement membrane containing elastic fibers and collagen fibers, which is surrounded by 3–4 layers of smooth muscle cells (myoid cells). This basement membrane thickens with age.

The process by which spermatogonia (first spermatogenic cells) divide, differentiate and mature to form spermatozoa is called spermatogenesis. In man spermatogenic cycle requires 64 days. Spermatogenesis does not occur simultaneously or synchronized in all seminiferous tubules, but rather occur in wave-like sequences of maturation, referred as cycles of the seminiferous epithelium. During spermatogenesis, daughter cells remain connected to each other via intercellular bridges. The resultant syncytium may be responsible for the synchronous development of germ cells along any one seminiferous tubule.

Each seminiferous tubule continues near the mediastinum into a straight tubule, a tubulus rectus, which enters in the mediastinum and form an anastomosing network of tubes, the rete testis. Straight tubule is lined by simple cuboidal epithelium whose cells resemble Sertoli cells. Rete testis is lined by single layer of cuboidal to low

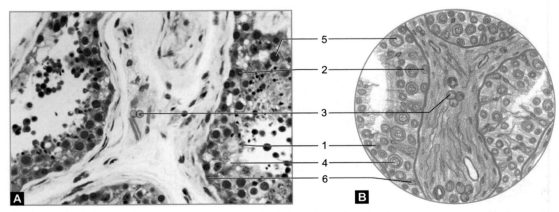

**Fig. 16.2:** Seminiferous tubules, (A) micrograph, (B) sketch, showing both spermatogenic and Sertoli cells (6). Spermatogenic cells are spermatogonia (2), spermatocyte (5) and spermatids (1). In between the seminiferous tubules (4) lies interstitial cells of Leydig (3)

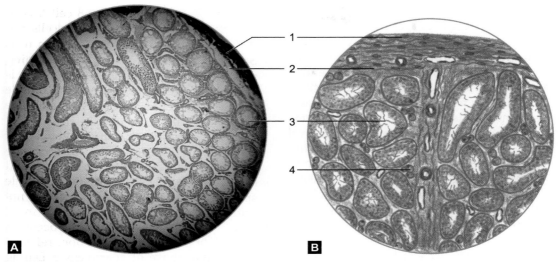

**Fig. 16.3:** Testis at low magnification, (A) micrograph, (B) sketch showing sections of seminiferous tubules (3). Each testis is enclosed in tunica albuginea (1) and beneath it lies tunica vasculosa (2). Interstitial cells (4) lie in between the seminiferous tubules

columnar cells (Fig. 16.4A, B). These cells have a single apical cilium and relatively a few short apical microvilli.

## SPERMATOGENESIS

It is the process by which spermatogonia divide and mature to form sperms. This process includes 2 phases: Spermatocytogenesis and spermiogenesis. Spermatogenesis is regulated by follicle stimulating hormone (FSH) and luteinizing-hormone (LH). FSH stimulates the seminiferous epithelium and LH stimulates testosterone production by Leydig cells in the interstitial tissue.

### A. Spermatocytogenesis

a. **Spermatogonia:** Primordial germ cells migrate from the yolk sac into the developing

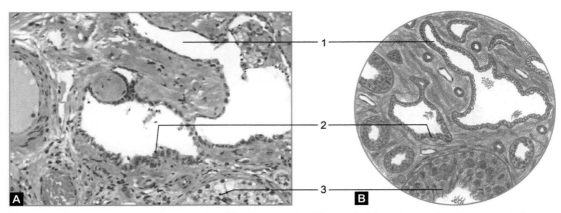

**Fig. 16.4:** Straight tubule and rete testis, (A) micrograph, (B) sketch. Near the mediastinum seminiferous tubules (3) continues into straight tubule (2), which form an anastomosing network in the mediastinum, called rete testis (1)

gonads, where they divide and differentiate into spermatogonia. Spermatogonia are the diploid germ cells (10–12 μm in diameter) and remain dormant until puberty. They are always in contact with the basement membrane of the tubule. These are of three types: Dark type A, pale type A and type B spermatogonia. Dark type A spermatogonia are dome-shaped cells. These cells have oval nuclei with abundant heterochromatin, giving a dense appearance to the nucleus. These cells are reserve cells, which are not entered in the cell cycle but may do so. Once they undergo mitosis, they form additional dark type A as well as pale type A spermatogonia. Pale type A spermatogonia are identical to the dark type A, except that their nuclei have abundant euchromatin, giving them a pale appearance. These cells are induced by testosterone to proliferate and divide by mitosis to give rise to additional pale type A and type B spermatogonia. Type B spermatogonia resemble the pale type A, but usually their nuclei are round rather than oval. These cells also divide mitotically to give rise to primary spermatocytes. Spermatogonia remain connected to each other by cytoplasmic bridges during spermatogenesis.

b. **Primary spermatocytes:** These diploid cells lie in the cell layer luminal to the spermatogonia and appear larger than that. They immediately enter the prophase of the first meiotic division and have a prolonged prophase (up to 22 days). Cell divisions, from the formation of primary spermatocytes and onwards, are incomplete. The cells remain connected by bridges of cytoplasm. The completion of the first meiotic division results in the formation of secondary spermatocytes.

c. **Secondary spermatocytes:** These haploid cells are smaller than primary spermatocytes. They rapidly enter and complete the second meiotic division, which results in the formation of spermatids. These cells are

present for only eight hours of the entire 64 days spermatogenic cycle; therefore, very few are present in a section.

d. **Spermatids:** These cells lie in the luminal part of the seminiferous epithelium. The spermatids are about one-half the size of the secondary spermatocyte. Initially, they have a very light eccentric nucleus. Early spermatids are spherical in shape, whereas late spermatids develop flagella and acrosomal caps. Spermatids do not divide but undergo cytodifferentiation to form spermatozoa. Intercellular cytoplasmic bridges now break down.

## B. Spermiogenesis

The terminal phase of spermatogenesis is called spermiogenesis and consists of the differentiation of the newly formed spermatids into spermatozoa. It occurs in 4 stages: Golgi, cap, acrosome and maturational (Fig. 16.5).

a. **Golgi stage:** During this stage the polarity of the spermatids is established. The acrosomal vesicle (rich in glycoproteins)

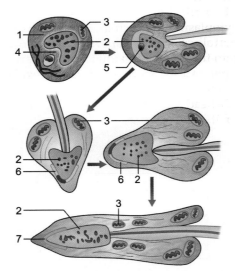

**Fig. 16.5:** Schematic diagram showing principal changes occurring in spermatid (1) during spermiogenesis. Nucleus (2), mitochondria (3), acrosome granules (4), acrosome vesicle (5), acrosomal cap (6) and acrosome (7)

develops from the Golgi complex. These vesicles come into contact with the nuclear envelope and bound to it and mark the anterior (head) pole of the sperm. Following this, the centrioles leave the vicinity of the nucleus. Then they migrate to the opposite end to establish the posterior pole and initiate the formation of flagellum.

b. **Cap stage:** During this stage the acrosomal vesicle spreads over the nucleus as the acrosomal cap. The portion of the nuclear envelope beneath the acrosomal cap loses its pores and become thicker. The nucleus also begins to condense and the flagellum starts to form.

c. **Acrosome stage:** During this stage the spermatid re-orients, so the flagellum projects into the lumen and the acrosome points towards the basal lamina. The nucleus flattens and elongates and the cytoplasm moves towards the posterior side to concentrate the mitochondria around the flagellum. The centrioles migrate again and come to the posterior surface of the nucleus and form the connecting piece (neck).

d. **Maturational stage:** During this stage excess cytoplasm is shed off and phagocytosed by Sertoli cells. The spermatids are released into the lumen as spermatozoa or sperm.

e. **Spermatozoa (sperm):** The newly released human sperm is nonmotile. It is composed of a head and a tail, which accounts for most of its length. The head of the sperm is flattened and surrounded by plasmalemma. The head contains the nucleus and the acrosome, which covers the anterior aspect of the nucleus. Acrosome contains various enzymes, like hyaluronidase, neuraminidase, acid phosphatase and a trypsin-like protease known as acrosin. These enzymes are essential for penetration of the zona pellucida of the ovum. As the sperm touches the egg, the acrosomal enzymes are released and this is known as acrosome reaction. This process facilitates sperm penetration and subsequent fertilization. The tail of the sperm is subdivided into four parts: Neck, middle piece, principal piece and end piece. The neck connects the head to the middle piece. It contains the centrioles and the connecting piece, which is attached to the nine outer dense fibers of the middle piece. The middle piece extends from the neck to the annulus, which is a ring-like, dense structure to which the plasmalemma adheres. It contains a spirally arranged sheath of mitochondria, which encircles the nine outer dense fibers and the central most axoneme. Axoneme consists of 9 + 2 arrangement of microtubules. The principal piece extends from the annulus to the end piece and contains the axoneme with its surrounding dense fibers, which in turn are encircled by a fibrous sheath. The end piece consists of the axoneme and the surrounding plasma membrane (Fig. 16.6).

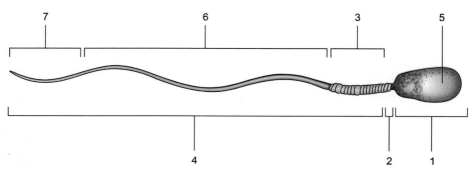

**Fig. 16.6:** Schematic diagram showing the structure of a mature spermatozoon. Head (1), neck (2), middle piece (3), tail (4), acrosome (5), principal piece (6) and end piece (7)

## C. Sertoli (Sustentacular) Cells

These are far less numerous than the sper-matogenic cells and are evenly distributed between them. These are columnar, non-replicating (post-mitotic) supporting cells that extend from the basement membrane to the lumen. The processes of the cells extend in between the spermatogenic cells. The nucleus is large oval or triangular in shape and its long axis is oriented perpendicular to the wall of the tubule (Fig. 16.7). Lateral processes of Sertoli cells are interconnected by tight junctions, which may be the structural basis for the blood–testis barrier.

Spermatogonia and primary spermatocytes are located in the basal compartment; other cellular stages of spermatogenesis are located in the luminal compartment. Because spermatogenesis begins after puberty, the newly differentiating germ cells, which have a different chromosome number as well as expressing different surface membrane receptors and molecules, it would be con-sidered "foreign cells" by the immune system. Thus the barrier protects the developing sperm cells from immunological attack. The passage of spermatogenic cells from the basal into the luminal compartment occurs via the formation of a new junctional complex between Sertoli cell processes that extend beneath the newly formed spermatocytes, followed by the breakdown of the junction above them.

a. **Functions of sertoli cells**

    i. These cells provide physical support, protection and nutrition for the different stages of spermatogenic cells.

    ii. These cells form blood–testis barrier, thus protect the spermatogenic cells from autoimmune destruction.

    iii. During spermiogenesis, excess cyto-plasm is shed as residual bodies. These cytoplasmic fragments are phagocytosed and digested by Sertoli cell lysosomes.

    iv. These cells serve as nurse cells and secrete a fructose-rich medium that nourishes and facilitates the transport of spermatozoa to the genital ducts.

    v. These cells control the release of mature sperm, into the lumen of seminiferous tubules.

    vi. These cells also secrete androgen-binding protein (ABP) into the luminal compartment under the influence of FSH to elevate the concentration of testosterone, where it is necessary for spermatogenesis. On the plasma membrane of Sertoli cells, receptors for follicle stimulating hormone (FSH) are present.

    vii. These cells secrete inhibin, a hormone that inhibits the synthesis and release of FSH by the anterior pituitary.

    viii. During embryonic development the Sertoli cells secrete a glycoprotein, the anti-Müllerian hormone (AMH) that promotes regression of the Müllerian ducts in males and inhibits the develop-ment of female reproductive organs.

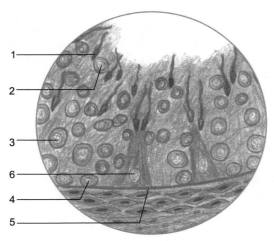

**Fig. 16.7:** Seminiferous tubules at high magnification. Sperm (1), spermatid (2), spermatocyte (3), spermatogonia (4), basement membrane (5) and sertoli cells (6)

## D. Stroma

It consists of collagen fibrils, capillaries, lymphatic, myoid cells and interstitial (Leydig) cells. The myoid cells are contractile cells that also produce the collagen of the stroma; their peristaltic contractions propel the newly formed spermatozoa through the seminiferous tubules. The Leydig cells are the testosterone producing endocrine cells located in the spaces between adjoining tubules. These cells are large, polyhedral or round in shape and found in clusters (Fig. 16.8A, B). The nucleus is large, round and often eccentric in position.

The cytoplasm is eosinophilic and possesses cytological features of steroid producing cells, such as extensive smooth endoplasmic reticulum, large numbers of lipid droplets and mitochondria with tubular cristae. As the lipid is removed during cell processing, so the cytoplasm stains lightly. The lipid droplets contain cholesterol esters, which are precursors of testosterone. In the cytoplasm rod-shaped crystalloids (Reinke's crystalloids) are also present.

Interstitial cells Both the activity and the number of the interstitial cells depends on hormonal stimuli. During pregnancy, placental gonadotropic hormone passes from the maternal blood to the male fetus, which stimulates the abundant fetal testicular interstitial cells to produce androgenic hormones. The presence of these hormones is required for the embryonic differentiation of the male genitalia. The embryonic interstitial cells remain fully differentiated up to 4 months of gestation; after that they regress, with an associated decrease in testosterone synthesis. They remain inactive throughout the rest of the pregnancy and up to the prepubertal period, when they restart testosterone synthesis in response to the stimulus of luteinizing hormone (LH) from the hypophysis.

## EXCRETORY GENITAL DUCTS

After production in the testis, spermatozoa pass through a series of ducts in their journey out of the male reproductive system. These ducts are:

### A. Epididymis

It is a 6 meters long highly coiled tube and lies along the superior and posterior surfaces of the testis. Along with connective tissue and muscle, it coils to form the head, body and tail of the epididymis, which then continues as the ductus deferens. 10–15 efferent ductules emerge from the mediastinum testis and unite the rete testis with the head of the epididymis. Efferent ductules are lined by ciliated tall columnar cells and cuboidal cells. Ciliated cells propel spermatozoa toward the epididymis, while cuboidal cells absorb testicular fluid. The lumen of ductule is irregular due to the difference in the height of the cells. One or two layers of smooth muscle fibers surround

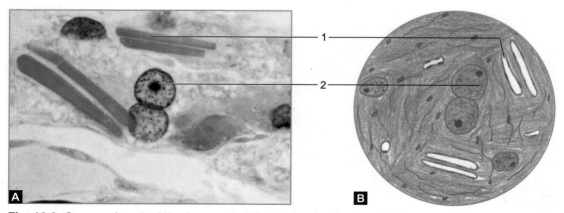

**Fig. 16.8:** Stroma of testis, (A) micrograph, (B) sketch, showing lymphatic capillary (1) and interstitial cells (2)

each ductule and help in the propulsion of spermatozoa (Fig. 16.9A, B).

Epididymis is lined by pseudostratified columnar epithelium consisting of basal and principal cells. The principal cells are columnar cells with basally placed oval nuclei. These cells have stereocilia projecting into the lumen. Stereocilia, decreases in height from head to tail regions. Basal cells lie in between the basement membrane and principal cells. These are pyramidal cells with rounded nuclei and act as stem cells to produce themselves as well as the principal cells as the need arises. The epithelium rests on the basal lamina. It is surrounded by a thin layer of circumferential smooth muscle that elaborates and thickens along the length of the duct so that in the tail it is tri-laminar (Fig. 16.10 A to C).

Epididymis absorbs excess testicular fluid and thus helps in movement of sperm towards the ductus deferens. In the proximal part of epididymis, spontaneous peristaltic contractions are present that slowly transport sperm through the epididymis. In the distal part the contractions are reduced, so this part stores the sperm while they undergo maturation to become mature sperm. Epididymis also phagocytose defective sperms and the residual bodies that were not removed by Sertoli cells. The principal cells secrete glycerophosphocholine, sialic acid and glycoproteins that help in the maturation of the sperm.

## B. Vas Deferens (Ductus Deferens)

It is the longest portion (45 cm) of the extra-testicular duct system and runs from the tail of the epididymis to the seminal vesicles. The mucosa of the vas deferens forms small longitudinal folds. It is lined by a pseudostratified columnar epithelium and cells have long stereocilia. Epithelium rest on a basal lamina, which separates it from the underlying loose fibroelastic connective tissue, which has numerous folds, thus making the lumen appears irregular. The muscle layer is well developed and consists of thin inner and outer longitudinal layers along with a thick middle circular layer of smooth muscle (Fig. 16.11). Muscle layer is surrounded by an adventitia, which is slightly denser than usual. At the termination, the ductus deferens is dilated to form the ampulla. Layers of smooth muscle fibers are unique, as the muscle fibers directly receive sympathetic innervation. This is responsible for the rapid, forceful contractions of the ductus deferens during ejaculation.

In the ampulla, the mucosa is much more folded and the muscular wall is thin. The longitudinal layers disappear near the origin of ejaculatory duct (formed by joining of ampulla and seminal vesicle). The ejaculatory duct is a short (2 cm), straight tubule that

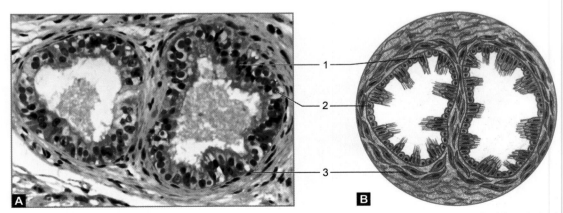

**Fig. 16.9:** Efferent ductules of testis, (A) micrograph, (B) sketch lined by ciliated columnar cells (1), cuboidal cells (2) and surrounded by smooth muscle fibers (3)

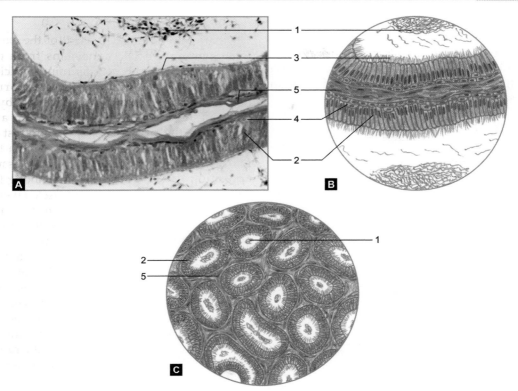

**Fig. 16.10:** Epididymis, (A) micrograph-LS, (B) sketch-LS, (C) sketch-TS. Pseudostratified epithelial (2) lining consists of columnar principal cells with stereocilia (3) and basal cells (4). Sperms (1) and smooth muscle fibers (5)

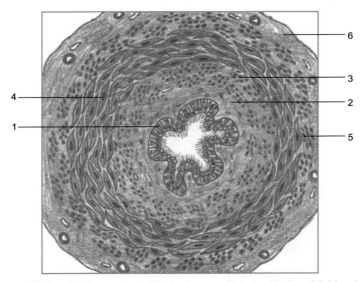

**Fig. 16.11:** Vas deferens-TS lined with pseudostratified columnar ciliated epithelium (1). Muscle coat is thick having inner longitudinal layer (3), middle circular layer (4) and outer longitudinal layer (5). Lamina propria (2) and adventitia (6)

enters the substance of and is surrounded by the prostate gland. Ejaculatory duct is lined by a simple columnar epithelium. The ejaculatory duct has no smooth muscle in its wall; the fibromuscular tissue of prostate substitutes for it.

## ACCESSORY GENITAL GLANDS

The products of these glands serve as the vehicle of transport of the spermatozoa in the female genital tract to ensure fertilization. During the transport the secretions also activate, nourish the sperm and clear the urethral tract prior to ejaculation. Three major accessory sex glands associated with the male reproductive system are:

### A. Seminal Vesicle

These are paired elongated, sac-like structures. Each seminal vesicle consists of a single (12–15 cm long) highly convoluted tube. These are located between the posterior aspect of the neck of the bladder and the prostate gland and join the ampulla of the ductus deferens just above the prostate gland. The mucosa shows thin, branching and anastomosing folds. The structure of the epithelium is variable appearing pseudostratified columnar. The columnar cells are secretory and the basal cells are stem cells. The lamina propria is fairly thin and loose. The muscle layer consists of inner circular and outer longitudinal layers of smooth muscle fibers (Fig. 16.12A to C).

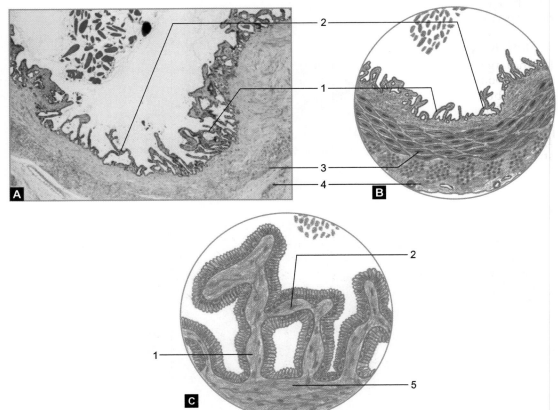

**Fig. 16.12:** Seminal vesicle, (A) micrograph at low magnification, (B) sketch at low magnification, (C) sketch at high magnification with primary (1) and secondary (2) mucosal folds. Muscle layers (3), adventitia (4) and lamina propria (5)

Outside the muscle layer, a layer of loose connective tissue with plenty of elastic fibers is present. The secretory product of the columnar cells can be seen in the lumen of the seminal vesicles and it is strongly acidophilic. It contains large amounts of fructose, which is utilized by the spermatozoa as a source of energy. Secretory activity is stimulated by testosterone. The seminal vesicle also forms large amounts of prostaglandins, which stimulate the activity of sperm in the female genital tract. The pale yellow color of semen is due to the lipochrome pigment released by the seminal vesicles. Contraction of the smooth muscle coats of the seminal vesicle during ejaculation discharges their secretion into the ejaculatory ducts and thus helps to flush sperms out of the urethra.

### B. Prostate

It is the largest accessory sex gland in men and weighs about 20 gm in adult males. It contains 30–50 tubuloalveolar glands, which empty into 15–25 independent excretory ducts. These ducts open into the urethra independently. The glands are embedded in a fibromuscular stroma, which mainly consists of smooth muscle separated by strands of connective tissue rich in collagenous and elastic fibers. The muscle forms a dense mass around the urethra and beneath the fairly thin capsule of the prostrate. The secretory alveoli of the prostate are very irregularly shaped because of papillary projections of the mucosa into the lumen of the gland. The epithelium is cuboidal or columnar. Basal cells are present and the epithelium may look pseudostratified where they are found. The secretory cells are slightly acidophilic and secretory granules may be visible in the cytoplasm. The secretory ducts of the prostate are lined by a simple columnar epithelium (Fig. 16.13A, B), which changes to a transitional epithelium near the openings of the ducts into the urethra.

In the lumen of the secretory alveoli prostatic concretions (corpora amylacea) are present, which are rounded eosinophilic bodies. Their number increases with age, particularly in past 50. They may undergo calcification. Corpora amylacea may appear in the semen. The secretion of the prostate contains citric acid, fibrinolysin (an enzyme that liquefies the semen), acid phosphatase and a number of other enzymes and lipids.

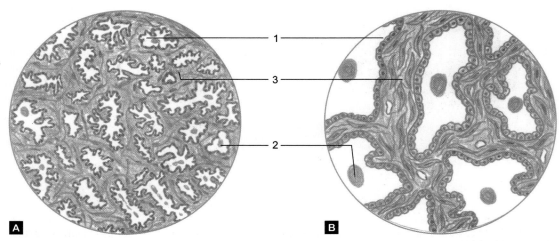

**A**  **B**

**Fig. 16.13:** Prostate, (A) low magnification, (B) high magnification showing prostatic acini (1) with prostatic concretions (2). Fibromuscular stroma (3) lies in between the prostatic acini

Prostate also produces a serine protease: prostate-specific antigen (PSA), which is used for diagnosis of some prostatic diseases. The secretory activity of the prostate is stimulated by testosterone.

Three concentric zones, which surround the prostatic part of the urethra, are:

a. The peripheral zone contains large glands (main prostatic glands) and their ducts run posteriorly to open into the urethra.

b. The internal zone consists of the submucosal glands.

c. The innermost zone contains mucosal glands.

## C. Bulbourethral (Cowper's) Glands

These are pair of small pea-sized glands placed bilaterally within the urogenital diaphragm. Their fibroelastic capsule contains not only fibroblasts and smooth muscle fibers but also skeletal muscle fibers derived from the muscles of the urogenital diaphragm. Septa derived from the capsule divide each gland into several lobules (Fig. 16.14).

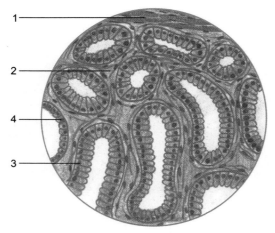

**Fig. 16.14:** Bulbourethral glands having secretory units (3) lined by simple columnar epithelium and excretory duct (4) lined by cuboidal cells. Skeletal muscle fibers (1) and connective tissue (2)

These compound tubuloalveolar glands are lined by simple columnar epithelium and their ducts open into the penile urethra. The glands secrete mucus, which contains galactose and sialic acid that lubricates the urethra prior to ejaculation. Secretory activity is stimulated by testosterone.

## D. Penis

It is copulatory organ that serves as an outlet for urine and semen. It is formed by three erectile bodies (corpora) surrounded by a fibrous capsule (tunica albuginea) and a subcutaneous connective tissue layer covered by a thin skin. Skin has only vellus type hairs (except at the base). The three erectile bodies are the dorsally positioned right and left corpus cavernosus and ventrally positioned unpaired corpus spongiosum. Tunica albuginea is thicker around the corpora cavernosa than around corpus spongiosum and it also forms an incomplete septum (pectiniform septum) between the corpora cavernosa. The corpus spongiosum contains the spongy urethra and at its end it dilates and forms the glans penis. The erectile tissue consists of numerous wide spaces lined with vascular endothelium and surrounded by smooth muscle (Fig. 16.15). These spaces are continuous with the arteries that supply them and with draining veins. Erection is mediated by vasodilation of the incoming arteries and constriction of the venous outflow; this results in the vascular space becoming engorged with blood.

For comparison between sperm and semen, *see* Table 32 given in Appendix I.

**Immotile Sperm** This is characterized by ultra-structural changes in the microtubules, causing immotility of cilia of the sperms. Males are often infertile in this syndrome.

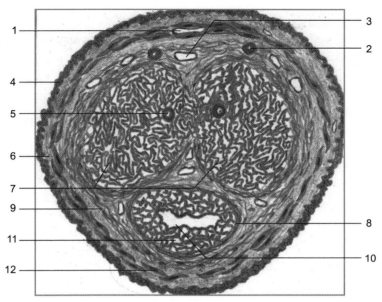

**Fig. 16.15:** Penis-TS consists of two corpora cavernosa (7) and one corpus spongiosum (11). Corpus spongiosum contains the spongy urethra (10). Superficial dorsal vein (1), dorsal artery (2), deep dorsal vein (3), epidermis (4), deep arteries (5), dermis (6), tunica albuginea (8), deep penile fascia (9) and dartos muscle (12)

## Summary

1. Testes serve as both exocrine (production of spermatozoa) and endocrine (production of testosterone) gland.

2. Testis is having 250 lobules and each lobule contains 1–4 convoluted seminiferous tubules, which are lined with stratified seminiferous epithelium.

3. Seminiferous epithelium consists of cells in different stages of spermatogenesis along with Sertoli cells.

4. In between seminiferous tubules testosterone secreting interstitial cells of Leydig are present.

5. Epididymis is lined by pseudostratified columnar epithelium consisting of basal cells and principal cells.

6. Epididymis absorbs excess testicular fluid and thus helps in movement of sperm towards the ductus deferens.

7. Vas deferens is lined by a pseudostratified columnar epithelium and cells have long stereocilia.

8. Muscle layer is well developed in the vas deferens and consists of thin inner and outer longitudinal layers along with a thick middle circular layer of smooth muscle.

9. Seminal vesicle is lined by pseudostratified columnar epithelium with thin lamina propria. The muscle layer consists of inner circular and outer longitudinal layer of smooth muscle fibers.

10. Prostate produces a serine protease: Prostate-specific antigen (PSA), which is used for diagnosis of some prostatic diseases.

11. Penis contains three erectile bodies, i.e. dorsally positioned right and left corpus cavernosus and ventrally positioned unpaired corpus spongiosum.

## Self Assessment

1. The number of seminiferous tubules in one testis is approximately:
   a. 100          b. 500
   c. 10,000       d. 1000

2. The fibromuscular stroma is present in the:
   a. Prostate
   b. Epididymis
   c. Seminal vesicle
   d. Testis

3. Testis is covered by all following layers EXCEPT:
   a. Tunica vaginalis
   b. Tunica adventitia
   c. Tunica vasculosa
   d. Tunica albuginea

4. Epididymis is lined by which type of epithelium?
   a. Stratified cuboidal
   b. Stratified columnar
   c. Pseudostratified
   d. Columnar

5. Blood–testis barrier is formed by which cells?
   a. Primary spermatocytes
   b. Secondary spermatocytes
   c. Leydig cells
   d. Sertoli cells

6. Which of the following organs is devoid of tunica albuginea?
   a. Penis
   b. Testis
   c. Ovary
   d. Epididymis

7. The secretion of seminal vesicle is rich in:
   a. Fructose
   b. Acid phosphatase
   c. Erythropoietin
   d. Citric acid

8. The corpora amylacea is seen in the:
   a. Penis
   b. Prostate
   c. Pineal gland
   d. Seminal vesicle

9. Ductus deferens is lined by which epithelium?
   a. Stratified cuboidal
   b. Stratified columnar
   c. Pseudostratified
   d. Columnar

10. Which of the following function is performed by Sertoli cells?
    a. Mechanical support
    b. Nutrition of developing sperm
    c. Synthesis of androgen binding proteins
    d. All of the above

## Answers

1. b,     2. a,     3. b,     4. c,     5. d,     6. d,     7. a,     8. b,     9. c,
10. d

# 17

# Female Reproductive System

The female reproductive system is composed of several distinct organs; begins with the paired ovaries, leads through the windings of the Fallopian tubes to the uterus and then opens through the cervix into the vagina. Special structures, like the placenta and the umbilical cord develop during pregnancy. The mammary glands are conventionally included in discussions of the female reproductive system, because they contribute to the same reproductive function and respond to the same set of hormone signals as the proper system. Several structures either show temporary changes during a particular phase or condition of the individual, such as uterine lining in menstrual cycle and/or develop new organs such as placenta during pregnancy and existing structure like mammary gland during menstrual cycle and pregnancy.

In the females at puberty, i.e. at the age of 10–14 years, ovaries, uterus and mammary glands undergo changes. This is the age of initiation of menstrual cycle, known as menarche. After this, uterus and ovaries undergo marked structural and functional changes in a cycle of 28–30 days. This is known as the menstrual cycle. Between the ages of 45–55 years, these cycles become irregular and finally ceases, known as menopause.

## OVARY

It is a paired organ situated on either side of the uterus and attached to the posterior layer of the broad ligament of the uterus by a fold of peritoneum, known as mesovarium. In nulliparous (women who have not borne children), ovary is about 3 cm in length, 1.5 cm in width and 1 cm in thickness. Before puberty, the surface of the ovary is smooth, but during reproductive life, it becomes progressively scarred and irregular due to repeated ovulations. In postmenopausal woman, the ovaries are about one-fourth of the size compared to the women in the reproductive period. Its surface is covered by a single layer of cuboidal epithelium, which is known as germinal epithelium. The term germinal epithelium is a misnomer; because the epithelium does not produce any germ cells. This layer is continuous with the peritoneal mesothelium. Immediately beneath the germinal epithelium, the dense fibrous connective tissue layer (tunica albuginea) forms a thin capsule. Tunica albuginea of the ovary is much thinner and less dense than that of the testis.

The ovary is divided into an outer cortex and an inner medulla. The cortex consists of a connective tissue stroma in which the ovarian follicles are embedded. The stroma is made up of an extensive network of reticular fibers among which lies a few collagen fibers and spindle-shaped fibroblasts (stromal or interstitial) cells. Scattered smooth muscle fibers are present in the stroma around the follicle (Fig. 17.1).

The follicles are present in different stages of development and depend upon a woman's age, number of pregnancies, health and whether or not she is currently pregnant. But the ovarian cortex of postmenopausal women mainly consists of stromal elements and scar tissue from degenerated follicles and only a few follicles are present. The two ovaries serve exocrine and endocrine functions. They perform their exocrine or cytogenic function by producing live cells; the secondary oocytes and their endocrine function by producing two steroid hormones—estrogen and progesterone. Estrogens produced by the ovarian follicles, stimulate development of the secondary sexual characteristics and also promote development of mammary glands. Progesterone, secreted by the corpus luteum, stimulates development of the uterus for the reception of the fertilized ovum and also prepares the breast for lactation.

## A. Ovarian Follicles

An ovarian follicle consists of one oocyte and the surrounding follicular cells. Follicular development can be divided into a number of stages:

a. **Primordial (quiescent) follicles:** These follicles first appear in the ovaries during the third month of fetal development and these are the only follicle present until puberty. They are located in a very large number in the cortex. These follicles contain primary oocyte, which is formed by the mitotic division of oogonia. The primary oocyte is 25–30 µm in diameter and it is surrounded by a single layer of flattened follicular cells (Fig. 17.2). Primary oocyte immediately begins the first meiotic division, which arrests in prophase.

b. **Primary follicle:** It is the first morphological stage that marks the onset of follicular maturation. The flattened follicular cells now form a cuboidal or columnar epithelium surrounding the primary oocyte. Oocyte

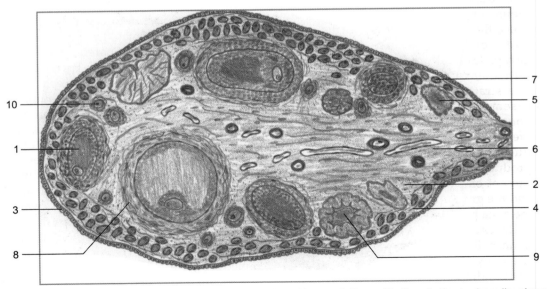

**Fig. 17.1:** Ovary, covered by germinal epithelium (3) and beneath the epithelium is the tunica albuginea (4). In the cortex (2) lie primordial follicles (7), primary follicle (10), secondary follicle (1), Graafian follicle (8), corpus luteum (9) and atretic follicles (5). Medulla (6) contains fibroblasts, smooth muscle and elastic fibers

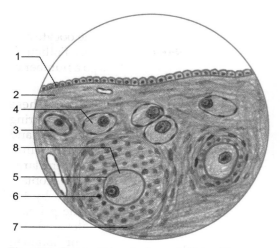

**Fig. 17.2:** Primordial and primary follicle of the ovary. In the primordial follicle (3) oocyte (4) is covered by a single layer of flattened follicular cells. In primary follicle (8) oocyte is surrounded by the zona pellucida (5) and granulosa cells (6), which are covered by theca folliculi (7). Germinal epithelium (1) and tunica albuginea (2)

enlarges and measures about 50–80 µm. Oocyte and follicular cells secrete a gel-like membrane that surrounds the oocyte, called the zona pellucida. Zona is refractile and rich in glycosaminoglycans and glycoproteins. The continued proliferation of follicular cells will result in the formation of a stratified epithelium (with a distinct basement membrane) surrounding the oocyte, called granulosa cells. The proliferative activity of the granulosa cells is due to the signaling molecule activin produced by the primary oocyte. Microvilli present on the surface of both the oocyte and the granulosa cells project deeply into the zona pellucida. Microvilli of granulosa cells can even completely cross the zona pellucida and contact the surface of the oocyte. Stromal cells of the ovary surrounding the growing follicle become organized in concentric sheaths, the theca folliculi (Fig. 17.2). The boundary between the thecal layers is not distinct. The theca folliculi further differentiates into a theca

interna and a theca externa. Theca interna is located just outside the basement membrane of the follicular cells and is composed of cuboidal secretory cells, which secrete the steroid hormone androgen. The theca externa is mostly collagenous. It contains a few muscle cells and many blood vessels, which provide nourishment to the theca interna. The boundary between the theca externa and surrounding stroma are even not distinct. Granulosa cells convert androgens, produced in theca interna, into estrogen.

c. **Secondary (antral or vesicular) follicle:** Small intercellular spaces become visible between the granulosa cells as the follicle reaches a diameter of about 400 µm. These spaces are filled with a fluid known as liquor folliculi. Continued proliferation of the granulosa cells of the secondary follicle depends upon FSH released by basophils of the anterior pituitary. Under the influence of FSH, the number of layers of the granulosa cells increases, as does the number of liquor folliculi-containing intercellular spaces. This fluid, an exudate of plasma, contains glycosaminoglycans, proteoglycans, and steroid-binding proteins produced by the granulosa cells. Moreover, it contains the hormone progesterone, estradiol, inhibin, folliculostatin, and activin, which regulate the release of LH and FSH. These spaces enlarge and fuse to form the follicular antrum. The granulosa cells become rearranged so that the primary oocyte is now surrounded by a small group of granulosa cells that project out from the wall into the fluid-filled antrum. These cells are called cumulus oophorus. The granulosa cells that attach the oocyte to the wall of the follicle are called discus proligerous (Fig. 17.3A, B).

d. **Mature (tertiary or preovulatory or Graafian) follicle:** It increases further in size (in particular in the last 12 hours before ovulation) and forms a small "bump" on

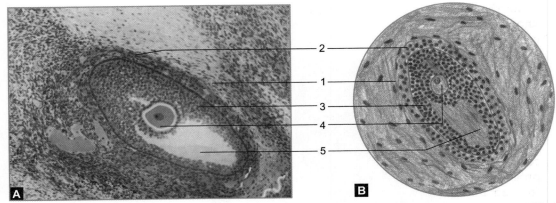

**Fig. 17.3:** Secondary follicle, (A) micrograph, (B) sketch having eccentric oocyte (4) and large fluid filled antrum (5). Oocyte is surrounded by granulosa cells (3). Theca folliculi differentiate in theca interna (2) and theca externa (1)

the surface of the ovary, known as the stigma (macula pellucida). The primary oocyte completes its first meiotic division and become secondary oocyte, which starts its second meiotic division and reaches the metaphase stage at the time of ovulation. Ovulation from either the right or left ovary is a random event; the ovaries do not have necessarily alternate months. Prior to ovulation the cumulus oophorus separates from the follicular wall (Fig. 17.4A, B). The oocyte is now floating freely in the follicular antrum. It is still surrounded by granulosa cells, which form the corona radiata. The follicle finally ruptures at the stigma and the oocyte is released from the ovary.

e. **Corpus luteum:** It is formed by both granulosa cells and thecal cells after ovulation has occurred. The wall of the follicle collapses into a folded structure, some of the ruptured blood vessels leak blood into the follicular cavity, forming a central clot. The resulting structure is known as the corpus hemorrhagicum. As the clot is removed by phagocytes, high levels of LH convert the corpus

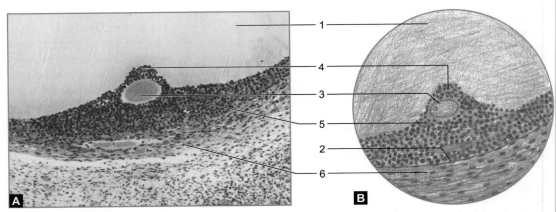

**Fig. 17.4:** Mature or Graafian follicle, (A) micrograph, (B) sketch. Antrum (1), zona pellucida (2), primary oocyte (3), cumulus oophorus (4), granulosa cells (5) and theca interna (6)

hemorrhagicum into a temporary structure known as the corpus luteum. Theca interna cells and granulosa cells triple in size and start accumulating lutein within a few hours after ovulation. They are now called as granulosa lutein cells and theca lutein cells (Fig. 17.5A, B).

Theca lutein cells manufacture progesterone and androgens and small amounts of estrogen. Granulosa lutein cells manufacture most of the body's progesterone and even convert androgens formed by the theca lutein cells into estrogens. Hormone secretion in the corpus luteum ceases within 14 days after ovulation if the oocyte is not fertilized and the absence of LH leads to degeneration of the corpus luteum, forming the corpus luteum of menstruation. If pregnancy occurs, human chorionic gonadotropin (hCG), secreted by the placenta, maintains the corpus luteum for 3 months and called corpus luteum of pregnancy.

f. **Corpus albicans:** As the corpus luteum degenerates, it is invaded by fibroblasts, it becomes fibrotic and are phagocytosed by macrophages. The fibrous whitish scar that forms in its place is known as the corpus albicans.

## B. Atretic Follicle

All types of follicles may undergo atresia or degeneration. Atresia can occur at any stage of follicular development and will begin in different layers of the follicle or oocyte depending on the follicle's stage of development. Many primordial follicles undergo atresia, before birth. Of the ~2 million primordial follicles and their primary oocytes present at birth, only about 450,000 oocytes/follicles remain at puberty and about 450 of those will be ovulated. The remainder degenerates, thereby producing more atretic than normal follicles. In humans, of the several follicles that begin growth each month, only one, as a rule, is destined for maturity and ovulation. The others undergo atresia. When follicles become atretic, the oocyte is the first structure of the follicle to show signs of dying. Its nucleus becomes pyknotic and its cytoplasm shrinks and then breaks. The zona pellucida thickens and becomes folded. Following the death of the oocyte, similar destructive changes occur in the follicular cells. The granulosa cells separate and degenerate; the thecal cells accumulate lipid and degenerate. The follicle eventually disappears as the ovarian stroma invades the degenerating follicles. After the menopause,

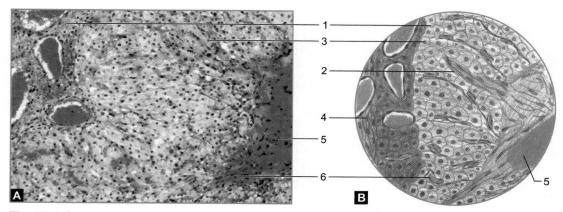

**Fig. 17.5:** Corpus luteum, (A) micrograph, (B) sketch showing granulosa lutein cells (3) and theca lutein cells (1). Connective tissue septum (2), theca externa (4), blood clot (5) and capillary (6)

primordial follicles are absent, so the cortex consists of the stroma and corpus albicans only, with no developing follicles.

## MEDULLA

The stroma of the medulla is looser than that of the cortex. Typical fibroblasts (lacking the potential to produce hormones), strands of smooth muscle (which accompany the blood vessels), and many elastic fibers are present. The demarcation between cortex and medulla is not well defined; however, they are showing different histological structure.

## FALLOPIAN TUBES

It is a typical tubular organ and functions as a conduit for the oocyte, from the ovaries to the uterus. It can be divided into four major parts:
1. The infundibulum
2. The ampulla
3. The isthmus
4. The intramural part

The infundibulum is the funnel-shaped segment of the tube. At proximal end it communicates with the ampulla and at distal end it opens into the peritoneal cavity. From the mouth of the infundibulum, finger-like extensions or fimbriae embrace the ovary. The ampulla is thin walled and forms lateral two-thirds of the tube. It is the longest segment of the tube and also the site of fertilization. The isthmus is thick walled and form medial one-third of the tube. The intramural part (interstitial part or isthmus) is about 1 cm in length, lies within the uterine wall and opens in the uterine cavity. The wall of the tube thickens progressively toward the uterus, whereas the lumen diminishes in size in this direction. Its wall consists of following three coats.

### A. The Mucosa

It is highly branched and folded, especially in the ampulla (Fig. 17.6A, B). It is formed by a simple columnar epithelium; some of the cells are ciliated. The non-ciliated cells are secretory in nature and referred as peg-cells, which produce nutritive fluid for the ovum. The ciliated cells are shorter than the secretory cells, making the epithelial surface irregular in outline. Cilia beat mostly toward the lumen of the uterus and may facilitate the transport of the developing embryo to the uterus. The number of ciliated cells and secretory cells varies along the fallopian tube. The numbers of ciliated cells are greatest in the infundibulum and ampulla and it is least in the isthmus. Secretory cells are most abundant in intramural part.

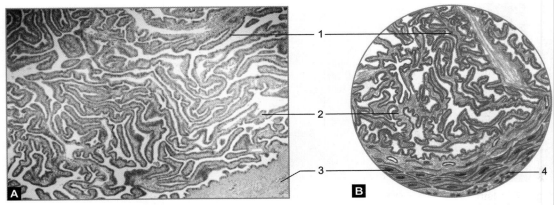

**Fig. 17.6:** Ampulla of fallopian tube, (A) micrograph, (B) sketch showing highly branched and folded mucosa (1). Lamina propria (2), inner circular layer (3) and outer longitudinal layer (4)

Secretory activity varies during the menstrual cycle. The epithelial cells undergo cyclic hypertrophy during the follicular phase and atrophy during the luteal phase in response to changes in hormonal levels, particularly estrogens. Also, the ratio of ciliated to nonciliated cells changes during the hormonal cycle. Estrogen increases the number of ciliated cells, while progesterone increases the number of secretory cells. The epithelium regresses in height towards the end of menstrual cycle and postmenopausally.

Epithelium rests on a lamina propria, as the basement membrane is inconspicuous. The lamina propria consists of loose connective tissue containing reticular fibers, fibroblasts, mast cells and lymphoid cells. Muscularis mucosa is absent. Submucosa is continuous with the lamina propria, forming a continuous connective tissue layer.

### B. Muscularis Externa

It has poorly defined inner circular and outer longitudinal smooth muscle layers, which are thinnest in the infundibulum. An additional inner longitudinal layer is present in the isthmus and the intramural part of the fallopian tube (Fig. 17.7A, B).

At the moment of ovulation, the fallopian tube shows active movement. The fimbriae come very close to the surface of the ovary where rupture will occur. As the oocyte is released, the ciliated cells sweep it towards the opening of fallopian tube. This movement is further promoted by peristaltic contraction. The cilia and peristaltic contractions also help in the movement of sperms, thus facilitates fertilization. The secretion of secretory cells contains nutrients for the oocyte. Unless it is fertilized, the oocyte remains viable for a maximum of about 24 hours.

### C. Serosa

The peritoneal surface of the fallopian tube is lined by mesothelium and a thin layer of connective tissue.

### UTERUS

It is a hollow pear-shaped, thick wall organ. It is divided into body (upper two-thirds) and cervix (lower one-third). The upper rounded part of the body, which lies above the attachment of the fallopian tubes is known as fundus. The fertilized ovum gets implanted and developed into a fetus in the uterus. The fetus is expelled from the uterus at full term. The lumen of the uterus (uterine cavity) is flattened and is continuous with the

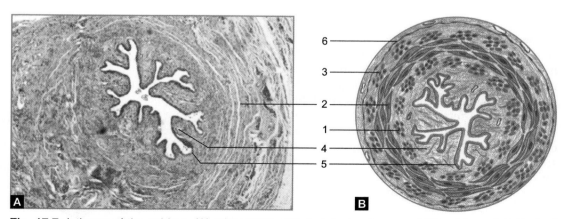

**Fig. 17.7:** Isthmus of the oviduct, (A) micrograph, (B) sketch showing an additional inner longitudinal layer (1). Middle circular layer (2), outer longitudinal layer (3), lamina propria (4), mucosal folds lined by simple columnar ciliated epithelium (5) and serosa (6)

fallopian tubes and the vagina. The wall of the body of the uterus is composed of three coats. From outer to inner surface, these are as follows.

## A. Perimetrium

It is the outermost protective serosal layer and consists of a single layer of mesothelial cells supported by a thin layer of elastic tissue. On each side, it is continuous with the broad ligament. Perimetrium is deficient over the lower half of the anterior surface, which is surrounded by adventitia. Large coiled blood vessels traverse the broad ligament to the perimetrium and penetrate the myometrium to reach the endometrium.

## B. Myometrium

It is the thickest layer of the uterus. It is dense and thick at the uterine midlevel and fundus, but thin at the openings of the fallopian tubes. It is composed of bundles of smooth muscle fibers separated by connective tissue. The bundles of muscle fibers form four layers, but the layers are ill-defined. The first and fourth layer consists of longitudinally arranged fibers, while middle layers contain the larger blood vessels. When the muscles contract, they compress the blood vessels and stop the bleeding from the endometrium. During pregnancy the myometrium becomes thicker to sustain and protects the fetus; the growth is due to the hypertrophy and hyperplasia of smooth muscle fibers. The amount of connective tissue also increases. As pregnancy proceeds, the uterine wall becomes progressively thinner as it stretches because of the growth of the fetus. After parturition, the uterus returns to almost its original size. The collagen produced during pregnancy to strengthen the myometrium is then degraded by the cells that secreted it. Near the end of pregnancy, the myometrium develops many gap junctions between its smooth muscle fibers. These junctions coordinate the contraction of the muscle fibers on stimulation by oxytocin and prostaglandins during parturition. After parturition, the myometrium is reduced in size because smooth muscle cells, deprived of estrogen, undergo apoptosis.

## C. Endometrium (Mucosa)

It consists of simple columnar epithelium (ciliated cells and secretory cells) and an underlying thick connective tissue stroma. The lining epithelium is invaginated to form many simple tubular uterine glands. The glands extend through the entire thickness of the stroma. The stromal cells of the endometrium are embedded in a network of reticular fibers. The endometrium is subject to cyclic changes, which is correlated with the maturation of the ovarian follicles. The end of each cycle is characterized by the partial destruction and sloughing of the endometrium, accompanied by bleeding from the mucosal vessels, and is known as menstruation or menstrual flow. Only the mucosa of the body of the uterus takes part in the menstrual cycle. The endometrium can be divided into two zones based on their involvement in the changes during the menstrual cycle: The basalis and the functionalis.

- The basalis is not sloughed off during menstruation, but functions as a regenerative zone for the functionalis after its rejection.
- The functionalis is the luminal part of the endometrium. It is sloughed off during every menstruation and it is the site of cyclic changes in the endometrium.

The blood vessels supplying the endometrium are of special significance in the periodic sloughing of most of its layers. The uterine arteries pierce the myometrium and give off 6 to 8 arcuate arteries. Branches from these vessels, the radial arteries, enter in the basalis layer of the endometrium. They give off small straight arteries, which supply to the basalis. The main branches of the radial artery continue upwards and known as coiled or spiral arteries, which supply to the functionalis.

## D. Cyclic Changes in Endometrium (Menstrual Cycle)

Beginning from puberty and ending at menopause, the endometrium undergoes cyclic changes. These cyclic changes are divided into a number of phases:

a. **Proliferative (follicular) phase (5–14 days):** After the menstrual phase, the uterine mucosa is reduced. It contains only basal portions of the uterine glands and lower portions of spiral arteries. Cellular proliferation continues during the entire proliferative phase, and reconstitutes both the glands and the surface epithelium. Secretions of the glands are watery and scanty. It also coincides with the development of ovarian follicles and production of estrogens. At the end of this phase, the endometrium is 2–3 mm thick and the glands, which consist of simple columnar epithelial cells, are straight tubules with a narrow lumen (Fig. 17.8A, B). Spiral arteries grow into the regenerating stroma.

b. **Secretory (luteal) phase (15–28 days):** This phase starts in response to the formation of the corpus luteum, which secretes progesterone. Stromal cells become large and pale; cytoplasm contains glycogen and lipid droplets. Tissue fluid accumulates in the stroma (edema). The endometrium increases in thickness to 4 mm or more in depth due to the hypertrophy of gland cells and increase of edema fluid. The glands swell and secrete profusely. At first, secretory material is present in the basal parts of the cells, later on material move to the apical zone. Secretion is thick and rich in glycogen. The glands become serrated (Fig. 17.9A, B). Spiral arteries grow nearer to the surface. Three zones in endometrium can be distinguished:

i. *Compact layer:* It is a comparatively narrow zone nearer to the surface and contains straight necks of the gland.

ii. *Spongy layer:* It is a relatively thick layer and contains tortuous portions of the gland.

The above two layers collectively form the functionalis, which is lost during menstrual bleeding.

iii. *Basal layer:* It is thin and contains blind ends of the gland and not lost during menstrual bleeding.

Last 2 (26–28) days of secretory phase are called ischemic part of secretory phase or

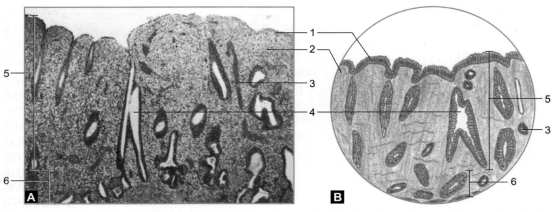

**Fig. 17.8:** Endometrium: Proliferative phase, (A) micrograph, (B) sketch showing straight uterine glands (4) with a narrow lumen. Simple columnar epithelium (1), lamina propria (2), coiled artery (3), functionalis layer (5) and basalis layer (6)

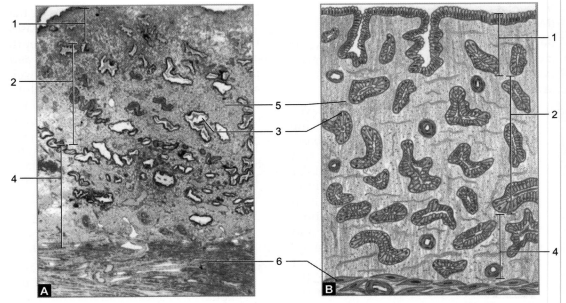

**Fig. 17.9:** Endometrium: Secretory phase, (A) micrograph, (B) sketch, can be distinguished into compact layer (1) with straight necks of the gland. Spongy layer (2) with tortuous parts of the gland filled with secretion (3) and basal layer (4) containing ends of the glands. Lamina propria (5) and myometrium (6)

premenstrual phase. Estrogen and pro-gesterone secretion from the corpus luteum decreases. As the endometrial glands begin to shrink, the spiral arteries are compressed, thereby reducing blood flow and causing ischemic damage.

c. **Menstrual phase (1–4 days):** The functionalis undergoes necrosis and is shed. After some time spiral arteries relax, the walls of the vessels near the surface break, and blood is added to the secretion of the glands. Patches of tissue separates and lost. Finally, the whole functionalis layer lost and only basalis remain (Fig. 17.10A, B). Normally menstrual blood does not clot because of release of local anticoagulant and contractions of the uterus also increase its expulsion. The surface epithelium quickly restored once the menstrual discharge ceases.

d. **Menopause phase:** The endometrium at menopause regresses and consists of only basal layer (Fig. 17.11A, B). The uterine glands also regress.

## CERVIX

It is the lowest cylindrical part of the uterus and in histological structure; it differs from the rest of the uterus. The mucosa of the cervix (endocerix) is continuous with the uterine endometrium and is lined by simple columnar epithelium with cilia (beat toward the vagina) and many mucus secreting cells (Fig. 17.12A, B). The part of the cervix (ectocervix) that pro-trudes into the vagina is covered by non-keratinized stratified squamous epithelium, similar to that of the vagina. The junction of this epithelium with the simple columnar epithelium is abrupt and is called external os. Mucosa is invaginated in the cavity of the cervix (cervical canal) and form longitudinal and oblique folds, known as plica palmatae. The folds are prominent along the middle dilated part of the cervical canal and diminish

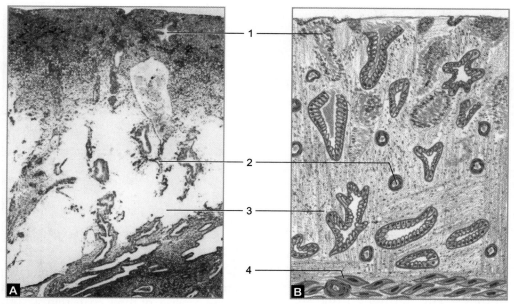

**Fig. 17.10:** Endometrium: Menstrual phase, (A) micrograph, (B) sketch, with uterine glands filled with blood (1) and basal layer (3) is intact. Coiled artery (2) and myometrium (4)

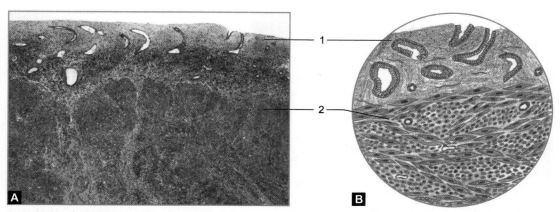

**Fig. 17.11:** Endometrium: Menopausal showing regression of uterine glands and only basal layer (1) is present. Thick myometrium (2) is present below the endometrium, (A) micrograph, (B) sketch

gradually until they disappear at the cervical opening into the vagina. The mucosa also contains the mucus cervical glands, which are extensively branched. The mucosa does not desquamate during menstrual cycle, although its glands undergo important functional changes that are related to the transport of spermatozoa within the cervical canal. The cervix produces cervical mucus that is mostly water, but also contains glycoproteins, glucose, and ions. At ovulation, cervical mucus is more hydrated and easier for spermatozoa to penetrate. After ovulation, when the corpus luteum is formed, cervical mucus is less hydrated, so it is more difficult for spermatozoa to penetrate. During pregnancy,

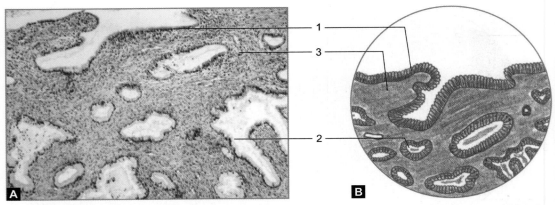

**Fig. 17.12:** Cervix of uterus, (A) micrograph, (B) sketch, illustrates cervical glands (2) present in the lamina propria (3) and lining of simple columnar epithelial cells (1)

a plug of cervical mucus forms and prevents bacteria present in the vagina from entering the uterus and attacking the fetus and fetal membranes. The hormone progesterone regulates the changes in the viscosity of the cervical gland secretions. The dilation of the cervix that precedes parturition is due to another luteal hormone; relaxin, which induces lysis of collagen and promotes its softening. The mucosa rests upon myometrium which is mainly composed of dense collagenous connective tissue containing many elastic fibers and only a few smooth muscle fibers (Fig. 17.13A, B).

## VAGINA

It is a fibromuscular tube that joins internal reproductive organs to the external environment. Its wall consists of three coats (Fig. 17.14).

### A. The Mucosa

It exhibits numerous transverse folds or rugae. It is lined with thick, stratified squamous non-keratinized epithelium. The surface cells continuously desquamate. Epithelium undergoes cyclic changes during the menstrual cycle. Under the influence of estrogen, during the follicular phase, the epithelial cells synthesize

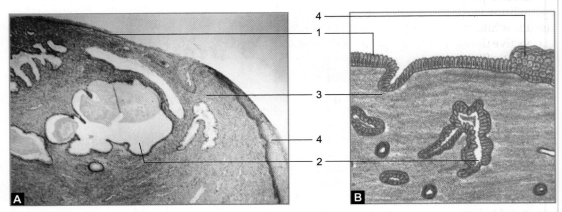

**Fig. 17.13:** Cervix and vagina, (A) micrograph, (B) sketch showing simple columnar epithelium of cervix (1) and stratified squamous nonkeratinized epithelium of the vagina (4). In the lamina propria (3) of cervix, cervical glands (2) filled with mucus can be seen

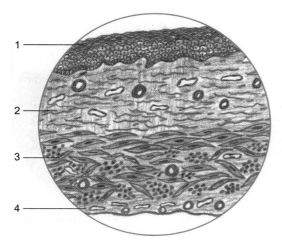

**Fig. 17.14:** Vagina, lined by mucosa consisting of stratified squamous nonkeratinized epithelium (1) and lamina propria (2). Outside this layer of smooth muscle fibers (3), adventitial layer (4) is present

and accumulate glycogen as they migrate towards the surface. Glycogen content diminishes towards the end of the cycle. The amount of glycogen is less, before puberty and after menopause. Glycogen is used by the vaginal bacterial flora (*Lactobacillus acidophilus*) to produce lactic acid, which lowers the pH during the follicular phase of the menstrual cycle and inhibits invasion by pathogens.

Lamina propria present just below the epithelium is a loose fibroelastic connective tissue, while in the deeper part it is dense connective tissue with numerous blood vessels and elastic fibers. This dense connective tissue layer can be regarded as submucosa. Glands are not present in the vagina and its surface is lubricated mainly by mucus produced by cervical glands. Muscularis mucosae is absent in the vagina.

## B. Muscularis Externa

It is composed of smooth muscle fibers, which are arranged in interlacing bundles. On the inner side, the fibers are mainly circularly arranged and thin, while on the outer side, fibers are longitudinally arranged and

thick. Longitudinal fibers are continuous with the corresponding layer of the uterus. Inferiorly, the striated, voluntary bulbo-spongiosus muscle forms a sphincter around the vagina.

## C. The Adventitia

The part of the adventitia bordering the muscularis is fairly dense and contains many elastic fibers. Loose connective tissue with a prominent venous plexus forms the outer part of the adventitia.

> The highly elastic lamina propria, muscle layers, and outer adventitia permit the distention of the vagina during parturition. On the contrary, after coitus involuntary contractions of smooth muscle fibers ensure that a pool of semen remains in the cervical region.

## EXFOLIATIVE CYTOLOGY (CYTOPATHOLOGY)

It is the microscopic examination of cells that have been shed from a lesion or have been recovered from a tissue for the diagnosis of disease. Examination of superficial epithelial cells scraped from the vaginal mucosa gives valuable information with respect to hormonal changes during the menstrual cycle and the microbial environment of the vagina. Certain infections cause inflammation of the vaginal mucosa. The abnormal cells shed from the epithelium are easily detected with a Pap smear examination. The Pap smear is an extremely effective and inexpensive screening method for cervical cancer.

## PLACENTA

It is a specialized extraembryonic tissue in which blood vessels of the fetus are brought into close intimacy with the maternal blood for the purpose of respiration, and metabolic activities during intrauterine life of the fetus. It weighs about 500 gm, measures 15–20 cm in diameter, and 3 cm in thickness. It consists of a fetal part (chorion) and a maternal part (decidua basalis). From the chorionic plate extend many villi (Fig. 17.15A, B).

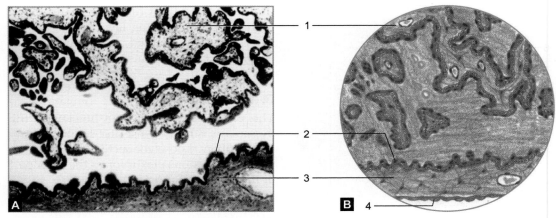

**Fig. 17.15:** Placenta, (A) micrograph: iron hematoxylin stain, (B) sketch: H and E, showing chorionic plate formed by trophoblast (2), mesenchyme (3) and amnion (4). The figure also shows placental villi (1)

The core of each villous contains a fetal capillary lined with typical endothelium. The decidual tissue sends incomplete projections (placental septa) towards the chorionic plate; they divide the placenta into lobules or cotyledons. A villous is lined with an inner cuboidal layer of cytotrophoblast (Langhans' layer) and outer layer of syncytiotrophoblast. Syncytiotrophoblast is variable in thickness and contains multiple nuclei with no intercellular boundaries (Fig. 17.16A, B).

In the second half of pregnancy, cytotrophoblast disappears and syncytiotrophoblast thins out over the fetal capillaries to form a narrow layer (Fig. 17.17). On the surface of the villi, irregular masses of an eosinophilic, homogenous substance called fibrinoid are

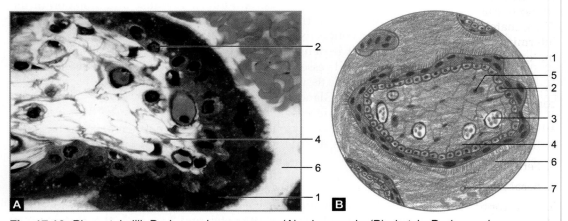

**Fig. 17.16:** Placental villi: During early pregnancy, (A) micrograph, (B) sketch. During early pregnancy each villus is lined by outer syncytiotrophoblast (1) and inner cytotrophoblast (2), but as pregnancy advances cytotrophoblast disappears. The core of each villus contains fetal blood vessels (3), mesnchyme (4) and macrophage (5). The intervillous space (6) contains maternal blood vessels (7)

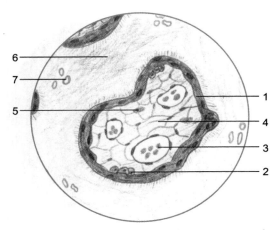

**Fig. 17.17:** Placental villi during late pregnancy. As pregnancy advances cytotrophoblast (2) present on the inner side of syncytiotrophoblast (1) disappears. The core of each villus contains fetal blood vessels (3), mesenchyme (4) and macrophage (5). The intervillous space (6) contains maternal blood vessels (7)

present. They become increasingly abundant in older placenta.

The maternal blood comes to intervillous space from spiral arteries of decidua. Fetal capillaries present in the villi are separated from the maternal blood by a placental barrier, which is formed by a slight amount of connective tissue and the syncytiotrophoblasts. Thus, maternal blood and fetal blood do not intermix; instead, nutrients and oxygen from maternal blood diffuse through this barrier to reach the fetal blood. In earlier stages of pregnancy (4–5 months) the placental barrier consists of:

1. Endothelium of fetal capillary
2. Basal lamina of fetal capillary
3. Fetal connective tissue
4. Basal lamina of cytotrophoblast
5. Cytotrophoblast
6. Syncytiotrophoblast

At full term, thickness of placenta reduces and now the placental barrier consists of:

1. Endothelium of fetal capillary
2. Basal lamina of fetal capillary
3. Thin layer of syncytiotrophoblast

In addition to being the site where nutritious substances, waste, and gases are exchanged between maternal and fetal circulation, the placenta (specifically the syncytiotrophoblast) also acts as an endocrine organ. The placenta synthesizes large amounts of hCG (human chorionic gonadotropin) which maintains the corpus luteum of pregnancy. Cells of syncytiotrophoblast secrete human chorionic somatomammotropin (hCS) or human placental lactogen (hPL), which is believed to stimulate the development of the mammary glands in preparation for lactation. The placenta also secretes progesterone and estrogens.

Measurement of hCG (human chorionic gonadotropin) is used to detect pregnancy and assess early embryonic development.

**UMBILICAL CORD**

It is the connecting cord from the developing fetus to the placenta. It measures about 50 cm in length and 1–2 cm in width. It is derived from connecting stalk of the embryo. The cord is covered by amniotic membrane, so lined by flattened amniotic epithelial cells. The umbilical cord is filled with gelatinous embryonic connective tissue, known as Wharton's jelly. The cells in this gelatinous tissue are mesenchymal cells with slender cell processes, which interconnect and form a meshwork. Embedded in this tissue are one umbilical vein and two umbilical arteries (Fig. 17.18A, B). Umbilical veins are thin walled with wide lumen and supplies the fetus with oxygenated, nutrient-rich blood from the placenta. On the contrary, umbilical arteries are thick walled with narrow lumen and return the deoxygenated, nutrient-depleted blood to the placenta. Umbilical arteries and veins are always strongly contracted after birth.

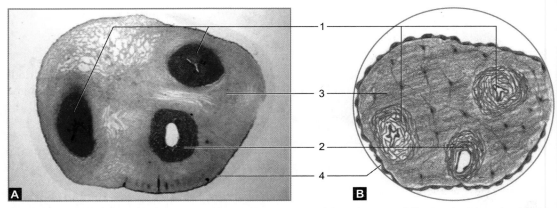

**Fig. 17.18:** Umbilical cord, showing two umbilical arteries (1) and one umbilical vein (2) embedded in Wharton's jelly (3). The cord is covered by flattened amnion (4). (A) micrograph, (B) sketch

## MAMMARY GLANDS (BREASTS)

These are compound branched alveolar, modified apocrine sweat glands. These glands are found in both sexes; but rudimentary in the males, and well developed in the females after puberty. These glands are made up of 15–25 lobes separated by interlobular connective tissue. Interlobular tissue is dense, irregular connective tissue with numerous fat cells. Lobes are further divided into lobules by intralobular connective tissue. Intralobular tissue is loose connective tissue with many plasma cells, lymphocytes, macrophages, and the fibroblasts. Each lobe is a cluster of alveoli (secretory unit) and drained by its own duct, known as lactiferous duct, which opens directly on the nipple. Near its termination on the nipple each lactiferous duct has a dilatation, known as lactiferous sinus. Several intralobular ducts join to form an interlobular duct, and several interlobular ducts join to form a single lactiferous duct. The alveoli are lined by cuboidal or columnar epithelium. Intralobular duct is lined by cuboidal epithelium, while interlobular duct is lined by cuboidal to low columnar epithelium. The lactiferous ducts are lined by two-layered stratified cuboidal epithelium and near their termination they are lined by stratified squamous keratinized epithelium. A layer

of myoepithelial cells is present in between the epithelium and the basement membrane of the branches of the lactiferous duct and the alveoli. The breasts reach their greatest development at the age of 20. The greatest changes occur during pregnancy and lactation. Atrophic changes start at the age of 40 and increase after menopause.

### A. Inactive (non-lactating) Gland

It mainly consists of ducts and their branches. The interlobular connective tissue makes up the majority of the gland (Fig. 17.19A to C). Alveoli, if present, are small buds and may be present in the form of masses of epithelial cells without lumen. An incomplete layer of myoepithelial cells are present.

### B. Active (lactating) Gland

Pregnancy induces a considerable growth leading to the formation of new terminal branches of ducts and of alveoli in the first half of pregnancy. Growth is initiated by the elevated levels of estrogen and progesterone produced in the ovaries and placenta. Concurrently, a reduction in the amount of intra- and interlobular connective tissue takes place. The continued growth of the mammary glands during the second half of pregnancy is due to increase in the

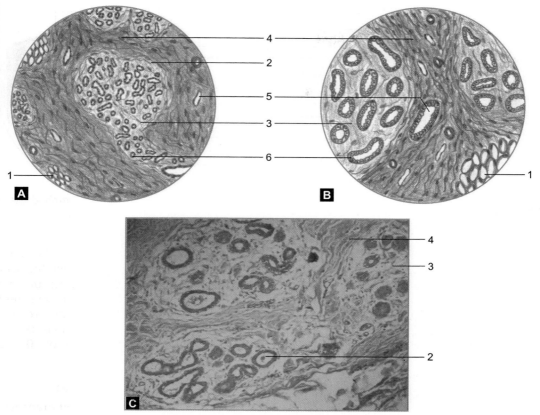

**Fig. 17.19:** Inactive mammary gland, (A) sketch at low magnification, (B) sketch at high magnification, (C) micrograph showing extensive intralobular (3) and interlobular (4) connective tissue. Alveoli (2) are poorly developed. The figure also shows adipose tissue (1), interlobular (5) and intralobular duct (6)

height of epithelial cells and an expansion of the lumen of the alveoli (Fig. 17.20 A to C). A complete layer of myoepithelial cells is present. As pregnancy progresses, mammary glands enlarge as a result of hypertrophy of the alveoli and distension with colostrums (premilk). Colostrum is an alkaline yellowish secretion, which is rich in proteins, and immunoglobulins. Within a few days after birth, when estrogen and progesterone secretions have droop, prolactin, secreted by acidophils of the anterior pituitary gland, activates the secretion of milk, which replaces the colostrum.

The alveolar cells secrete two distinct products: Lipids and proteins. Lipids arise as droplets within the cytoplasm. The small droplets coalesce to form larger and larger droplets, then move to the apical region of the cell. They are released from the alveolar cells through the apocrine mode of exocytosis. Proteins are synthesized in the rough endoplasmic reticulum, then packed into membrane-bound secretory vesicles and finally transported to Golgi apparatus. They are released by the alveolar cells through the merocrine mode of exocytosis.

The act of suckling initiates sensory impulses from receptors in the nipple to the hypothalamus. Then

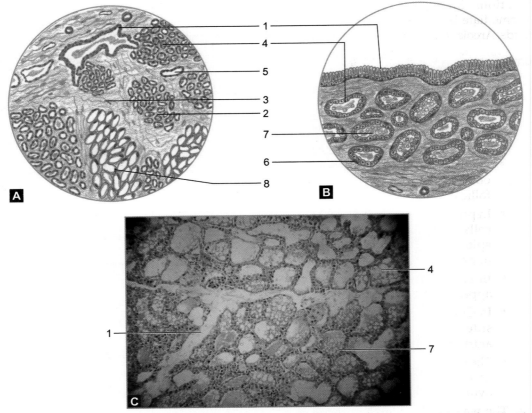

**Fig. 17.20:** Active mammary gland, (A) sketch at low magnification, (B) sketch at high magnification, (C) micrograph showing extensive glandular alveoli (4). The intralobular (2) and interlobular (3) connective tissue is reduced in amount. The figure also shows adipose tissue (8), interlobular duct (5), lactiferous duct (1), myoepithelial cells (6) and secretions rich in fatty droplets (7) in the lumen of glands

concomitant with the production of prolactin, oxytocin is released from the posterior lobe of the pituitary. Oxytocin initiates the milk ejection reflex by stimulating the myoepithelial cells present around the alveoli, causing them to contract and ejection of milk.

For comparison between non-lactating mammary gland and lactating mammary gland, *see* Table 33 given in Appendix I.

## C. Nipple and Areola

These are covered by highly pigmented skin. Nipple is a conical projection present just below the center of the mammary gland and contains the openings of the lactiferous ducts. It is composed of dense collagenous connective tissue interlaced with smooth muscle fibers The smooth muscle fibers are arranged circularly around the nipple and longitudinally along the lactiferous ducts. The contraction of these muscle fibers allows the nipple to be erected in response to various stimuli. Numerous sensory nerve endings are present in the nipple. The circular area surrounding the nipple is the areola. It contains sweat glands, sebaceous glands, and modified mammary glands (glands of Montgomery). Glands of Montgomery lie in the areolar margin and produce small elevations. Structurally, these glands are intermediate between sweat and mammary glands. Areola has a few sensory nerve endings.

## Summary

1. Ovary
   - The ovary is divided into an outer cortex (connective tissue with ovarian follicles) and an inner medulla (connective tissue with blood vessels).
   - In the primordial follicles primary oocyte is surrounded by squamous follicular cells.
   - In primary follicle flattened follicular cells form a cuboidal or columnar epithelium. Zona pellucida is formed in primary follicle.
   - In secondary follicle small cavities appear in between follicular cells.
   - In Graafian follicle ovum lies on one side of the follicle and one large antrum is present.
   - The corpus luteum is formed by both granulosa cells and thecal cells after ovulation has occurred.
2. The wall of the fallopian tube consists of 3 layers: Mucosa, muscularis externa and serosa.
3. The wall of the uterus is composed of three coats from outer to inner surface- perimetrium, myometrium and endometrium.
4. Beginning from the puberty and ending at menopause, the endometrium undergoes cyclic changes—proliferative phase (5–14 days), secretory phase (15–28 days) and menstrual phase (1–4 days).
5. The cervix produces cervical mucus that is mostly water, but also contains glycoproteins, glucose and ions.
6. Wall of vagina consists of 3 coats: Mucosa, muscularis externa and adventitia.
7. Placenta consists of fetal part (chorion) and a maternal part (decidua basalis).
8. The umbilical cord is the connecting cord from the developing fetus to the placenta.
9. In the umbilical cord, 2 umbilical arteries and 1 umbilical vein are embedded in Wharton's jelly.
10. Mammary glands are compound branched alveolar, modified sweat glands.
11. Inactive mammary glands contain interlobular connective tissue and alveoli are poorly developed.
12. During lactation, a few alveoli are distended with secretory material containing fatty droplets.

## Self Assessment

1. The ovary is lined by which epithelium?
   a. Simple cuboidal
   b. Simple columnar
   c. Stratified cuboidal
   d. Stratified columnar

2. Fertilization takes place at:
   a. Ampulla of uterine tube
   b. Uterine cavity
   c. Cervix
   d. Vagina

3. The vagina is lined by which epithelium?
   a. Stratified squamous nonkeratinized
   b. Stratified squamous keratinized
   c. Stratified cuboidal
   d. Stratified columnar

4. The lactating mammary gland is characterized by:
   a. Well developed glandular tissue
   b. Well developed alveoli containing milk
   c. Less amount of connective tissue
   d. All of the above

5. Umbilical cord contains:
   a. Two umbilical arteries
   b. Two umbilical veins
   c. One umbilical artery
   d. Three umbilical veins

6. The wall of the uterus is made by all of the following EXCEPT:
   a. Endometrium    b. Myometrium
   c. Perimetrium     d. Exometrium

7. Granulosa lutein cells of corpus luteum secrete:
   a. Progesterone
   b. Human chorionic gonadotropin
   c. Luteinizing hormone
   d. Estrogen

8. The primary oocyte completes its first meiotic division at the time of:
   a. Puberty
   b. Ovulation
   c. Fertilization
   d. None of the above

9. Uterine tube is lined by which type of epithelium?
   a. Simple cuboidal
   b. Simple columnar
   c. Pseudostratified
   d. Simple squamous

10. Syncytiotrophoblast layer is:
    a. Uninucleated
    b. Binucleated
    c. Multinucleated
    d. None of the above

## Answers

1. a,    2. a,    3. a,    4. d,    5. a,    6. d,    7. a,    8. b,    9. b,
10. c

# 18

# Endocrine System

Endocrine glands are highly vascular ductless glands whose secretion (hormones) is delivered directly into the blood–vascular system. However, some hormones are secreted directly into the intercellular space (paracrine hormone) to obtain a local effect on adjacent cells (e.g. prostaglandin) and some hormones act on the same cells (autocrine hormone) where they are synthesized (e.g. interleukin-2 produced by T cells). Along with the autonomic nervous system, the endocrine glands coordinate and control the metabolic activities and the internal environment of the body. The major endocrine glands are the pituitary gland, pineal gland, thyroid gland, parathyroid gland and adrenal (suprarenal) glands. Endocrine glands may appear as distinct organs (e.g. hypophysis and adrenal glands), may be found associated with exocrine glands (e.g. pancreatic islets and the interstitial cells of the testis), or may have isolated endocrine cells in the epithelial lining (e.g. argentaffin cells of the digestive and respiratory systems). In addition, numerous organs, which are not endocrine completely also secrete hormones, including the kidney, liver, thymus and placenta. In endocrine glands endothelial lining of the capillaries is mostly fenestrated to facilitate the entry of the hormone into the blood–vascular system and even cells are usually arranged in plates or cords to maximize surface contact with blood vessels.

Cells of endocrine system elaborate more than 100 hormones, which on the basis of their chemical nature belong to three main types:

- **Steroids:** Progesterone, estradiol, testosterone, and cortisol.
- **Proteins and polypeptides:** Insulin, glucagon, paratharmone, thyroid stimulating hormone (TSH), antidiuretic hormone (ADH), oxytocin, and follicle-stimulating hormone (FSH).
- **Amino acid derivatives:** Epinephrine, norepinephrine, and thyroxin.

Hormones act only on selected cells, called as target cells, which have specific receptors for it. Hormone receptors can be present on the surface of the cells, in the cytoplasm, or in the nucleus of the target cells. Protein and polypeptide hormones generally have their receptors on the surfaces of the cell, because they cannot penetrate the cell membrane. When hormone binds with these receptors, they activate and produce a large number of small intracellular molecules, known as secondary messengers. These messengers then initiate specific responses. Receptors for steroid and thyroid hormones are mainly present within the nucleus, because they can cross both cell membrane and nuclear membrane.

## PITUITARY GLAND (HYPOPHYSIS)

It is a small pea shaped structure located in the sella turcica (hypophyseal fossa) of the sphenoid bone. It weighs about 0.5 gm and in multiparous women it is larger (1.5 gm). It is attached to the inferior surface of the brain by an extension of the nervous tissue of the tuber cinereum of the hypothalamus, called infundibulum. Pituitary is regarded as "master endocrine gland" because some of the hormone secreted by it controls the secretory activity of other endocrine glands. However, its own activity is under the direct influence of hormones produced by the hypothalamus and by the pineal body.

The hypophysis has two parts: Adenohypophysis and neurohypophysis, which are different in the development, structure and function (Fig. 18.1).

An ectodermal diverticulum of the roof of stomodeum ascends into the cranial cavity and surrounds a down growth (infundibulum) from the neuroectoderm of the diencephalon. This diverticulum is known as Rathke's pouch. During further development, pouch loses its connection and lies in close contact with the infundibulum. The anterior wall of Rathke's pouch forms the adenohypophysis and the posterior wall develops into the pars

intermedia. The infundibulum gives rise to the neurohypophysis (Fig. 18.2).

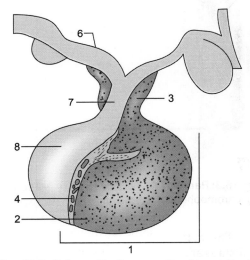

**Fig. 18.2:** Schematic diagram showing parts of a pituitary gland. Adenohypophysis (1) consists of pars distalis (2), pars tuberalis (3) and pars intermedia (4). The neurohypophysis (5) includes the median eminence (6) of the tuber cinereum, the infundibular stalk (7) and the pars nervosa (8)

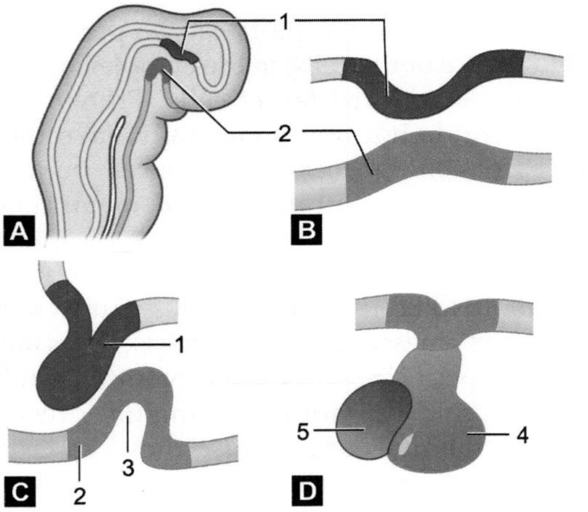

Pituitary gland is surrounded by a thin connective tissue capsule and the capsule is thickest where it encloses the pars distalis.

## A. Adenohypophysis

It has three subdivisions:

a. **Pars distalis:** It accounts for about 75% of the hypophyseal tissue. In this, glandular cells are arranged in irregular clumps or cords in between thin walled fenestrated sinusoids. Glandular cells are subdivided into chromophobes and chromophils (acidophil and basophil). This subdivision is based on their differential staining with H&E. The contents of the secretory vesicles are responsible for the staining characteristics of the chromophils (Fig. 18.3A, B). Along with these two types of cells, one more type is present, which is known as folliculostellate cells.

**Fig. 18.1:** Schematic diagram showing the development of the pituitary gland. Neuroectoderm (1), oropharynx ectoderm (2), Rathke's pouch (3), anterior lobe (4) and posterior lobe (5)

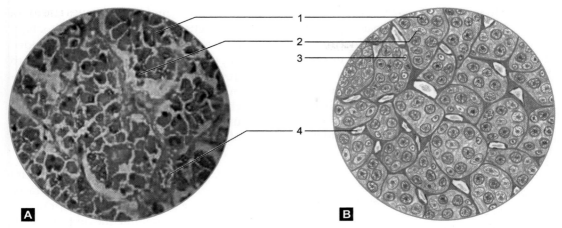

**Fig. 18.3:** Pars distalis—at high magnification, (A) micrograph, (B) sketch showing acidophils (1), basophils (2), chromophobes (3) and sinusoids (4)

The activities of the cells of the pars distalis are mainly controlled through peptide hormones produced by neurons in the hypothalamus. These hormones either stimulate or inhibit hormone secretion from their target cells in the pars distalis. These are stored in the median eminence. When released, they are transported to the pars distalis through the capillary plexuses and then they act upon specific cells of the pars distalis.

i. *Acidophils (alpha cells)*: These are oval or polygonal cells and typically smaller than basophils. These account for roughly 65% of the cells in the adenohypophysis and their granules are stain with acidophilic eosin. The most frequent subtype of acidophils is the somatotrophs, and other subtype is mammotrophs (lactotrophs).

• **Somatotrophs:** These are medium-sized, oval cells with centrally placed, rounded nucleus. These cells produce growth hormone (GH or somatotrophic hormone or STH or somatotropin); thus, they are stimulated by SRH (somatotropin-releasing hormone) and inhibited by somatostatin produced by the hypothalamus. Growth hormone stimulates liver cells to produce somatomedin C (insulin-like growth factor-1 [IGF-1]), which promotes the cell division in the cells of the growth plates and in skeletal muscles and thus results in the growth of the body.

• **Mammotrophs (lactotrophs):** These are large, polygonal cells with centrally placed, oval nucleus. The number of these cells increases significantly in late pregnancy and the early months of lactation. These cells produce prolactin (PRL, mammotropin, or luteotropin). Dopamine produced by the hypothalamus inhibits the secretion of prolactin, and the hormones estrogen and oxytocin enhance prolactin secretion. Prolactin stimulate the development of mammary glands during pregnancy and initiates milk formation.

ii. *Basophils (beta cells):* Its granules are basophilic so stain with hematoxylin. These are divided into three subtypes on the basis of their hormone products: Thyrotrophs, gonadotrophs, and corticotrophs.

- **Thyrotrophs:** These are large, polygonal cells with eccentrically placed, rounded nucleus. These cells produce thyroid stimulating hormone (TSH or thyrotropin), which stimulates the activity of the thyroid gland. The secretion of TSH is stimulated by thyrotropin-releasing hormone (TRH) and inhibited by the level of $T_3$ and $T_4$ in the blood.

- **Gonadotrophs:** These are small, oval cells with eccentrically placed, rounded nucleus. These cells secrete follicle stimulating hormone (FSH), and luteinizing hormone (LH). In males, FSH stimulates the spermatogenesis in association with testosterone and in females, it stimulates early follicular growth. In males, LH stimulates production of testosterone by Leydig cells and thus known as interstitial cell stimulating hormone (ICSH). In females, it stimulates late follicular maturation, estrogen secretion and formation of the corpus luteum. Secretion of Gonadotrophs is stimulated by Gonadotropin-releasing hormone (GnRH) produced by the hypothalamus and is inhibited by various hormones that are produced by the ovaries and testis.

- **Corticotrophs:** These are medium-sized, polygonal cells with eccentrically placed, rounded nucleus. These cells secrete adrenocorticotropic hormone (ACTH or corticotropin) and lipotropin (LPH). ACTH stimulates the secretion of some hormones of the adrenal cortex. Secretion of corticotrophs is stimulated by corticotropin-releasing hormone (CRH) produced by the hypothalamus. LPH has no known functions in humans.

iii. *Chromophobes (C cells)*: These cells are smaller and poorly staining than chromophils. These are also known as reserve or chief cell. The cytoplasm of these cells is scanty and devoid of (or have only a few) granules. Cells are rounded or polygonal and are frequently arranged in groups or clumps. Sometimes chromophobes resemble degranulated chromophils, suggesting that they are undifferentiated cells, which are capable of differentiation into various types of chromophils.

iv. *Folliculostellate cells*: These cells account for 5–10% cells in the pars distalis. These are stellate shaped supporting cells, which resemble the dendritic cells of lymphoid organs. These cells are probably derived from neuroectodermal cells. These cells regulate the paracrine regulation of functioning of cells of the pars distalis via cytokines and growth factors.

b. **Pars intermedia:** It is rudimentary in man and accounts only for 2% of the hypophyseal tissue. It contains colloid-filled cysts (Rathke's cysts) that are lined by cuboidal cells, and along with these some basophils, and chromophobes are also present (Fig. 18.4A, B). These basophils synthesize the prohormone proopiomelanocortin (POMC), which forms melanocyte-stimulating hormone (MSH), corticotropin, β-lipotropin, and β-endorphin. MSH in some species (amphibia) stimulate melanin production.

c. **Pars tuberalis:** It forms a collar of cells around the infundibular stalk. It is a highly vascular region containing veins of the hypothalamo-hypophyseal system. The cuboidal cells, in close association with numerous blood vessels, are arranged in groups or longitudinally oriented short cords or in the follicles filled with colloid. Cytoplasm is weakly basophilic, and contains fine granules (Fig. 18.5). The function of pars tuberalis is unknown in humans.

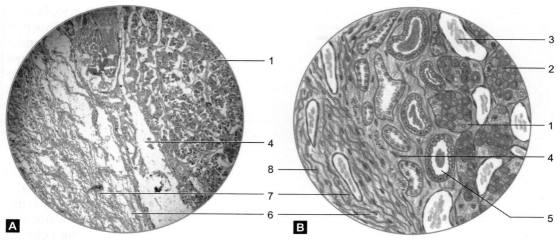

**Fig. 18.4:** Pituitary gland, (A) micrograph (B) sketch showing its parts. Pars distalis (1) is the largest part of the gland and composed of glandular cells (2) and sinusoids (3). Pars intermedia (4) is composed of colloid filled cysts (5). Neurohypophysis (6) is composed of unmyelinated nerve fibers (7) and pituicytes (8)

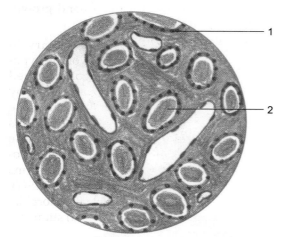

**Fig. 18.5:** Pars tuberalis—at high magnification. This part of the adenohypophysis is composed of basophilic cuboidal cells (1) surrounding colloid-filled vesicles (2)

## B. Neurohypophysis

The neurohypophysis includes the median eminence of the tuber cinereum, the infundibular stalk and the pars nervosa. Some 10,000 unmyelinated nerve fibers, forming the hypothalamo-hypophyseal tract by their axons pass into the neurohypophysis. Their cell bodies lie in the supraoptic and para-ventricular nuclei of the hypothalamus. The cells of neurohypophysis, pituicytes, are small cells with short branching processes which either end in relation to blood vessels or end into the connective tissue septa. These cells occupy approximately 25% of the volume of the pars nervosa. Pituicytes resemble astrocytes and provide support to axons in this region (Fig. 18.6A, B). These cells contain lipid droplets, intermediate filaments, and pigments. Neurohypophysis is associated with the release of two hormones in the blood: Anti-diuretic hormone (ADH or vasopressin) and oxytocin.

These hormones are synthesized by neurons of supraoptic and paraventricular nuclei and they reached through the axons of the neurons in the neurohypophysis. The endings of some axon become extremely dilated with stored secretions. Such dilatations are known as Herring bodies. During axonal transport each hormone is joined to a binding protein called neurophysin. The hormone-neurophysin complex is synthesized as a single protein and constitutes a major part of the Herring bodies. From axons, these hormones are then released in the capillaries. Cell bodies of neurons that

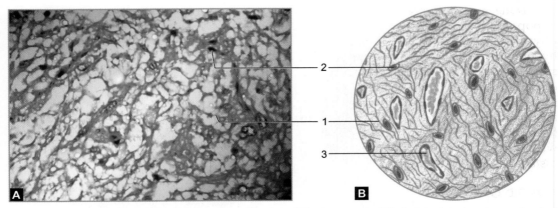

**Fig. 18.6:** Neurohypophysis—at high magnification, (A) micrograph, (B) sketch showing unmyelinated nerve fibers (1), pituicytes (2) with short branching processes and sinusoids (3)

secrete vasopressin are located mainly in the supraoptic nucleus of the hypothalamus, and cell bodies of neurons that secrete oxytocin are located mainly in the paraventricular nucleus of the hypothalamus.

The main effect of ADH is to increase the permeability of collecting tubules of the kidney for water, so more water is reabsorbed instead of being eliminated in the urine. Oxytocin stimulates contraction of the myoepithelial cells that surround the alveoli and ducts of the mammary glands during nursing and of the smooth muscle of the uterine wall during copulation and childbirth. The secretion of oxytocin is stimulated by nursing or by distention of the vagina or the uterine cervix. This occurs via nerve tracts that act on the hypothalamus. The neurohormonal reflex triggered by nursing is called the milk-ejection reflex.

### C. Blood Supply of Pituitary Gland

The pituitary gland receives its blood supply from the superior and inferior hypophyseal branches of internal carotid artery. Branches of superior hypophyseal arteries supply the median eminence and stalk; and inferior hypophyseal arteries supply mainly to pars nervosa. Superior hypophyseal arteries first form a primary capillary plexus in the median eminence and pars tuberalis. The vessels of these plexus give rise to a network of portal venules. These venules run downward around the stalk and drain into a secondary plexus of sinusoid in the pars distalis. Small efferent hypophyseal veins drain into the cavernous sinuses surrounding the gland (Fig. 18.7). All

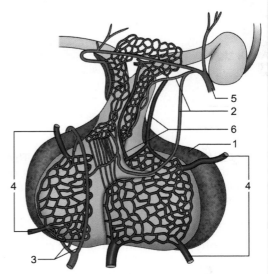

**Fig. 18.7:** Schematic diagram showing the blood supply of pituitary gland (1). Superior hypophyseal arteries (2), inferior hypophyseal arteries (3), hypophyseal veins (4), internal carotid artery (5) and hypophyseal portal veins (6)

this arrangement is referred to as hypothalamo-hypophyseal portal system. Inferior hypophyseal arteries carry blood to the neurohypophysis and drain into the plexus of the sinusoid, which takes the blood through efferent hypophyseal veins to the cavernous sinus. Some branches of superior hypophyseal arteries bypass the portal circulation and form capillary plexus in the pars intermedia, which anastomose with capillaries in the pars distalis.

## THYROID GLAND

It is situated on the lateral sides of the lower part of the larynx and upper part of the trachea. The gland is having two lateral lobes, which are connected by a narrow isthmus in front of the trachea. The gland weighs about 25–40 gm and it is heavier in females (enlarges during pregnancy and menstruation). The gland consists of rounded follicles and each follicle is supported by a reticular network that contains a huge capillary plexus, and numerous nerve fibers.

The follicle is the structural and functional building block of the gland. In the follicle a lumen filled with a viscous substance (colloid) is lined by epithelial cells (Fig. 18.8A to D). The colloid is the secretary product of the follicular cell. The height of the cells and the

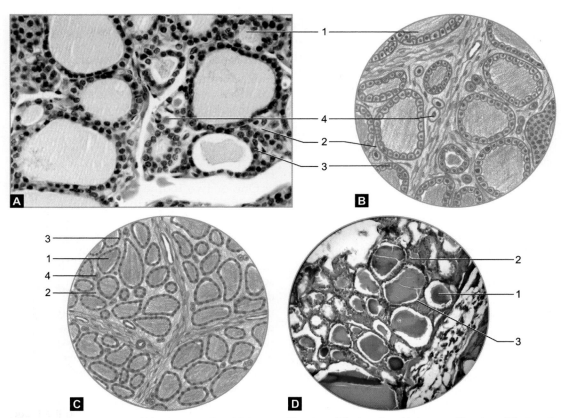

**Fig. 18.8:** Thyroid gland, (A) micrograph at high magnification, (B) sketch at high magnification, (C) sketch at low magnification, (D) micrograph at low magnification, illustrating rounded colloid filled follicles (1) separated by interfollicular connective tissue (2). Follicles are lined by simple cuboidal epithelium (3). Groups of parafollicular cells (4) are present in the connective tissue

amount of colloid varies according to the functional activity. When the cells are squamous and the lumen is filled with colloid, the follicles are referred to as "inactive". If the cells are cuboidal or low columnar and colloid is moderate, then they are referred to as "active". When the cells are columnar and colloid is scanty, the follicles are referred to as "hyperactive".

Follicular cells possess short, blunt microvilli, which extend into the colloid. The basal parts of these cells are rich in rough endoplasmic reticulum. The apical part has a discrete Golgi apparatus and small secretory granules whose content are similar to that of the follicular colloid. Lateral cell membranes of follicular cells are united at the apex by junctional complexes. These complexes prevent the colloid from leaking into the adjacent glandular stroma. The main component of colloid is thyroglobulin, which consists of triiodothyronine ($T_3$) and tetraiodothyronine ($T_4$ or thyroxin).

T$_3$ and T$_4$ hormones increase the basal rate of oxygen consumption, heat production and cardiac output. These hormones also increase gluconeogenesis and glycogen degradation. These hormones stimulate cartilage growth, endochondral ossification and linear growth of bone. These hormones play a crucial role in central nervous system development (a deficiency of $T_4$ and $T_3$ results in permanent brain damage).

Apart from follicular cells the gland also contains C cells (clear cells or parafollicular cells). These cells are found either as single cell in between the follicular epithelium and the basement membrane or as clusters in the interfollicular connective tissue. Parafollicular cells are larger than follicular cells, but lightly stained and never directly border the follicular lumen. C cells produce the hormone calcitonin, which decreases blood calcium concentration by acting on the osteocytes and osteoclasts of bone to inhibit resorption of bone and release of calcium into the blood.

## A. Control of the Thyroid

The secretory activity of the thyroid gland is controlled by interactions between two organs, i.e. hypothalamus and adenohypophysis. Levels of $T_4$ and $T_3$ in the blood provide feedback to the hypothalamus, which releases thyrotropin releasing hormone (TRH). TRH then stimulates thyrotrophs present in the pars distalis to release thyroid stimulating hormone (TSH). TSH stimulates follicular cells of the thyroid gland to phagocytose stored thyroglobulin, degrading it intracellularly and then releasing it into the blood stream as $T_4$ and $T_3$. The cell membrane of the basal portion of follicular cells is rich in receptors for TSH. Secretion of TSH is also increased by exposure to cold and decreased by heat and stressful stimuli.

## B. Synthesis and Release of Thyroid Hormones

Iodide from the blood is taken up by the follicular epithelial cells using $Na^+ - I^-$ cotransporter. Iodide ion then actively diffuses towards apical cell membrane where they are oxidized to iodine, an active form of iodide. This process is catalyzed by the thyroid peroxidase enzyme.

One or two iodine atoms then added to tyrosine residues of thyroglobulin within the colloid, and also catalyzed by thyroid peroxidase. The addition of one iodine atom to a single tyrosine residue form the monoiodotyrosine (MIT). The addition of a second iodine atom to MIT residues forms diiodotyrosine (DIT). Then iodotyrosine molecules are coupled together. If two diiodotyrosine molecules couple together, the result is the formation of thyroxin ($T_4$). If a diiodotyrosine and a monoiodotyrosine are coupled together, the result is the formation of triiodothyronine ($T_3$).

When stimulated by TSH, thyroid follicular cells take up colloid by endocytosis. The colloid within the endocytic vesicles is then digested by lysosomal enzymes. Hydrolysis of thyroglobulin results in $T_4$, $T_3$, DIT, and MIT, which are liberated into the cytoplasm. The free $T_4$ and $T_3$ cross the basolateral cell membrane and are discharged into the capillaries. Monoiodotyrosine and diiodotyrosine are not secreted into the blood, and their iodine is removed by a deiodinase. The products of this enzymatic reaction are iodine and tyrosine, which are reused by the follicular cells.

$T_4$ is the most abundant compound, constituting 90% of the circulating thyroid hormone. $T_3$ is quick and short lasting in action, whereas $T_4$ is slower and long lasting in its effects on the various tissues of the body. The major production of $T_3$ actually occurs outside of the thyroid gland.

## PARATHYROID GLANDS

These are four small oval bodies located at the posterior surface of the thyroid gland and they total weigh about 0.4 gm. Each gland is surrounded by a thin connective tissue capsule. Delicate connective tissue trabeculae containing blood vessels, lymphatics and nerves extend from the capsule, enter in the gland and subdivide it. A considerable number of fat cells infiltrate the gland (beginning around puberty) and may account for about half of the weight of the parathyroid glands in adults. Two cell types can be distinguished in the parathyroid glands (Fig. 18.9A, B).

### A. Chief (Principal) Cells

These are the most numerous small rounded cells with light and centrally placed nucleus. Cytoplasm is very weakly acidophilic and contains large accumulations of glycogen and lipid droplets. Lipofuscin granules are also present in the cytoplasm. These cells synthesize parathyroid hormone (PTH or parathormone).

### B. Oxyphilic (Eosinophil) Cells

These polyhedral cells are less frequent, entirely lacking in small children; occurring first in children six to seven years old and afterwards increasing in number with age. Cytoplasm is strongly acidophilic because of large amounts of mitochondria. The nucleus is small and basophilic. The function of these cells is unknown.

There are plenty of transitional cells, i.e. cells that morphologically represent transitions between chief cells and oxyphilic cells.

### C. Action of Parathyroid Hormone

PTH is essential for life. It binds to receptors in osteoblasts to produce an osteoclast-

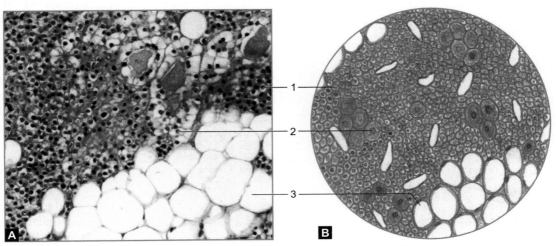

**Fig. 18.9:** Parathyroid gland, (A) micrograph, (B) sketch, showing small rounded chief cells (1) and large oxyphilic cells (2). Adipose tissue (3) can also be seen in the figures

stimulating factor (OSF). OSF increases the number and activity of osteoclasts and thus promotes the absorption of the calcified bone matrix and the release of Ca⁺⁺ into the blood. The resulting increase in the concentration of $Ca^{++}$ in the blood suppresses the production of PTH. Along with the calcitonin from the thyroid gland this hormone constitutes a dual mechanism to regulate blood levels of $Ca^{++}$, an important factor in homeostasis. It also acts directly on the distal convoluted tubules of kidneys to promote the absorption of $Ca^{++}$ and inhibits the absorption of $PO_4^-$ from the glomerular filtrate. PTH indirectly increases the absorption of $Ca^{++}$ by influencing the kidneys to form hormone calcitriol (active form of vitamin D). Calcitriol increases calcium absorption from the gastrointestinal tract into the blood stream.

## SUPRARENAL (ADRENAL) GLANDS

These paired glands are flattened and triangular-shaped, situated at the apical pole of each kidney and together they weigh about 8 gm. Their weight and size vary with the age and physiological condition of the individual. They are enclosed within a connective tissue capsule and have an outer cortex and inner medulla that are developmentally and functionally distinct from each other (Fig. 18.10A, B). The cortex is derived from mesoderm, while medulla is derived from neural crest cells (ectoderm). The medulla is surrounded by the cortex except at the hilum through which the vein comes out and it forms only one-tenth of the entire suprarenal gland. Vessels and nerves reach the medulla by way of connective tissue trabeculae which extend from the capsule towards the medulla.

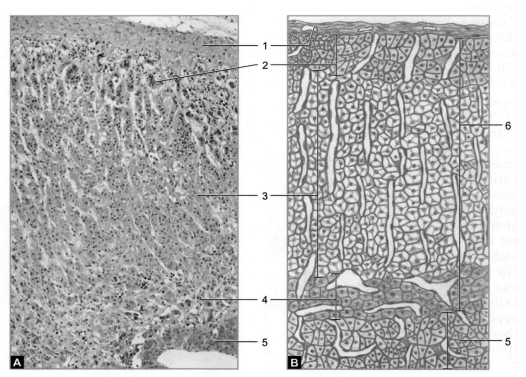

**Fig. 18.10:** Suprarenal gland, (A) micrograph, (B) sketch, showing collagenous capsule (1). Three zones of the cortex (6) are—zona glomerulosa (2), zona fasciculata (3) and zona reticularis (4) clearly distinguishable in the figure. Medulla (5) is present in the lower part of the figures

## A. Cortex

The cells of the cortex do not store their secretory products in granules; rather, they synthesize and secrete steroid hormones upon demand. Steroids, being low-molecular weight, lipid-soluble molecules, diffuse through the plasma membrane and do not require the specialized process of exocytosis for their release. It is divided into three concentric zones which from the surface inwards are:

a. **Zona glomerulosa:** It accounts for about 15% of the cortical thickness. Cells are organised into small rounded groups or curved columns. Cells are polyhedral or columnar and smaller than in the other two zones, their nuclei are dark and rounded, and the cytoplasm is slightly basophilic. A rich network of fenestrated sinusoidal capillaries surrounds each cell group. Cells of zona glomerulosa have abundant sER, multiple Golgi apparatus, large mitochondria, free ribosomes, and some rER. It acts as a chief regenerative zone for cells of the zona fasciculata.

b. **Zona fasciculata:** It accounts for about 75% of the cortical thickness. It consists of radially arranged cell cords of one or two cells thick, which are separated by fenestrated sinusoidal capillaries. The cords sometimes branch to form an anastomosis with adjacent cords. Cells are polyhedral and larger than the cells of zona glomerulosa and zona reticularis. Nuclei are light and centrally located. Cells have highly developed sER and mitochondria. The cytoplasm is also slightly acidophilic and contains numerous lipid droplets. Cells have a characteristic foamy or spongy appearance (extraction of lipid during tissue processing), therefore also called spongiocytes. Cells contain lipofuscin pigment granules.

c. **Zona reticularis:** It accounts for about 5–7% of the cortical thickness. It consists of anastomosing cell cords separated by sinusoids. Cells are typically smaller than the cells of zona fasciculata. Their cytoplasm is eosinophilic, less spongy than that of other cells in the cortex and the nucleus is rather light and large. Lipofuscin accumulates in the cells with age. These accumulations have an orange tinge in H&E stained preparations.

## B. Hormones Produced in the Cortex

All hormones produced in the cortex are steroids and as they are synthesized in the cortex, they are known as corticosteroids. Corticosteroids are further subdivided into mineralocorticoids and glucocorticoids. The most important mineralocorticoids are aldosterone and deoxycorticosterone, which regulates the reabsorption of sodium and excretion of potassium in the tubules of the kidney. Glucocorticoids are named so because of their role in regulating gluconeogenesis (glucose synthesis) and glucogenesis (glycogen polymerization). The most important glucocorticoids are cortisol (dihydrocortisone) and cortisone, which has a wide range of effects on most cells of the body. These hormones regulate carbohydrates, protein, amino acids and fat metabolism. It is also important in the body's response to stress and in reducing inflammatory, allergic and immune response. Small amounts of androgens, estrogens and progesterone (sex hormones) are also produced by cortical cells, which induce weak masculinizing effect.

Mineralocorticoids are produced in the zona glomerulosa, glucocorticoids are produced in the zona fascicularis and reticularis, and sex hormones are produced in the zona reticularis.

## C. Control of the Adrenal Cortex

The zona fasciculata and zona reticularis depend on adenocorticotropic hormone (ACTH or corticotropin) to sustain their function and survival. The zona glomerulosa is not influenced by ACTH. The secretion of ACTH is controlled through the release of corticotropin-releasing hormone in the median eminence. Aldosterone secretion is controlled primarily by renin-angiotensin and secondarily by ACTH.

### D. Medulla

It is not sharply delimited from the cortex. Cells are arranged in strands or small clusters. Cells are columnar or polyhedral and store their hormones in granules. Capillaries and venules are present in the intervening spaces. The cytoplasm of the cells is weakly basophilic. They are called chromaffin cells because the granules of these cells stained yellow with potassium bichromate. This is called the chromaffin reaction. Chromaffin cells cor-respond to the adrenaline or epinephrine (80%) and noradrenaline or norepinephrine (20%) producing cells of the medulla. These two cell groups cannot be distinguished using routine histology. Epinephrine increases cardiac output, elevates the level of blood glucose and increases the basal metabolic rate. Norepinephrine, on the other hand, acts primarily to elevate and maintain blood pressure by causing vasoconstriction in the peripheral segments of the arterial region. The medullary cells arise from neural crest cells, as do the postganglionic neurons of sympathetic and parasympathetic ganglia. Thus, the cells of the adrenal medulla can be considered modified sympathetic postganglionic neurons that have lost their axons and dendrites during embryonic development and have become secretory cells.

### E. Blood Supply of Suprarenal Gland

The suprarenal glands have profuse blood supply. Each suprarenal gland is supplied by three separate arteries, which arise from three separate sources:

- Superior suprarenal arteries which originate from the inferior phrenic arteries,
- Middle suprarenal arteries which originate from the aorta,
- Inferior suprarenal arteries which originate from the renal arteries.

These arteries branch before entering the capsule, to produce many small arteries that penetrate the capsule, and form a subcapsular plexus. The cortical arteries arise from the plexus and form a network of fenestrated cortical sinusoidal capillaries, which drain into the fenestrated medullary sinusoidal capillaries. Small venules arising from these capillaries drain into a suprarenal vein, which emerges from the hilum. In addition, some arteries (medullary arteries) pass unbranched through the cortex and enter into the medulla, where they form capillaries networks (Fig. 18.11).

Thus, the medulla receives a dual blood supply: (1) an arterial supply from the medullary arteries and (2) numerous vessels from the cortical sinusoidal capillaries. This arrangement of vessels facilitates the

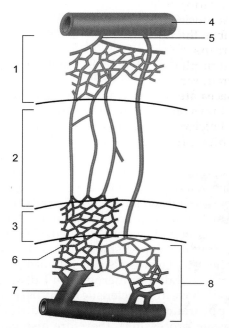

**Fig. 18.11:** Schematic diagram showing the blood supply of the suprarenal gland. Zona glomerulosa (1), zona fasciculata (2), zona reticularis (3), capsular artery (4), cortical arteriole (5), medullary sinusoidal capillaries (6), medullary vein (7) and medulla (8)

cortical hormones to influence the activity of medullary cells.

## PINEAL GLAND (EPIPHYSIS CEREBRI)

It is a flattened, conical endocrine gland of neuroectodermal origin and lies at the posterior wall of the third ventricle near the center of the brain. It weighs about 120 mg. It is covered by pia matter in the form of a thin connective tissue capsule. From this capsule trabeculae extend, which divide it into incomplete lobules. In the lobules lie large pale-staining pinealocytes and neuroglial (interstitial) cells (Fig. 18.12A, B).

Pinealocytes are pale-staining cells with numerous long processes that end in dilatations near capillaries. Pinealocytes secrete melatonin and peptides that are similar to the peptide form in hypothalamo-hypophyseal axis. Neuroglial (interstitial) cells resemble astrocytes, with elongated processes and a small, dense nucleus. Neuroglial cells are fewer in number than pinealocytes. The gland also contains basophilic accumulations of calcium phosphates and carbonates, known as brain sand or corpora arenacea. Corpora arenacea are radiopaque, and can be seen in the X-rays of the skull, so are a useful guide for clinicians. Synthesis of pineal hormones exhibits circadian (diurnal) and seasonal rhythms; its level rises during darkness and falls during the day. Melatonin helps to regulate LH levels. The pineal gland also contains substantial levels of GnRH and has a role in the onset of puberty. The gland also plays an important role in adjusting the sudden changes in day length in travellers suffering from jet lag.

> **Pheochromocytoma** It is the tumor of the adrenal gland, which produces excess adrenaline. Pheochromocytomas arise from the central portion of the adrenal gland which is called the adrenal medulla. This results in transient elevations of blood pressure. These tumors can also develop in the extramedullary sites.

## Summary

1. Pituitary gland:

   • Adneohypophysis:

     Pars distalis:

     i. Acidophils—somatotrophs (GH) and mammotrophs (PRL)

     ii. Basophils—thyrotrophs (TSH), gonadotrophs (FSH and LH), corticotrophs (ACTH, LPH)

     iii. Chromophobes—folliculostellate cells

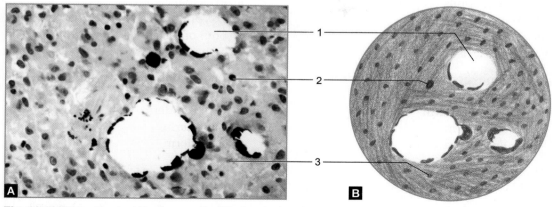

**Fig. 18.12:** Pineal body, (A) micrograph, (B) sketch showing empty spaces where brain sands are stored (1), glial cells (2) and pinealocyte (3)

Pars intermedia:

i. Basophils (MSH, corticotropin, β-lipo-tropin, β-endorphin)

Pars tuberalis

- Neurohypophysis—ADH and oxytocin

2. Thyroid—Colloid in the follicle is thyro-globulin.

3. Parafollicular cells produce hormone calcitonin.

4. Parathyroid gland—chief cells (PTH) and oxyphil cells.

5. Suprarenal gland:
- Cortex (corticosteroids)—zona glomerulosa, zona fasciculata and zona reticularis
- Medulla—chromaffin cells—adrenaline and noradrenaline

6. Pineal gland—pinealocytes (melatonin).

## Self Assessment

1. The corpora arenacea are seen in the:
   a. Thyroid
   b. Parathyroid
   c. Pineal
   d. Suprarenal

2. Which cells of pituitary gland secrete thyroid stimulating hormone?
   a. Acidophils
   b. Basophils
   c. Chromophobes
   d. Pituicytes

3. Neurohypophysis is derived from:
   a. Neuroectoderm
   b. Oral ectoderm
   c. Mesoderm
   d. Endoderm

4. Follicles are present in which endocrine gland?
   a. Suprarenal     b. Thyroid
   c. Parathyroid    d. Adrenal

5. Calcitonin is produced by which cells?
   a. Acidophils
   b. Basophils
   c. Parafollicular
   d. Pituicytes

6. Suprarenal cortex is characterized by:
   a. Presence of chromaffin cells in medulla
   b. The cortex is having 3 zones
   c. Lies on upper pole of kidney
   d. All of the above

7. Aldosterone is produced by cells of which zone of adrenal cortex?
   a. Zona glomerulosa
   b. Zona fasciculata
   c. Zona reticularis
   d. None of the above

8. Parafollicular cells are present in which endocrine gland?
   a. Thyroid
   b. Parathyroid
   c. Suprarenal
   d. Pituitary

9. Cells present in the parathyroid gland are:
   a. Principal cells
   b. Oxyphilic cells
   c. Both of the above
   d. None of the above

10. Adenohypophysis is derived from:
    a. Neuroectoderm
    b. Oral ectoderm
    c. Mesoderm
    d. Endoderm

## Answers

1. c,    2. b,    3. a,    4. b,    5. c,    6. d,    7. a,    8. a,    9. c,
10. b

# 19

# Nervous System

The nervous system is developed entirely from ectoderm. The nervous system manifests optimally the two properties of protoplasm; irritability and conductivity and is one of the most highly differentiated tissues in the body. The human nervous system is formed by a network of more than 100 million nerve cells (neurons), assisted by many more glial cells. Each neuron has, on average, at least 1,000 interconnections with other neurons, forming a very complex system for communication network. The nervous system is divided anatomically into the central nervous system and the peripheral nervous system. Functionally, the nervous system is divided into the somatic nervous system (SNS) and autonomic nervous system (ANS). SNS is involved in the control of voluntary functions. It provides sensory and motor innervations to all parts of our body except smooth and cardiac muscle, glands and viscera. ANS is involved in control of involuntary functions and it is further having three subdivisions: Sympathetic, parasympathetic, and enteric nervous system. It provides afferent sensory innervation from the viscera and also provides efferent involuntary motor innervation to smooth muscle and glands.

For comparison between nervous and endocrine system, *see* Table 34 given in Appendix I.

## CENTRAL NERVOUS SYSTEM

The central nervous system includes the cerebrum, cerebellum, and the spinal cord. It consists of grey and white matter without any intervening connective tissue and is therefore a relatively soft, gel-like organ and its support comes from the three meninges that surround it. Grey matter consists of aggregations of neuronal cell bodies, dendrites, and unmyelinated portions of axons as well as glial cells; the absence of myelin causes these regions to appear grey in living tissues. White matter is composed mostly of myelinated nerve fibers along with some unmyelinated fibers and glial cells; its white color results from the abundance of myelin surrounding the axons.

## A. Cerebrum

In the cerebral hemispheres, grey matter is located on the surface as the cerebral cortex and white matter is present in the more central regions. Grey matter is also embedded in the white matter as nuclei. The surface of hemispheres is uneven due to the presence of certain folds (gyri) with intervening depressions (sulci). The composition of the cortex is complex with many different types of nerve cells. These include many local interneurons (stellate cells and granule cells) as well as the much larger and more conspicuous pyramidal cells; axons of some of them enter the underlying white matter and travel to other cortical areas or to other regions of the brain. Cells of the cerebral cortex are related to the integration of sensory information and the initiation of voluntary motor responses. The white matter is composed of bundles of myelinated fibers passing in all directions.

The cortex is described as having six layers; however, the distinction between these layers is not well marked (Fig. 19.1). These layers are distinguished on the basis of the predominance of cell type and arrangement of fibres. From superficial to deep these layers are:

a. **Layer I (the molecular or plexiform layer):** This layer is situated just beneath the pia mater. It mainly consists of fibers and two kinds of nerve cells, i.e. horizontal cells of Cajal and stellate cells. The peripheral portion consists largely of fibers, which travel parallel to the surface. In its deeper part lie the horizontal cells of Cajal, whose cell body and processes are disposed horizontally.

b. **Layer II (the outer granular layer):** This layer consists of two types of nerve cells, i.e. small pyramidal and granule or stellate cells. Their apical dendrites extend in the layer I and axons end into the deeper layer. Axons of these nerve cells will form association fibers that interconnect different parts of a hemisphere.

c. **Layer III (the outer pyramidal layer):** This layer consists of cell bodies of small pyramidal cells. Axons of these nerve cells will form commissural fibers that interconnect the two hemispheres via the corpus callosum.

d. **Layer IV (the inner granular layer):** This layer consists of densely packed granule cells with a white horizontal fiber layer called the external band of Baillarger. This layer provides connections between nerve cells of different layers.

e. **Layer V (the inner pyramidal or ganglionic layer):** This layer consists of cell bodies of large pyramidal cells (giant pyramidal cells of Betz) (Fig. 19.2). Axons from these cells

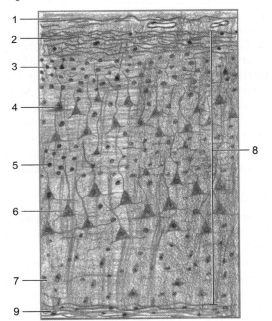

**Fig. 19.1:** Cerebrum at low magnification showing the pia mater with blood vessels (1) and the layers of cerebral cortex (8) are—molecular layer (2), outer granular layer (3), outer pyramidal layer (4), inner granular layer (5), inner pyramidal layer (6), polymorphic layer (7). White matter (9) can be seen in the lower part of the figure

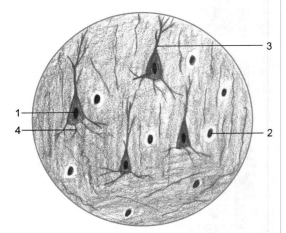

**Fig. 19.2:** Pyramidal cells of cerebrum at high magnification showing large pyramidal cells (1) and neuroglial cells (2). In pyramidal cells apical dendrites (3) are most prominent processes and axon (4) arises from the base of the cell body

typically project to more distant cortical regions, to other parts of the brain, or to lower centers (such as spinal motor neurons). The horizontal fibers in the deeper part are called internal band of Baillarger.

f. **Layer VI (the polymorphic or fusiform cell layer):** This layer mainly consists of spindle-shaped fusiform cells and a few stellate cells. The fusiform cells are located in the deeper part of the cerebral cortex. Deep to this layer lies white matter.

## B. Cerebellum

In the cerebellum, grey matter is located on the surface as cerebellar cortex and white matter is present in the center as the medulla. The cortex is responsible for maintaining equilibrium, balance, muscle tone, and coordination of skeletal muscles. The cortex is thrown into numerous folds or folia. The cortex consists of three very well-defined layers: Molecular layer, Purkinje layer, and granular layer (Fig. 19.3A, B). Deep to the granular layer lie lightly stained region of white matter, which contains nerve fibers, and supporting neuroglial cells.

a. **Molecular layer:** This layer is situated just beneath the pia mater. It stains lightly with eosin and is featureless as it consists of a few cells and more of myelinated and

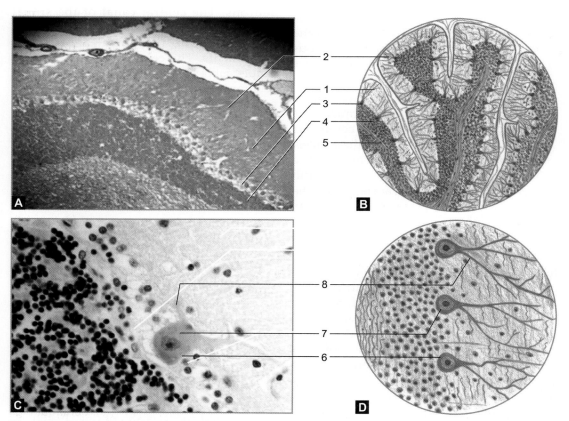

**Fig. 19.3:** Cerebellum, (A) micrograph—at low magnification, (B) sketch—at low magnification, (C) micrograph—at high magnification, (D) sketch—at high magnification, showing outer grey matter (1) having molecular layer (2), Purkinje cell layer (3) and granular layer (4). The core is formed by white matter (5). Purkinje cells (6) have large flask shape cell body (7), the apex of which gives rise to dendritic tree (8)

unmyelinated nerve fibers. This layer consists of a few scattered stellate cells in the superficial part and a few basket cells in the deeper part. However, dendritic processes of Purkinje cells and the axons of granule cells occupy most of the molecular layer.

b. **Purkinje cell layer:** This layer consists of Purkinje cells, which are arranged in a single row in between the molecular and the granular layer. Purkinje cell is a large flask shape neuron, the apex of which gives rise to many dendrites in a plane perpendicular to the long axis of the folium. These dendrites branch repeatedly to form dendritic arborization. Purkinje cells give a single thin axon, which passes through the granular layer to end in the deeper nuclei of the cerebellum and thus represent the beginning of outflow fibers from the cerebellum (Fig. 19.3C, D).

c. **The inner granular layer:** This layer stains deeply with hematoxylin because it is packed with nuclei of many cerebellar granule cells. These are among the smallest and most numerous neurons in the body. This layer also consists of glomeruli (cerebellar islands), which are regions of the cerebellar cortex where incoming fibers synapse with granule cells.

## C. Spinal Cord

It is invested by a protective coating, the three-layered meninges, which are identical to the meninges of the brain. The most intimate is the pia mater, surrounded by the arachnoid, which in turn, is invested by the thick, collagenous dura mater. The arachnoid has fewer trabeculae in the spinal cord, so it can be more clearly distinguished from the pia mater. The spinal cord itself is organized into white matter and grey matter. The white matter is located peripherally and does not contain nerve cell bodies. It is composed of nerve fibers, most of which are myelinated (Fig. 19.4A, F) along with various types of glial cells. The white matter is subdivided into anterior and posterior funiculi. The grey matter contains the cell bodies of the neurons, as well as the initial and terminal end of their processes, many of which are usually not myelinated. These nerve cell processes and those of numerous glial cells form an interwoven network of fibers known as neuropil. The grey matter is subdivided into regions, namely the dorsal horn, the ventral horn, and the grey commissure. Dorsal horn contains neurons that receive, process, and retransmit information from the sensory neurons whose cell bodies are present in dorsal root ganglion, while the ventral horn contains the large cell bodies of motor neurons. The central canal of the spinal cord passes through the grey commissure, dividing it into the dorsal and ventral components. The central canal is lined by simple cuboidal ependymal cells and it is a remnant of the lumen of the embryonic neural tube. Central canal contains CSF and communicates with the ventricles of the brain. Processes of neurons enter and leave the spinal cord as ventral and dorsal roots, respectively.

The structure of spinal cord varies at different levels:

a. **Cervical:** The maximum white matter lies at this level. The posterior funiculus is divided by a posterolateral septum into fasciculus gracillis and cuneatus. The ventral horn is wide (Fig. 19.4B).

b. **Thoracic:** The grey matter is very less and the ventral and dorsal horn looks similar. Lateral horn is present at this level. Lateral horn contains the cell bodies of autonomic neurons (Fig. 19.4C).

c. **Lumbar:** The grey matter is more in comparison to the white matter. The posterolateral sulcus is absent (Fig. 19.4D).

d. **Sacral:** The grey matter is more and ventral and dorsal horns are equal in size (Fig.19.4E).

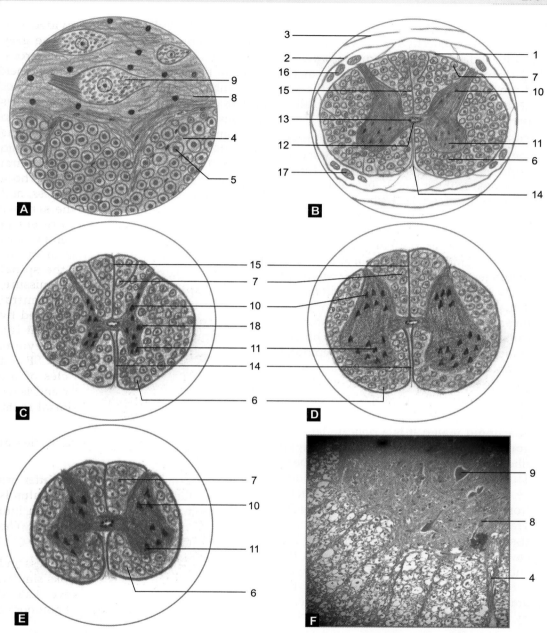

**Fig. 19.4:** TS of spinal cord at different levels, (A) high magnification, (B) cervical level, (C) thoracic level, (D) lumbar level, (E) sacral level and (F) high magnification. The spinal cord is invested by pia mater (1), arachnoid (2) and dura mater (3). White matter (4) is located peripherally and composed of myelinated nerve fibers (5). It is divided into anterior (6) and posterior (7) funiculi. Grey matter (8) is composed of cell bodies of neurons (9) and divided into the dorsal horn (10), ventral horn (11) and grey commissure (12). Central canal (13) passes through the commissure. The figure also shows the anterior median fissure (14), posterior median sulcus (15), dorsal root (16), ventral root (17) and lateral horn (18)

## D. Meninges

These are the connective tissue coverings of the brain and spinal cord. From superficial to deep these are: Dura mater, arachnoid mater and pia mater. The arachnoid and the pia mater are linked together, so commonly called as pia-arachnoid or leptomeninges.

a. **Dura mater:** It is composed of dense fibrous connective tissue consisting of interlacing bundles of collagen and elastic fibers associated with flattened fibroblasts. In the brain, dura mater is further having two layers: Outer endosteal and inner meningeal. The endosteal layer is continuous with the periosteum of the skull and gets attached to the margin of the foramen magnum. The meningeal layer continues in the spinal cord. The dura mater that envelops the spinal cord is the meningeal layer and it is not adhere to the walls of the vertebral canal, instead separated from it by the epidural space. This space contains epidural fat and a venous plexus. The dura mater is always separated from the arachnoid by the thin subdural space containing a small amount of serous fluid.

b. **Arachnoid mater:** It is a delicate layer of connective tissue formed by collagen fibers, fibroblasts and a few elastic fibers. This layer is avascular although blood vessels travel through it. Trabeculae extend from this layer and connect it to the pia mater. Trabeculae are composed of loose connective tissue containing elongated fibroblasts. The cavities between the trabeculae form the subarachnoid space, which is filled with cerebro-spinal fluid. Both surfaces of the arachnoid mater and trabeculae are covered by squamous epithelial cells.

c. **Pia mater:** It is composed primarily of loose connective tissue containing many blood vessels. It follows all the irregularities of the surface of the central nervous system. Arteries enter the central nervous system with a sleeve of pia attached to them, but it disappears from the arteries as the capillaries are formed.

## E. Blood–Brain Barrier

It is a functional barrier present between specific blood–borne substances and the neural tissue of the CNS. It prevents the passage of some substances, such as antibiotics, chemical, and toxic matter, from the blood to the nervous tissue. This barrier is formed by the occluding junctions of endothelial cells lining the continuous capillaries that course through the CNS. These endothelial cells of capillaries in the brain are different from the capillaries present in the peripheral tissues in following ways:

- These endothelial cells are joined by occluding junctions, retarding the flow of materials between cells.
- These endothelial cells have relatively a few pinocytotic vesicles.
- These capillaries are invested by well-defined basal lamina, which in turn are almost completely surrounded by the end-feet of numerous astrocytes.

The blood–brain barrier does not exist in some areas of the CNS, such as the median eminence, neurohypophysis, lamina terminalis, pineal gland, area postrema, and choroid plexus.

## THE PERIPHERAL NERVOUS SYSTEM

The peripheral nervous system includes cranial and peripheral nerves and associated ganglia. The nerves, which carry sensory input from the cutaneous areas of the body and also from the viscera, back to the CNS for processing, are called afferent or sensory nerves. The nerves, which originate in the CNS and carry motor impulses to the effector organs, are called efferent or motor nerves.

## A. Ganglia

A collection of nerve cell body outside the central nervous system is called a ganglion. Two types of ganglia can be distinguished on the basis of difference in morphology and function: Dorsal root (sensory) ganglia, and autonomic (sympathetic) ganglia. In ganglia, the body of each ganglion cell is enveloped by a layer of small cuboidal glial cells called satellite cells. The entire ganglion is covered by the connective tissue capsule.

a. **Dorsal root ganglia (sensory ganglia):** These ganglia are located in the dorsal roots of the spinal nerves and in the paths of V, VII, IX, and X cranial nerves. Each ganglion is surrounded by a connective tissue capsule, which is formed by epineurium of the dorsal root. Under the capsule lie groups of large cell bodies. In between and around the groups of neurons lie bundles of myelinated nerve fibers. The neurons are pseudounipolar and the cell bodies are spherical in shape with centrally placed nucleus. Unlike autonomic ganglia, these ganglia do not have synapses (Fig. 19.5).

b. **Autonomic ganglia:** The sympathetic ganglia lie along the sympathetic chain, whereas parasympathetic ganglia are located within certain organs, especially in the walls of the digestive tract, where they constitute the intramural ganglia. The neurons are multipolar, so cell bodies are irregular in shape. The nucleus is eccentric in position and neurons are frequently covered by an incomplete layer of satellite cells. The neurons are smaller as compared to the sensory ganglia and even they are not arranged in groups rather than that they are scattered. The nerve fibers are thin and non-myelinated. Nissl substances are better defined here in comparison to sensory ganglia (Fig. 19.6). These ganglia are motor ganglia in which axons of preganglionic neurons synapse on postganglionic neurons.

For comparison between dorsal and autonomic ganglia, *see* Table 35 given in Appendix I.

## B. Peripheral Nerves

In the peripheral nervous system, the axons are grouped into bundles to form the nerves. Each axon may be myelinated or unmyelinated, or may be sensory, motor or a mixture of both types. Except for a few thin nerves made up of myelinated nerve fibers, nerves have a whitish appearance because of their myelin content. Myelin is produced by Schwann cells. There are no neuronal cell bodies within the nerves. The bulk of a peripheral nerve consists of nerve fibers and their supporting Schwann cells. The individual nerve fibers and their associated Schwann cells are held together by connective tissue organized into three

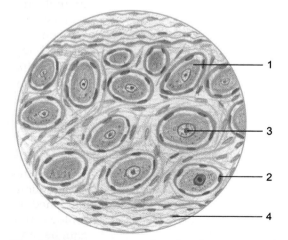

**Fig. 19.5:** Sensory ganglia, showing groups of pseudounipolar neurons (1) separated by bundles of myelinated nerve fibers (4). The neurons have many satellite cells (2) and central nucleus (3)

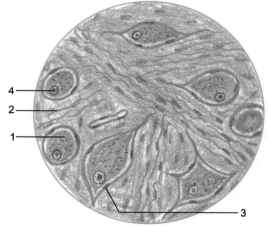

**Fig. 19.6:** Autonomic ganglia, showing scattered multipolar neurons (1) separated by thin unmyelinated nerve fibers (2). The neurons have an incomplete layer of satellite cells (3) and eccentric nucleus (4)

distinctive components. Nerves have an external fibrous coat of dense irregular collagenous connective tissue called epineurium. It is thickest where it is continuous with the dura covering the CNS at the spinal cord or brain, and where the spinal or cranial nerves originate, respectively. Each bundle is surrounded by a dense connective tissue sheath called the perineurium, but it is thinner than the epineurium (Fig. 19.7A, B). Inner surface of perineurium consists of layers of flattened epithelial-like cells joined by tight junctions that prevent passage of most macromolecules. In between these layers lie collagen fibers and a few elastic fibers. Each nerve fiber is surrounded by loose connective tissue containing collagen fibrils with a few fibroblasts, mast cells and macrophages. This layer is called endoneurium, produced mainly by Schwann cells.

## CONDUCTIVE TISSUE

It consists of two principal types of cells, neurons and supporting cells.

### A. Neuron

The neuron is the basic structural and functional unit of the nervous system. It consists of the cell body (perikaryon or soma)

and its processes (dendrites and axon) (Fig. 19.8). In the central nervous system, cell bodies are present only in the grey matter and white matter contains only neuronal cell

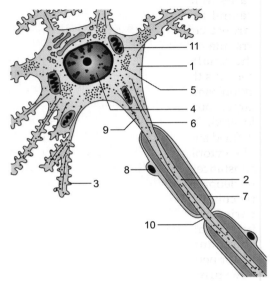

**Fig. 19.8:** Schematic diagram of neuron showing soma (1), axon (2) and dendrites with spines (3). Nucleus (4), Nissl substances (5), neurofilaments (6), myelin sheath (7), Schwann cell (8), axon hillock (9), nodes of Ranvier (10) and mitochondria (11)

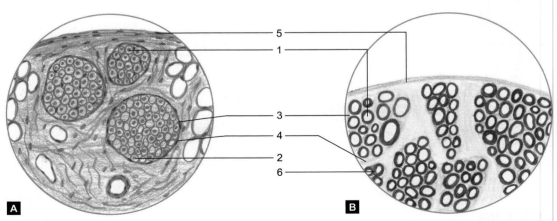

A

B

**Fig. 19.7:** Peripheral nerve, (A) H and E stain, (B) osmic acid stain, showing myelinated nerve fibers (1) and their axons (2). Each nerve fiber is surrounded by endoneurium (3) and each bundle of nerve fibers is surrounded by perineurium (4) and nerve is surrounded by epineurium (5). Myelin sheaths (6) are stained black by osmic acid

processes. In the peripheral nervous system, cell bodies are found in the ganglia and in some sensory regions (olfactory mucosa).

a. **Nerve cell body:** Size of cell body depends on the type and functions of the cell and varies from 5 to 150 μm. Motor neurons of ventral horn of the spinal cord have the largest cell body in the CNS, whereas granule cells in the cerebellar cortex have the smallest cell body. The cell body contains the nucleus with the surrounding cytoplasm. Nuclei of neurons are usually large, rounded, euchromatic and centrally located. They are characterized by well-defined and strongly RNA-positive nucleoli. The cytoplasm of neurons is rich in Nissl substances, which are composed of ribonucleoprotein bound to rough endoplasmic reticulum. The number of Nissl substances varies according to neuronal type and functional state. They are particularly abundant in large nerve cells, such as motor neurons and help in the synthesis of new protein. Nissl substances extend into the proximal portions of dendrites but is absent from axons and axon hillocks (Fig. 19.9). Nissl substances disintegrate in

response to axonal injury (chromatolysis). In addition to the Nissl substances, neuronal cytoplasm is rich in mitochondria and contains a prominent perinuclear Golgi apparatus. Mitochondria are especially abundant in the axon terminals. Microtubules, microfilaments, and neurofilaments form the cytoskeleton of a neuron. Microfilaments are involved in the rapid transport of protein molecules through axons and dendrites. Neurofilaments are made up of structural proteins similar to the intermediate filaments of other types of cells. In addition, neuronal cytoplasm may contain lipid droplets, glycogen and pigment granules. Some types of neurons, such as Purkinje cells of the cerebellum, do not contain pigment granules. Neurons do not divide; however, in some areas of the brain, such as olfactory bulb and the dentate gyrus of the hippocampus, neural stem cells are present and are able to differentiate and replace damaged nerve cells.

> Dark brown to black melanin granules are found in neurons of certain regions of the CNS such as substantia nigra and locus ceruleus. Lipofuscin is a yellowish brown pigment granule and is more common in the neuronal cytoplasm of older adults. This pigment is thought to be the remnant of lysosomal enzymatic activity and increase in number with advancing age. This pigment is also called wear and tear pigment.

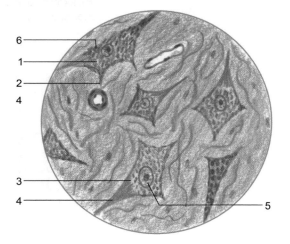

**Fig. 19.9:** Neurons showing cell body (1), dendrites (2), axon hillock (3), axon (4) and nucleus (5). The Nissl substance (6) can also be seen in the figure, but not in the axon hillock and axon

b. **Nerve cell processes:** Neuronal processes are extensions of the cell body and serve to initiate or conduct nerve impulses. Dendrites generally receive and then conduct impulses toward the cell body, whereas axons conduct them away from the cell body. Separation of a process from the cell body results in the death of that process.

   i. *Dendrites:* It repeatedly branch and becomes thinner. Its surfaces are studded with spines or gemmules, thus expanding the receptive cell surface. Some neurons can receive as many as 100,000 axon terminals on their dendritic expansion. Bipolar neurons, with only one dendrite, are found in special sites only. Dendrites are devoid of the Golgi apparatus. In the dendrites of most neurons, neurofilaments are reduced to small bundles or single filaments. Mitochondria are abundant in dendrites.

ii. *Axons:* These are more slender than dendrites and are more uniform in diameter. The region of origin of the axon of a nerve cell is termed the axon hillock and it is devoid of Nissl substances. Distally, each axon breaks up into simple or complex arborizations, the telodendria, which end on other neurons, glands, or muscles. The plasma membrane of the axon is called axolemma and the cytoplasm is called axoplasm. Axon cytoplasm (axoplasm) lacks a Golgi apparatus, but contains smooth endoplasmic reticulum, rough endoplasmic reticulum, and elongated mitochondria. Axons invariably acquire sheaths along their course. The axon and its sheath are referred to as a nerve fiber. Nerve fibers that run together in a bundle and share a common origin and destination in the central nervous system constitute a tract. Bundles of axons in the peripheral nervous system constitute a peripheral nerve. Nerve fibers may be myelinated or unmyelinated. Myelin sheaths are elaborated and maintained by oligodendrocytes in the central nervous system, and by Schwann cells in the peripheral nervous system. The region of the axon between the apex of the axon hillock and the beginning of the myelin sheath is known as the initial segment. It is the site at which an action potential is generated in the axon. At initial segment, the stimuli, whether inhibitory or stimulatory are summated and the resulting nerve stimuli are generated. The myelin sheath around an axon is interrupted at regular intervals known as the nodes of Ranvier. The nodes are the site of voltage-gated sodium channels and ionic movement of impulse conduction. The flow of an electrical impulse along the nerve fiber thus skips from one node of Ranvier to the next. Myelin sheaths serve to insulate axons between nodes and thus speed up conduction of the nerve impulse between nodes of Ranvier (saltatory conduction). Myelin is made up of a lipid-protein complex. Large and heavily myelinated fibers conduct faster than small, unmyelinated ones.

There is a bidirectional transport of small and large molecules along the axon. Macromolecules and organelles that are synthesized in the cell body are transported continuously by an anterograde flow along the axon to its terminals. Simultaneously with anterograde flow, a retrograde flow in the opposite direction transports several molecules, including material taken up by endocytosis (including viruses and toxins), to the cell body.

For comparison between axon and dendrite, *see* Table 36 given in Appendix I.

### B. Types of Neuron

a. **Neurons are of three types on the basis of number of processes (Fig. 19.10):**

i. *Unipolar (Pseudounipolar):* These neurons have spherical cell bodies with single processes that later bifurcate, both branches are structurally axon-like. One branch extends to the periphery and other branch extends to the CNS. Unipolar are also sensory neurons. Cell bodies of unipolar neurons are found in numerous dorsal root ganglia of the spinal nerves and cranial nerve ganglia.

ii. *Bipolar:* These neurons are spindle-shaped, with one process at each end. These neurons are rare and are purely sensory neurons. These neurons are mostly associated with the receptors for

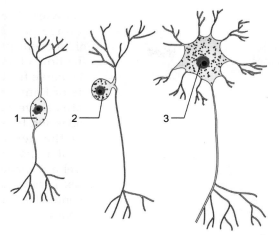

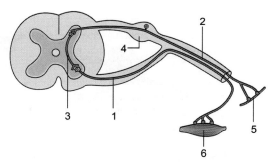

**Fig. 19.10:** Schematic diagram showing types of neurons on the basis of number of processes. Bipolar (1), pseudounipolar (2) and multipolar (3)

**Fig. 19.11:** Schematic diagram showing types of neurons on the basis of their function. Afferent (1), efferent (2), interneurons (3), dorsal root ganglia (4), skin (5) and muscle (6)

the special senses (taste, hearing, smell, sight and equilibrium).

iii. *Multipolar:* These neurons have polygonal cell bodies with many dendrites and only one axon. These are the most common type in the CNS and include all motor neurons and interneurons of cerebrum, cerebellum and spinal cord.

b. **Neurons are of three types on the basis of their function (Fig. 19.11):**

  i. *Motor (efferent):* These neurons convey impulses from the CNS or ganglia to effector cells. Processes of these neurons are included in somatic efferent and visceral efferent nerve fibers.

  ii. *Sensory (afferent):* These neurons convey impulses from receptors to the CNS. Processes of these neurons are included in somatic afferent and visceral afferent nerve fibers.

  iii. *Interneurons (internuncial):* These neurons establish the interrelationships among other neurons, forming complex functional chains or circuits.

## C. Supporting or Neuroglial Cells

These cells can be seen only with special gold and silver stains. In the central nervous system supporting cells are: Astrocytes, oligodendrocytes, microglia, and ependymal cells. In the peripheral nervous system supporting cells are: Schwann cells and satellite cells (Fig. 19.12).

a. **Astrocytes:** These are largest of neuroglial cells. These are star-shaped cells with relatively lightly staining nuclei. Many of their processes are closely applied to capillary blood vessels (perivascular end-feet or footplates). The cytoplasm of astrocytes contains bundles of intermediate filaments made up of glial fibrillary acidic protein (GFAP). Astrocytes play a role in the metabolite transfer within the central nervous system. Astrocytes scavenge ions and debris from neuron metabolism and supply energy for metabolism. They also provide a covering for the "bare areas" of myelinated axons, e.g. at the nodes of Ranvier and at synapses.

Two varieties are distinguished on the basis of the morphology of their processes:

  i. *Protoplasmic:* These are found mostly in grey matter. These cells have short and abundant cell processes that branch repeatedly. Processes of these astrocytes are present at the periphery of brain and spinal cord, forming a layer under the

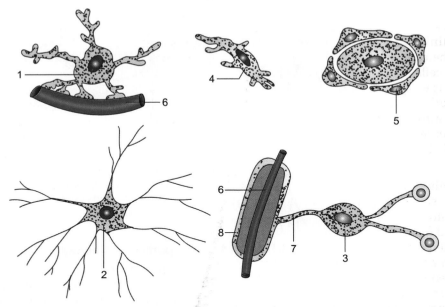

**Fig. 19.12:** Schematic diagram showing the types of neuroglial cells. Protoplasmic astrocyte (1), fibrous astrocyte (2), oligodendrocyte (3), microglia (4), satellite cell (5), blood capillary (6), axon (7) and myelin sheath (8)

pia mater. These astrocytes help to establish the blood-brain barrier and may contribute to its maintenance.

ii. *Fibrous:* These are found mostly in white matter. These cells have more slender but well-defined and a fewer cell processes. These astrocytes are longer and straighter in comparison to the protoplasmic variety. Intermediate filaments are much more numerous in these astrocytes. These cells play a role in healing and scar formation after injury in the central nervous system.

b. **Oligodendrocytes:** These are smaller than astrocytes and have a small spherical darkly stained nucleus and cytoplasm. These glial cells are seen adjacent to myelinated nerve fibers in the white matter or forming satellite cells to the neurons in the grey matter. These cells have a few delicate processes and form and maintain the myelin sheaths in the central nervous

system. Each cell is able to send out processes which wrap around up to twelve axons. These cells are necessary for the survival of neurons.

c. **Microglia:** These are the smallest of the neuroglia and these are dense cells with deeply staining elongated nuclei. These cells are frequently seen in the grey matter in close proximity to the neurons. These cells are quiescent under normal circumstances and with age they slowly accumulate pigment. In some disease or injury states the microglia become active and proliferates. The active cells become antigen-presenting cells and secrete cytokines. Astrocytes and oligodendrocytes are derived from ectoderm; while microglia originates in the bone marrow and are part of the mononuclear phagocytic system.

For comparison among protoplasmic astrocytes, fibrous astrocytes, oligodendrocytes and microglia, *see* Table 37 given in Appendix I.

d. **Ependymal cells:** These cells are epithelial cells lining the ventricles of the brain and the central canal of the spinal canal. These cells are low columnar to cuboidal in shape and their apical surface is ciliated. These cells take part in the elaboration of cerebro-spinal fluid and also serve as a barrier between fluid and neural elements.

e. **Schwann cells:** Schwann cells are flattened cells whose cytoplasm contains flattened nuclei, small Golgi apparatus and only a few mitochondria. Although these cells are derived from neural crest cells, they are still considered as neuroglial cells. These cells protect and insulate neurons of the PNS as oligodendrocytes work in the CNS. Schwann cells form either unmyelinated or myelinated coverings over neurons and are separated from each other by the nodes of Ranvier. A myelin sheath consists of several Schwann cell plasmalemma wrapped around a single axon.

f. **Satellite cells:** These cells surround the nerve cells of ganglia (dorsal root ganglia and autonomic ganglia). These cells are flattened and have prominent nuclei. These cells provide support and insulation to the neurons of ganglia.

## D. Synapses

These are the specialized junctions between neurons and at the synapse the nerve impulse is transmitted from one neuron (presynaptic) to another (postsynaptic). Synapses function by altering the membrane potential of neurons and other effector cells. It is composed of a terminal membrane (presynaptic membrane), a region of extracellular space (synaptic cleft: 20–30 nm wide), and a postsynaptic membrane. The pre- and postsynaptic membranes may show increased density, indicating the active site. In the presynaptic element a collection of presynaptic vesicles are present, which contain a neurotransmitter substance.

a. **Classification:** Synapses are classified according to the site of synaptic contact and the method of signal transmission.

i. *Site of synaptic contact*
   - Axodendritic synapses: These synapses are most common and are located between an axon and a dendrite.
   - Axosomatic synapses: These synapses are located between an axon and a soma.
   - Axoaxonic synapses: These synapses are located between axons.
   - Dendrodendritic synapses: These synapses are located between the dendrites.

ii. *Method of signal transmission*
   - Chemical synapses: These synapses involve the release of a chemical substance (neurotransmitter or neuro-modulator) by the presynaptic neuron, which acts on the postsynaptic neuron to generate an action potential. Chemical synapses are the most common neuron-neuron synapse and the only neuron-muscle synapse. Signal transmission across these synapses is delayed by about 0.5 milli-seconds, which is the time required for secretion and diffusion of neuro-transmitter from the presynaptic membrane of the first neuron into the synaptic cleft and then to the postsynaptic membrane of the second neuron. Neurotransmitters do not affect the change; they only activate a response in the second neuron. With the arrival of an action potential at the presynaptic terminal, synaptic vesicles fuse with the presynaptic membrane at special "release sites", discharging their contents into the synaptic cleft. The transmitter, then passes to the postsynaptic membrane to interact there with receptor molecules. This causes a change in membrane potential of the postsynaptic neuron and thus transmission of the impulse.

- Electrical synapses: These synapses involve movement of ions from one neuron to another via gap junctions, which transmit the action potential of the presynaptic neuron directly to the postsynaptic neuron. Electrical synapses are uncommon in mammals, but they are present in the brain stem, retina, and the cerebral cortex. Signal transmission across these synapses is almost immediate.

## Summary

1. The central nervous system includes the cerebrum, cerebellum, and the spinal cord.

2. Cerebrum—the cerebral cortex (grey matter) is having six layers from superficial to deep, these layers are:
   - Molecular layer
   - Outer granular layer
   - Outer pyramidal layer
   - Inner granular layer
   - Inner pyramidal layer
   - Polymorphic layer

3. Cerebellum—the cerebellar cortex (grey matter) consists of three very well-defined layers—molecular layer, Purkinje layer, and granular layer.

4. Spinal cord:
   - It is organized into the peripheral located white matter and centrally located grey matter.
   - Grey matter is subdivided into dorsal horn, ventral horn and the central grey commissure (contain central canal).
   - White matter is subdivided into anterior and posterior funiculi.

5. Brain and spinal cord are covered by three meninges from superficial to deep—dura mater, arachnoid mater, and pia mater.

6. The blood–brain barrier is formed by occluding junctions of endothelial cells.

7. Ganglion: Two types:
   - Dorsal root ganglion—large cell bodies of pseudounipolar neurons separated by bundles of myelinated nerve fibers.
   - Autonomic ganglion—smaller multipolar neurons separated by thin, non-myelinated nerve fibers.

8. Types of neurons:
   - Pseudounipolar—neurons of dorsal root ganglion
   - Bipolar—ganglia of acoustic and olfactory systems
   - Multipolar—autonomic ganglia

9. Neuroglial cells:
   - Astrocytes—it is of two types: protoplasmic and fibrous and takes part in the blood–brain barrier.
   - Oligodendrocytes—form and maintain myelin sheath in the central nervous system.
   - Microglial cells are phagocytic cells.
   - Schwann cells—form myelin sheath in peripheral nervous system.
   - Ependymal cells—take part in elaboration of CSF.
   - Satellite cells—support and insulation to the neurons of ganglia.

## Self Assessment

1. The Nissl substance is:
   a. Absent in the dendrites
   b. Composed of neurofibrils
   c. Absent in the axon hillock
   d. Present only in the perinuclear region in the neuron

2. All of the following cells are present in the cerebral cortex EXCEPT:
   a. Pyramidal     b. Stellate
   c. Purkinje     d. Basket

3. Which of the following form the blood–brain barrier?
   a. Fenestrations between brain capillary endothelial cells
   b. Microglial activity

c. Astrocytic foot processes surrounding blood vessels

d. Occluding junctions between brain capillary endothelial cells

4. Myelin sheath in the CNS is formed by which cells?
   a. Astrocytes
   b. Schwann cells
   c. Oligodendrocytes
   d. Microglia

5. Myelin sheath in the peripheral nervous system is formed by which cells?
   a. Astrocytes
   b. Schwann cells
   c. Oligodendrocytes
   d. Microglia

6. The ventricles are lined by which cells?
   a. Astrocytes
   b. Schwann cells
   c. Ependymal cells
   d. Microglia

7. Sympathetic ganglion contains which type of neurons?
   a. Multipolar       b. Bipolar
   c. Unipolar         d. Pseudounipolar

8. Dorsal root ganglion contains which type of neurons?
   a. Bipolar
   b. Unipolar
   c. Pseudounipolar
   d. Multipolar

9. Nissl substance is composed of:
   a. rER
   b. sER
   c. Lysosomes
   d. Mitochondria

10. Cerebellar cortex is made from all cell layers EXCEPT:
    a. Molecular
    b. Purkinje
    c. Pyramidal
    d. Granular

## Answers

1. c,      2. c,      3. d,      4. c,      5. b,      6. c,      7. a,      8. c,      9. a,
10. c

# 20

# Eye

The human eyes are present within the bony orbit of the skull and are approximately 25 mm in diameter. Its movements in the bony orbit are controlled by six extrinsic muscles. A thick layer of adipose tissue partially surrounds the eye and work as a cushion for the eye. The wall of the eye is formed by three layers, or tunics. From the outside to the inside of the eyeball these three tunics are:

1. Fibrous tunic, which forms a capsule and subdivided into the cornea and the sclera. The cornea is slightly thicker than the sclera.
2. Vascular tunic consists of choroid, ciliary body and iris. This tunic is also called the uveal tract.
3. Neural tunic consists of the retina, which forms the photoreceptive layer of the eye (Fig. 20.1). The lens is a specialized

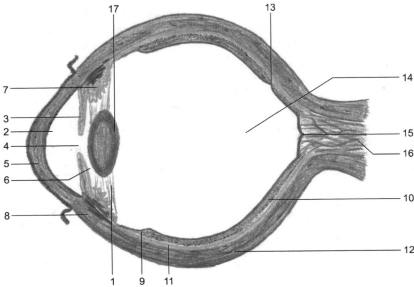

**Fig. 20.1:** Whole eye (sagittal section) at low magnification and showing three tunics of its wall: Outer fibrous, which is composed of cornea (5) and the sclera (12); middle vascular, which is composed of choroid (11), ciliary body (7) and iris (3) and the inner most retina (10). The figure also shows the zonular fibers (1), anterior chamber (2), pupil (4), posterior chamber (6), limbus (8), ora serrata (9), macula (13), vitreous body (14), optic papilla (15), lens (17) and optic nerve (16)

epithelial structure, suspended behind the pupil. In between the iris and the cornea; a space filled with aqueous humor, the anterior chamber lies. Similarly, a space is present in between the posterior surface of the iris and anterior surface of the lens, called the posterior chamber. The anterior surface of the eye is covered by folds of skin called eyelids.

The anterior portion of the eye up to the cornea and internal surface of the eyelids is covered by conjunctiva. The lacrimal (tear) gland is present beneath the conjunctiva on the upper lateral side of the orbit whose secretion, lacrimal fluid (tears) moistens the anterior surface of the eye.

## FIBROUS TUNIC

### A. The Cornea

It projects forward from the sclera and only 0.5 mm thick at its center and 1 mm thick at its periphery. The cornea is colorless, avascular, and transparent, and it forms the anterior one-sixth of the eye. It consists of three cellular layers, which are separated from each other by two thin, acellular layers. The anterior surface of the cornea is lined by a stratified squamous nonkeratinized epithelium (50 µm thick). The surface cells of this stratified epithelium present microvilli which help in the retention of an unbroken film of tear fluid. Numerous free nerve endings present in the corneal epithelium make it extremely sensitive to touch and pain. Damage to the cornea is repaired rapidly; as the cells divide by mitosis and migrate to the defect to cover the injured region. The basement membrane of this epithelium rests on the acellular anterior limiting lamina or Bowman's membrane (8–10 µm thick). It separates the epithelium from the underlying corneal stroma and consists of densely packed type I collagen fibers embedded in amorphous ground substance. This membrane may be synthesized by both; the corneal epithelium and cells of the underlying stroma. It gives some strength to the cornea and also acts as a barrier to the spread of infections. If damaged, it cannot regenerate; healing of it results in the formation of opaque scar, which interferes with vision. The corneal stroma (substantia propria) is the thickest layer of the cornea, constituting about 90% of its thickness (Fig. 20.2A, B). It consists

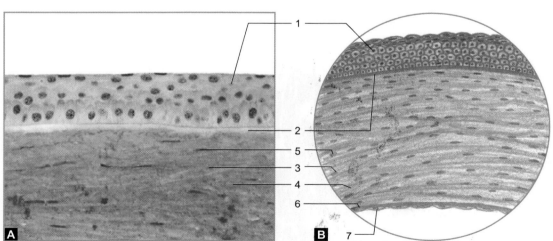

**Fig. 20.2:** Cornea, (A) micrograph, (B) sketch, showing stratified squamous nonkeratinized epithelium (1) covering the anterior surface of cornea. It rests on the acellular Bowman's membrane (2) just beneath the membrane lie corneal stroma (3) formed by collagen fibers (4) and fibrocytes (5). The figure also shows the endothelium (7) covering the posterior surface of the cornea and separated from stroma by Descemet's membrane (6)

of 200–250 layers of regularly organized collagen fibers embedded in a ground substance rich in chondroitin sulphate and keratin sulphate. Collagen fibers within each layer runs parallel to each other, but at large angles to collagen fibers in the next layer. Flattened fibrocytes (keratocytes) are located between the layers of collagen fibers. The small diameter of collagen fibers and their regular arrangement accounts for the transparency of the cornea. The posterior surface of the cornea is lined by an endothelium (squamous or low cuboidal). The endothelium and the stroma are separated from each other by the acellular posterior limiting lamina or Descemet's membrane (10 μm thick), which corresponds to the basement membrane of the endothelium. Descemet's membrane is formed by an interwoven network of fibers and regenerates after injury. The endothelial cells are joined by tight junctions and these are responsible for the synthesis of proteins that are necessary for secreting and maintaining Descemet's membrane. The endothelial cells also pump out excessive fluid from the cornea to ensure its transparency. The lateral margins of the cornea are continuous with the conjunctiva (anterior corneal epithelium) and sclera (corneal stroma). The corneoscleral junction or limbus is highly vascularized area. Cornea gets its nutrition from aqueous humor and blood vessels of the limbus.

## B. The Sclera

It is white of the eye and its thickness ranges from 0.6 mm to 1 mm. Distended by the intraocular pressure, the sclera maintains the shape of the eyeball. The sclera is also the site of attachment of the extraocular muscles. The sclera is pierced by blood vessels, nerves and optic nerve. It consists of three ill-defined layers, which from outside to inside, are:

a. **Episclera:** It consists of loose connective tissue. The tendons of the extraocular muscles pierce this layer and get attached to the underlying stromal layer.

b. **Substantia propria (stroma or Tenon's capsule):** It consists of a dense network of thick collagen fibers.

c. **Lamina fusca (suprachoroid lamina):** It consists of loose connective tissue. Along with fibroblasts and other connective tissue cells macrophages are also present in this layer (Fig. 20.3A, B).

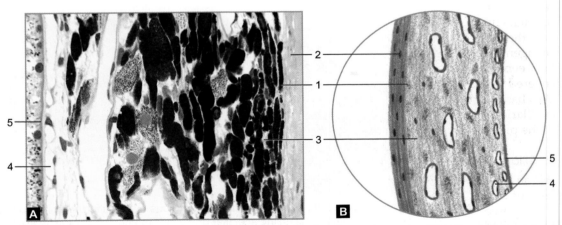

**Fig. 20.3:** Sclera and choroid, (A) micrograph, (B) sketch showing melanocytes (1) in the deeper parts of sclera (2). The figure also shows the suprachoroid lamina (3). Choroid (4) separates from the retina by Bruch's membrane (5)

**Aqueous humor:** It is a clear watery fluid similar in composition to CSF. It is produced by the ciliary processes. It first enters in the posterior chamber and reaches the anterior chamber through opening between the iris and the lens. In close proximity to the iridocorneal angle in the sclera lies endothelial lined channel known as canal of Schlemm. The aqueous humor from anterior chamber reaches this canal of Schlemm, which is the main exit route for the aqueous humor and drains the humor through minute veins into the plexus of episcleral veins that leaves the eye and delivers the fluid to the venous circulation.

## VASCULAR TUNIC

### A. The Choroid

It is the posterior part of the middle coat of eye and lies between the sclera externally and retina internally. It is thin and highly vascular. It consists of loose connective tissue, which contains thinner collagen and elastic fibers. Connective tissue cells and pigment cells (melanocytes) are numerous. Medium and large size blood vessels are present in the deeper parts, also called choriocapillary layer. In between the blood vessels in the connective tissue lies melanocytes, which is responsible for the dark color of the choroid. Inner to the choriocapillary layer, a single layer of small blood vessels is present, which supplies the retina with nutrients. Bruch's membrane (lamina vitrea) is located between the choroid and the retina. It consists of two layers of collagen fibers and a network of elastic fibers between them. Each collagen fiber layer is covered on its outer side by a basal lamina. This basal lamina on one side belongs to the capillaries, while on the other side, it belongs to the pigment epithelium of the retina.

### B. Ciliary Body

It is an inward extension of the choroid at the level of the lens. The bulk of the ciliary body is composed of three groups of smooth muscle fibers called the ciliary muscle. These groups are: (1) Longitudinal muscle fibers, which stretch the choroid to open the iridocorneal angle to facilitate drainage of the aqueous humor; (2) radial muscle fibers, whose contraction causes the lens to flatten and thus allows the eyes to focus for distant vision; (3) circular muscle fibers, which reduce the tension on the lens and cause the lens to become more convex to accommodate for near vision. A small amount of loose connective tissue containing numerous elastic fibers, blood vessels and melanocytes is present in between the bundles of smooth muscle fibers. 60–70 ciliary processes extend from the anterior one-third of the ciliary body towards the lens. The ciliary processes contain a dense network of fenestrated capillaries. Ciliary body and processes are lined by the pars ciliaris (pigment layer composed of two layers of cuboidal cells) of the retina. The inner cell layer, which faces the posterior chamber of the eye, is a nonpigmented cuboidal epithelium (nonpigmented ciliary epithelium). The outer cell layer is composed of a pigmented simple cuboidal epithelium (pigmented ciliary epithelium), which is rich in melanin (Fig. 20.4A, B). The cells of the inner non-pigmented layer generate the aqueous humor of the eye. Zonular fibers (suspensory ligament) extend from the ciliary processes towards the lens and tension in this ligament flattens the lens.

### C. Iris

It arises from the ciliary body and partially covers the lens, leaving a rounded aperture in the center called pupil. Pupil regulates the amount of light passing into the eye. The anterior surface of the iris is rough and irregular due to the numerous ridges and grooves. It is formed by an incomplete layer of fibroblasts and melanocytes. Beneath this layer is a highly vascularized connective tissue stroma, which is covered on its posterior surface by highly pigmented cells. The basal lamina of these cells, faces towards the posterior chamber of the eye. Located beneath this layer is a layer of myoepithelial cells, whose apical parts contain melanin granules. The basal part of these cells possess processes

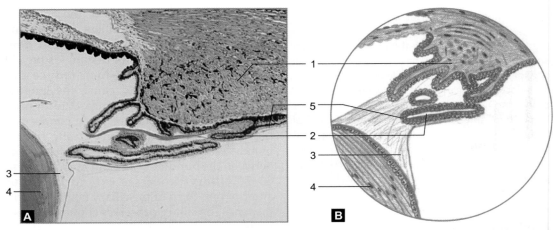

**Fig. 20.4:** Ciliary body and ciliary zonules, (A) micrograph, (B) sketch. The figure shows the ciliary body (1) which is an extension of the choroid and gives rise to the ciliary processes (2). Zonule fibers (3) extend from the ciliary processes towards the lens (4). Ciliary processes are lined by two layers of cuboidal cells (5)

with contractile property arranged radially and known as dilator pupillae muscle of the iris. The stroma of iris consists of a vascularized loose connective tissue rich in melanocytes in addition to macrophages and fibrocytes, which are all surrounded by a loose meshwork of fine collagen fibers. The large number of melanocytes presents in the epithelium and stroma of the iris not only blocks the passage of light into the eye (except at the pupil) but also provides color to the eye. In the stroma of the iris near the pupillary margin circumferentially oriented smooth muscle fibers are present known as sphincter or constrictor pupillae muscle (Fig. 20.5 A to D). These two muscles regulate the size of the pupil, i.e. the constrictor pupillae reduces the size of the pupil in response to bright light, while dilator pupillae increases the size of the pupil in response to dim light. The posterior surface of the iris is covered by the retina.

## NEURAL TUNIC

### A. Retina

It is the inner coat of the eyeball. It has several layers and from outside to inwards the layers are (Fig. 20.6A, B):

a. **Pigment epithelium:** It consists of a single layer of cuboidal pigmented cells containing melanin granules. These cells are connected with the junctional complex made up of gap junctions, zonula occludens and zonula adherens. Pigment cells have large microvilli which projects in spaces between the processes of rods and cones. These cells absorb light and prevent back reflection. These cells also destroy (phagocytic) the used-up tips of rods and cones. These cells also isolate the retinal cells from blood-borne substances, i.e. serves as a major component of the blood–retina barrier. These cells also play an active role in vision by esterifying vitamin A derivatives in their smooth endoplasmic reticulum. Pigment epithelium is separated from the choroid by Bruch's membrane.

b. **Layers of rods and cones:** This layer contains outer rod and cone-shaped processes of rods and cones.

c. **External limiting membrane:** It is formed by outer terminal processes of Muller cells and lies at the level of the inner segments of the photoreceptors, to which the Muller cells tightly attach by junctional complexes. It is believed that this layer acts as metabolic

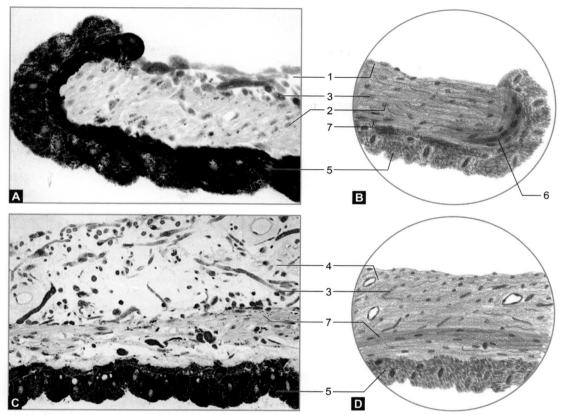

**Fig. 20.5:** Iris, (A) micrograph of the free edge, (B) sketch of free edge, (C) micrograph of the central part, (D) sketch of the central part, showing the two-layered posterior epithelium (5). Anterior surface (1) is covered by condensation of fibrocytes (2) and melanocytes (3). Sphincter pupillae muscle (6) can be seen in the stroma (4) near the free edge and dilator pupillae (7) in the central part

barrier that restricts the passage of large molecules into the inner layers of the retina.

d. **Outer nuclear layer:** This layer contains cell bodies and nuclei of rods and cones. This layer is thicker and nuclei are more densely packed in comparison to the inner nuclear layer (Fig. 20.6A, B).

e. **Outer plexiform layer:** This layer contains only nerve fibers that form a plexus. It contains synapses between rods and cones with the dendritic processes of bipolar, amacrine, and horizontal cells.

f. **Inner nuclear layer:** This layer contains nuclei and bodies of bipolar cells, Muller cells, horizontal cells and amacrine cells.

g. **Inner plexiform layer:** This layer contains axons of bipolar cells synapsing with dendrites of ganglion cells and amacrine cells.

h. **Ganglion cell layer:** This layer contains nuclei and the bodies of multipolar ganglion cells.

i. **Nerve-fiber layer:** This layer contains axons of ganglion cells, which pass over the internal surface of the retina as the nerve fiber layer to converge on the optic papilla, where they pass out unmyelinated through

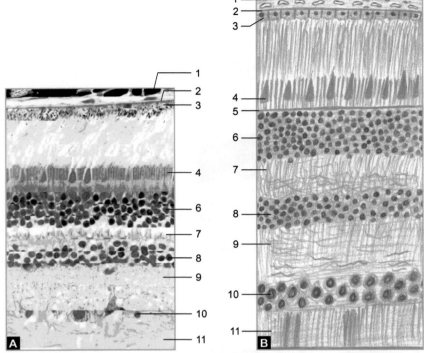

**Fig. 20.6A, B:** Retina showing the choriocapillary layer (1), Bruch's membrane (2) and along with these all ten layers of the retina: pigment epithelium (3) formed by cuboidal cells; a layer of rods and cones (4); external limiting membrane (5); outer nuclear layer (6); outer plexiform layer (7); inner nuclear layer (8); inner plexiform layer (9); ganglion cell layer (10) and nerve fiber layer (11)

the eye's other two coats (choroid and sclera) to form the optic nerve.

j. **Inner limiting membrane:** It is a basal lamina, which separates the inner processes of Muller cells from the vitreous body.

## B. Photoreceptor Cells

The rod and cones are photoreceptor cells. In each retina about 6–7 million cones are present, while rods are more numerous (100–120 million). Rods are about 120 μm long and 2 μm in diameter, while cones are about 75 μm long and 5 μm wide. Rods are more sensitive to light and come into play in dim light. Cones are color sensitive and are used for vision in bright light. Rods and cones share some common cytoarchitectural structures. Each cell consists of a cell body, outer segment, inner

segment, inner fibers, spherule (rods) and pedicle (cones) (Fig. 20.7A, B). Outer segment

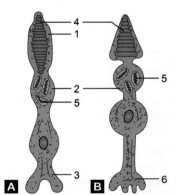

**Fig. 20.7A, B:** Schematic diagram showing fine structure of rod and cone. Outer segments (1), inner segments (2), spherule (3), stacked cell membranes (4), mitochondria (5) and pedicle (6)

(dendrite) is the real photo-receptor element. It contains a large number of stacks of membranous discs, which are enclosed within a cylindrical extension of the cell membrane.

These discs are oriented at right angles to the long axis of the cell and are rich in photosensitive pigments. Pigment of rods is known as rhodopsin, which are the sensors of black, grey and white color. Pigment of cones is known as iodopsin, which are the sensors of blue, green and red color. Outer segment is connected to the inner segment by a thin connecting stalk, which has a cilium composed of nine peripheral microtubule doublets extending from a basal body. The outer segment is longer in rods than in cones, so rods contain more rhodopsin and respond more slowly than cones. The inner segment contains the nucleus, the cell body of the bipolar neuron and its apical pole. The apical pole tapers gradually to form the ellipsoid. The ellipsoid is a football-shaped body, filled with many long mitochondria that provide ATP for the bioenergetically demanding process of photoelectric sensory transduction that occurs in the outer segment. Inner fibers of rods and cones resemble axon. In case of rods it terminates in spherule, while in cones it terminates in pedicle. Spherule and pedicle make synapses with dendrites of bipolar cells and processes of horizontal neurons.

## C. Specializations of the Retina

The fovea defines the center of the retina and it is the region of highest visual acuity. In the fovea there are almost exclusively cones and they are at their highest density. The area in and around the fovea has a pale yellow pigmentation (xanthophyll) and is known as the macula. The ganglion cell axons all leave the eyeball at one location, the optic disk. At the optic disk all photoreceptors and accessory cells are pushed aside, so the axons can penetrate the choroid and the sclera. This creates a hole in our vision, the blind spot. Normally, each eye covers for the blind spot of the other and the brain fills in missing information with whatever pattern surrounds the hole. Therefore, we are not conscious of the blind spot.

## LENS

It is a transparent crystalline biconvex structure. It is made up of lens capsule, subcapsular epithelium and lens fibers (Fig. 20.8A, B). Lens capsule is transparent and homogenous and made up by type IV collagen fibers along with glycoprotein. The lens capsule measures about 10–20 μm. Just beneath the capsule on the

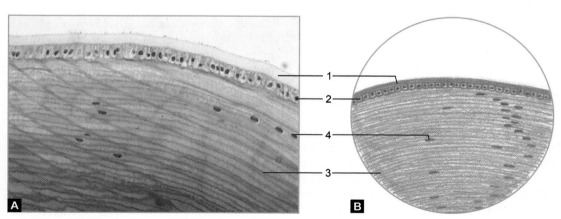

**Fig. 20.8:** Lens, (A) micrograph, (B) sketch showing capsule (1) of the lens. Just beneath the capsule lies anterior cuboidal epithelium (2). The figure also shows the lens fibers (3) which are nucleated (4)

anterior surface lies the simple cuboidal epithelium. Towards the equator (where the fibers of the zonule are attached to lens) the epithelial cells become columnar and then they further elongate to form long lens fibers. The epithelial cells are mitotically active. The lens fibers are made up of crystalline proteins. Lens fibers are about 10 μm long, 10 μm wide and 2 μm thick. Their shape is like hexagon in cross sections. Lens transparency is due to the regular arrangement of the lens fibers. Lens fibers develop in successive waves from the embryonic period and its elaboration continues throughout life in the equator. The younger fibers are nucleated, whereas old fibers lose their nuclei. Lens does not contain blood vessels or nerves. The lens is not of uniform hardness. The central harder part is called the nucleus, while the peripheral part is called the cortex. It is elastic and its shape can be changed during accommodation through changing the tension in the ligaments of the ciliary muscles.

## ACCESSORY STRUCTURES OF THE EYE

### A. Conjunctiva

It is a thin, transparent mucous membrane, which covers the internal surface of the eyelids (palpebral conjunctiva) and sclera of the anterior portion of the eye (bulbar conjunctiva). It is composed of a stratified columnar epithelium containing numerous goblet cells. Epithelium rests on a lamina propria made up of loose connective tissue. The secretion of goblet cell is a part of the tears which helps in lubrication and protection of the epithelium.

### B. Eyelids

These are movable folds of tissue that covers the anterior surface of the eye. Eyelids protect the eyes from injury with the foreign objects and also maintain a thin film of moisture on the surface of the cornea to prevent it from drying out. The outer surface of eyelids is covered by skin, whereas inner surface is covered by palpebral conjunctiva (Fig. 20.9).

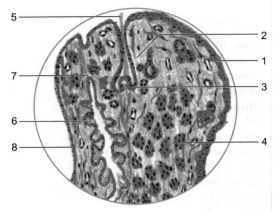

**Fig. 20.9:** Eyelid. Epidermis (1), dermis (2), hair follicle (3), orbicularis oculi (4), eyelash (5), tarsal glands (6), tarsus (7) and palpebral conjunctiva (8)

The dermis of the eyelids is thinner than in most skin. Loose connective tissue is present deep to the skin, which is devoid of fat. Within each eyelid is a flexible support, the tarsal plate, consisting of dense fibrous and elastic tissue.

Overlying the tarsal plate lies a thin sheet of skeletal muscle, known as orbicularis occuli. Fibers of levator palpebrae superioris muscle are also present in the connective tissue of the eyelids. The margin of the eyelids contains eyelashes arranged in rows of three or four, but they are without arrector pili muscles. In addition to eccrine sweat glands, the eyelids also contain three other major types of glands. These are the tarsal glands (Meibomian glands), sebaceous glands of eyelashes (glands of Zeis) and apocrine glands of eyelashes (glands of Moll). The Meibomian glands are long sebaceous glands, which are embedded in the tarsal plate. The oily secretion of these glands forms a layer on the surface of the tears and thus retards their evaporation. Glands of Zeis are smaller, modified sebaceous glands that are connected to and empty their secretion into the follicles of the eyelashes. Glands of Moll are unbranched sweat glands and form a simple spiral before opening into the follicles of the eyelashes.

## C. Lacrimal Apparatus

The lacrimal apparatus consists of the lacrimal gland, lacrimal canaliculi, lacrimal sac and nasolacrimal duct. The lacrimal gland is a tear-secreting gland present beneath the conjunctiva on the upper lateral side of the orbit. The lacrimal gland is a tubuloalveolar gland that usually has distended lumen and is composed of column-shaped cells of the serous type. Well-developed myoepithelial cells surround the secretory portions of the lacrimal gland (Fig. 20.10).

These cells help in the expulsion of secretion of lacrimal gland into the duct system, which drains into the conjunctiva. Approximately 8–12 ducts drain from the lacrimal gland into the superior conjunctival fornix (conjunctiva lined recess present just beneath the upper eyelid). Tears drain from the eye through lacrimal puncta, the small opening of the lacrimal canaliculi, located at the medial angle. The upper and lower canaliculi join to form the common canaliculi that open into the lacrimal sac. The sac is continuous with the nasolacrimal duct that opens into the inferior nasal meatus. A pseudostratified columnar ciliated epithelium lines the lacrimal sac and nasolacrimal duct. The lacrimal glands secrete a fluid rich in lysozyme, an enzyme that hydrolyzes the cell walls of certain species of bacteria, facilitating their destruction.

**Lamellar keratoplasty:** It involves replacement of damaged or diseased anterior corneal stroma and Bowman's membrane with donor material. Most of the bottom three layers of the cornea can be preserved. The donor corneal disc becomes repopulated with host cells, and the recipient epithelium usually covers the anterior corneal surface.

**Eye donation:** In this case, through surgery the damaged whitish cornea should be replaced by a crystal-like healthy cornea, which has been donated by a healthy person. This can restore vision to those who have become blind due to the cataract or those whose cornea has been affected. This occurs due to the fact that the cornea is an avascular tissue and hence, an antibody that may cause rejection of transplanted cornea does not enter the transplanted tissue.

**Glaucoma:** It occurs due to prolonged increased intraocular pressure caused by failure of drainage of the aqueous humor from the anterior chamber of the eye. It is one of the leading causes of blindness. In chronic glaucoma, the continued increasing intraocular pressure causes progressive damage to the eye, particularly in the retina; if left untreated, blindness develops.

**Retinal detachment:** As the optical ends of rods and cone cells are not firmly attached to the pigment epithelium, the retina may get separated from the pigment epithelium. This condition is called the detachment of the retina. Most commonly it occurs due to the formation of a hole or tears in the retina through which fluid seeps behind the retina displacing it from its normal position. This is a common but serious condition. It may be treated by laser surgery. However, if this condition is left unattended, the rods and cones die because they will have lost the metabolic support normally provided from chorio-capillary layer of choroid.

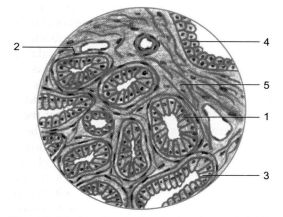

**Fig. 20.10:** Lacrimal gland showing acini (1), myoepithelial cells (2), intralobular duct (3), interlobular duct (4) and connective tissue (5)

## Summary

1. Each eyeball is surrounded from outside to inside by three tunics: Fibrous tunic (cornea and sclera), vascular tunic (choroid, ciliary body and iris) and neural tunic (retina).

2. Cornea—it is transparent and forms anterior one-sixth of the eye. It consists of the following layers (from anterior to posterior):
   - Stratified squamous nonkeratinized epithelium
   - Bowman's membrane (anterior limiting membrane)
   - Stroma (substantia propria)
   - Descemet's membrane (posterior limiting membrane)
   - Endothelium (simple squamous or low cuboid)

3. Retina—it consists of ten layers (from outside to inside):
   - Pigment epithelium
   - Layer of rods and cones
   - External limiting membrane
   - Outer nuclear layer
   - Outer plexiform layer
   - Inner nuclear layer
   - Inner plexiform layer
   - Ganglion cell layer
   - Nerve fiber layer
   - Inner limiting membrane

4. Rods and cones are photoreceptor cells. Rods function in dim light, while cones are color sensitive and sensitive to bright light.

## Self Assessment

1. Eyeball is lined by all of the following tunics EXCEPT:
   a. Fibrous          b. Muscular
   c. Vascular         d. Neural

2. Sclera is mainly composed by which fibers?
   a. Collagen         b. Elastic
   c. Reticular        d. Nerve

3. Which of the following layer is not present in cornea?
   a. Bowman's membrane
   b. Substantia propria
   c. Pigment layer
   d. Endothelium

4. Lacrimal gland contains which type of acini?
   a. Serous           b. Mucous
   c. Mixed            d. None of the above

5. Anterior surface of lens is lined by which type of epithelium?
   a. Simple cuboidal
   b. Simple squamous
   c. Simple columnar
   d. Stratified columnar

6. Retina contains all of the following cells EXCEPT:
   a. Rods             b. Cones
   c. Bipolar          d. Pyramidal

7. Tarsal glands are:
   a. Modified sweat gland
   b. Modified sebaceous gland
   c. Mixed gland
   d. None of the above

8. Fovea centralis:
   a. Contains only cones
   b. Contains only rods
   c. Contains rods and cones
   d. Does not contain both rods and cones

9. How many layers are present in retina?
   a. 5                b. 6
   c. 8                d. 10

10. Cornea is lined by which epithelium?
    a. Stratified squamous nonkeratinized
    b. Stratified squamous keratinized
    c. Stratified cuboidal
    d. Pseudostratified

## Answers

1. b,    2. a,    3. c,    4. a,    5. a,    6. d,    7. b,    8. a,    9. d,
10. a

# 21

# Ear

The ear is an extraordinarily complex organ with two functions: Sound reception and maintenance of positional equilibrium. It is made up of three main parts: External, middle and internal ear.

## EXTERNAL EAR

The external ear comprises the auricle (pinna), external acoustic meatus and tympanic membrane. The auricle projects from the lateral surface of the head and collects sound waves from the exterior. The entire auricle, except the lobule is made up of an irregularly shaped plate of elastic cartilage, which is covered by thin skin. The lobule consists of fibrofatty tissue.

The external acoustic meatus (Fig. 21.1) is an air-filled canal that follows a gentle

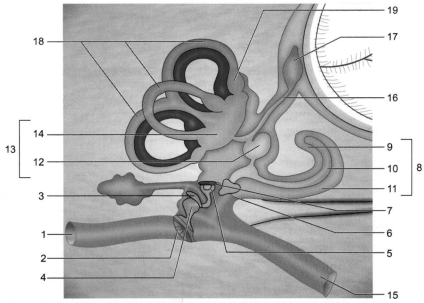

**Fig. 21.1:** Schematic diagram of the ear showing external acoustic meatus (1), tympanic membrane (2), incus (3), malleus (4), stapes (5), round window (6), oval window (7), cochlea (8), scala vestibuli (9), scala media (10), scala tympani (11), saccule (12), vestibule (13), utricle (14), auditory tube (15), endolymphatic duct (16), endolymphatic sac (17), semicircular ducts (18), and ampulla (19)

S-shaped course. It extends from the auricle to the external surface of the tympanic membrane. The wall of the lateral one-third is cartilaginous and is continuous with the elastic cartilage of auricle. The medial two-thirds of the canal is present within the temporal bone. The meatus is lined by thin skin, which is tightly attached to the perichondrium or periosteum. The skin of the meatus contains hair follicles, sebaceous glands, and ceruminous glands. The ceruminous glands resemble the apocrine glands and their secretion mixes with the secretions of the sebaceous gland, and desquamated keratinocytes to form a waxy material called cerumen (earwax). Cerumen act as an agent that protects against damage from moisture trapped inside the canal. Coarse hairs can be found at the opening of the acoustic meatus (external acoustic pore), which prevent the entrance of foreign particles.

The tympanic membrane separates the external acoustic meatus from the middle ear. The tympanic membrane is lined from outside to inside by:
1. Skin of the external acoustic meatus
2. A connective tissue core made up of collagen, and elastic fibers along with fibroblast cells
3. Mucous membrane of the middle ear

This membrane receives sound waves transmitted to it by air through the external acoustic meatus, which cause it to vibrate and thus, the sound waves are converted into mechanical energy that is transmitted to the ear ossicles present in the middle ear.

## MIDDLE EAR (TYMPANIC CAVITY)

It is an air-filled space present in the petrous part of the temporal bone and contains three ear ossicles: The malleus, incus, and stapes. This space communicates anteriorly with the pharynx via the auditory tube (Eustachian tube) and posteriorly, with the mastoid air cells. Laterally, it is bounded by tympanic membrane and medially, by the bony wall of the internal ear.

The middle ear is lined with simple squamous epithelium resting on a thin lamina propria, which is adherent to the subjacent periosteum. Near the auditory tube and in its interior, the simple epithelium becomes pseudostratified ciliated columnar epithelium. Located within the medial wall of the tympanic cavity are the oval window (fenestra vestibuli) and the round window (fenestra cochleae), which connect the middle ear cavity to the internal ear. The ear ossicles are articulated by synovial joints and lined with simple squamous epithelium. The malleus is attached to the tympanic membrane, with the incus interposed between it and the stapes is attached to the oval window. The ossicles transmit the mechanical vibrations generated in the tympanic membrane to the internal ear.

The auditory tube connects the middle ear to the nasopharynx and it is lined by pseudostratified columnar ciliated epithelium with plenty of goblet cells. Cilia beat toward the pharynx. The auditory tube is usually collapsed, but opens during swallowing to equilibrate air pressure.

## INTERNAL EAR

It is composed of two labyrinthine compartments: The bony labyrinth, and membranous labyrinth. The membranous labyrinth lies within the bony labyrinth.

### A. Bony Labyrinth

It is an irregular, hollow cavity present within the petrous part of the temporal bone. It is filled with perilymph, which is similar in ionic composition to extracellular fluids elsewhere, but has very low protein content. It has three components: Three semicircular canals, the vestibule, and the cochlea.

a. **Semicircular canals:** Three canals (anterior, posterior, and lateral) lie at 90 degrees to each other within the temporal bone and enclose the semicircular ducts. Each semicircular canal forms about three quarters of a circle. Each circle arises and returns to the vestibule. One end of each canal lying close to the vestibule is enlarged and known as ampulla. The three canals open in the vestibule by five orifices; as anterior and posterior semicircular canals join at one end.

b. **Vestibule:** It is a small oval chamber present in the center of the bony labyrinth and contains the utricle and saccule of the membranous labyrinth. It lies in between the anterior positioned cochlea and the posterior positioned semicircular canals. Its lateral wall contains the oval window and the round window. The footplate of the stapes is attached to the oval window. The vestibule contains the utricle in an elliptical recess and the saccule in a spherical recess.

c. **Cochlea:** It is a hollow bony spiral of about 35 mm, which is connected to the vestibule and it contains cochlear duct. The basic shape of the cochlea is that of a snail-shell, or tapering helix. It makes two and three-quarter turns around a central bony column known as the modiolus (Fig. 21.2A, B).

The modiolus projects into the cochlea with a thin bony ridge known as the osseous spiral lamina. Through this lamina blood vessels, and the cell bodies and processes of the acoustic branch of the eighth cranial nerve (spiral ganglion) traverses (Fig. 21.3A, B).

## B. Membranous Labyrinth

It consists of a series of communicating sacs and ducts containing endolymph. It lies within the bony labyrinth and it is surrounded by perilymph. Thin strands of connective tissue attached to the endosteum of the bony labyrinth pass through the perilymph to be inserted into the membranous labyrinth. In addition to anchoring the membranous labyrinth to the bony labyrinth, these connective tissue strands carry blood vessels that nourish the epithelia of the membranous labyrinth. It is composed of two divisions: Vestibular labyrinth (with saccule, utricle, and three semicircular ducts), and cochlear labyrinth (with the cochlear duct).

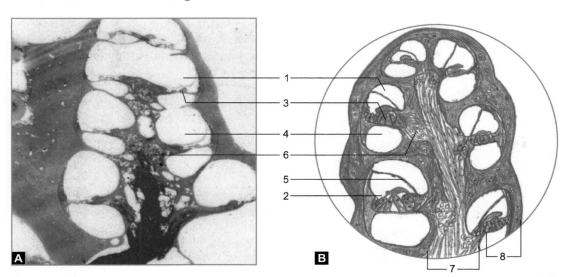

**Fig. 21.2:** Cochlea, (A) micrograph, (B) sketch showing the bony labyrinth (8) around a central bony modiolus (7). Embedded in the modiolus is the spiral ganglion (6). Cochlear canal is subdivided into two large compartments lower scala tympani (4) and upper scala vestibuli (1). The Reissner's membrane (5) separates the scala vestibuli from the scala media (2). The organ of Corti (3) extends from the base of the cochlea to its apex

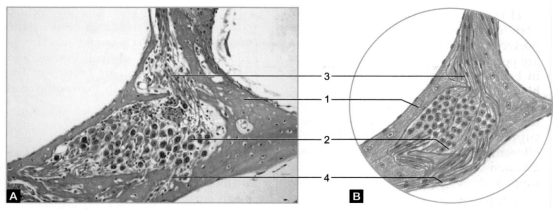

**Fig. 21.3:** Spiral ganglion, (A) micrograph, (B) sketch. The figure shows the modiolus (1) containing spiral ganglion (2). Afferent fibers (3) enter in the ganglion and numerous bundles of efferent fibers (4) pass to the center of modiolus

a. **Saccule and utricle:** These two are sac-like structures and in this saccule lies in a spherical recess of vestibule, while utricle lies in an elliptical recess of the vestibule. They are connected to each other by a small duct, the ductus utriculosaccularis. Small ducts from each join to form the endo-lymphatic duct, whose dilated blind end is known as the endolymphatic sac. The saccule also communicates with the cochlear duct, via a small duct known as the ductus reuniens. The saccule and utricle are made up by a thin connective tissue layer lined on the inner side by simple squamous epithelium.

Specialized regions of the saccule and utricle act as sensory receptors for orientation of the head relative to gravity and acceleration, respectively. These receptors are called the macula sacculi (Fig. 21.4A, B) and the macula utriculi. The macula of the saccule occupies the lateral wall (detect linear vertical

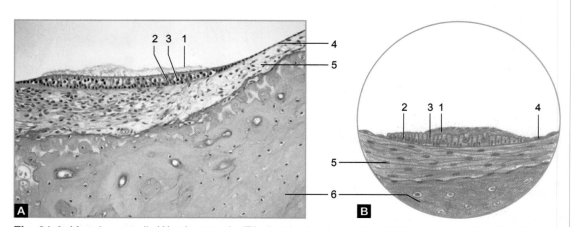

**Fig. 21.4:** Macula sacculi, (A) micrograph, (B) sketch showing hair cell (3) in between the tall columnar supporting cell (2). Jelly with otoliths (1) can be seen on the top of the hair cells. The figure shows the continuity of the simple squamous epithelium of membranous labyrinth (4) with the macula sacculi. Nerve fibers (5) and the bony wall of the vestibule (6) can be seen in the figure

acceleration), whereas the macula of the utricle lies on its floor (detect linear horizontal acceleration) so the maculae are perpendicular to one another. Maculae in both locations have the same basic histological structure. The maculae are composed of two types of neuroepithelial cells (type I and type II hair cells), some supporting cells and the afferent and efferent nerve endings. The vestibular division of the vestibulocochlear nerve supplies these neuroepithelial hair cells.

Each hair cell has 40 to 90 long, rigid stereocilia, and one cilium. Stereocilia are arranged in rows of increasing length, with the longest located adjacent to the cilium. The cilium has a basal body and the usual 9 + 2 arrangement of microtubules in its proximal portion, but the two central microtubules soon disappear. This cilium is usually called a kinocilium. Type I hair cells are rounded cells with a rounded base that narrows toward the neck, while type II hair cells are columnar in shape. The rounded bases of the type I hair cells are almost entirely surrounded by a cup-shaped afferent nerve fiber. Type II hair

cells exhibit many afferent fibers synapsing on the basal area of the cell. Both cell types have efferent nerve endings that are probably inhibitory. The supporting cells lie in between the hair cells and are columnar in shape, with few microvilli. Maculae are covered by a thick gelatinous glycoprotein layer, known as the otolithic membrane. The surface region of this membrane contains small crystals of calcium carbonate, known as otoliths (earstones or earsand or otoconia).

b. **Semicircular ducts:** Each duct is housed within its semicircular canal and has the same form as the semicircular canal. Each duct is dilated at its lateral end and these expanded regions are known as ampulla (Fig. 21.5A, B). Within each ampulla is a ridge or crest containing receptor areas called the crista ampullaris. The cristae are oriented perpendicular to the wall of semicircular canal. The free surface of crista is also covered by sensory epithelium containing neuroepithelial hair cells and supporting cells. Cristae are structurally similar to maculae, but their glycoprotein layer is thicker and this layer has a conical

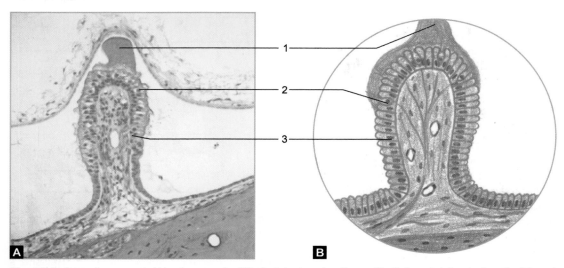

**Fig. 21.5:** Ampullary crest, (A) micrograph, (B) sketch showing the epithelial containing hair cells (2) and supporting cells (3). Cupula (1) rests on the hair cells

form called a cupula. It does not contain otoliths.

c. **Cochlear duct:** It is a diverticulum of the saccule and lies in the bony cochlea. It divides the cochlea into three compartments or scalae: The scala vestibuli, the scala media, and the scala tympani. The scala media or cochlear duct contains endolymph and is continuous with the lumen of the saccule. It contains specialized sound receptors known as the spiral organ of Corti. The scala vestibuli lies above, and scala tympani lie below the scala media and both are perilymph containing spaces. These two compartments communicate with each other at the apex of the cochlea via an opening known as the helicotrema. The scala vestibuli begins at the oval window, while scala tympani end at the round window. The roof of the scala media (cochlear duct) is the vestibular (Reissner's) membrane, whereas the floor of the scala media is the basilar membrane.

The vestibular membrane consists of two layers of squamous epithelium, separated from each other by a basal lamina. One layer is derived from the scala media and the other is derived from the lining of the scala vestibuli. Cells of both layers are joined by numerous tight junctions, thus make a high ionic gradient across the membrane. The basilar membrane extends from the spiral lamina at the modiolus to the lateral wall and the organ of Corti rests on this membrane.

The stria vascularis is an unusual vascularized pseudostratified columnar epithelium located in the lateral wall of the cochlear duct. Unlike most epithelia, it contains an intraepithelial plexus of capillaries and produces endolymph for the scala media.

d. **The spiral organ of Corti:** It is a complex epithelial layer and lies on the floor of the scala media. It is formed by: Hair (neuro-epithelial) cells, phalangeal cells, and pillar cells.

Hair cells are of two types: Inner hair cells and outer hair cells. The inner hair cells form a single row of cells throughout the cochlear duct. The outer hair cells form three to five rows, depending on the distance from the base of the organ. All hair cells have stereocilia, but kinocilium is absent. In the outer hair cells stereocilia have a w-shaped arrangement and in inner hair cells stereocilia have a linear arrangement. Inner hair cells are short and exhibit a centrally located nucleus. The outer hair cells are elongated cylindrical cells whose nuclei are located near their bases. The inner hair cell stereocilia may only touch the tectorial membrane, while the outer hair cell stereocilia are firmly attached to it (Fig. 21.6).

Phalangeal cells are supporting cells for both types of hair cells. The inner phalangeal cells are associated with inner hair cells and completely surround these cells. Outer phalangeal cells are associated with outer hair cells and their apical portions are cup-shaped and only

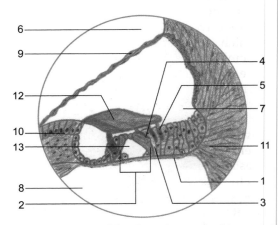

**Fig. 21.6:** Organ of Corti, resting on the basement membrane (1). Pillar cells (2), phalangeal cells (3), inner hair cell (4), outer hair cells (5). Scala vestibuli (6), scala media (7), scala tympani (8). Reissner's membrane (9), spiral limbus (10), spiral ligament (11), tectorial membrane (12), and tunnel of Corti (13)

support the basilar portions of the outer hair cells.

Inner and outer pillar cells are tall cells with wide bases and apical ends; thus, they are shaped like an elongated "I." They are attached to the basilar membrane, and between them they form a triangular tunnel, the inner spiral tunnel.

e. **Vestibular function of the internal ear:** A change in the position of the head causes a flow of the endolymph in the semicircular ducts (circular movement) or in the saccule and utricle (linear movement). Movement of the endolymph in the semicircular ducts displaces the cupula overlying the crista ampullaris, causing bending of the stereocilia of the hair cells. Movement of the endolymph in the saccule and utricle displaces the otoliths. This deformation is transmitted to the maculae via the overlying gelatinous layer, causing bending of the stereocilia of the sensory hair cells. In both cases, movement of the stereocilia is transduced into electrical impulses, which are transmitted to the brain via vestibular nerve fibers.

f. **Auditory function of the internal ear:** Sound waves collected by the external ear, pass into the external acoustic meatus and are received by the tympanic membrane, which is set into motion. The tympanic membrane converts sound waves into mechanical energy. Vibrations of the tympanic membrane set the malleus, and consequently the remaining two ossicles, into motion. Movement of the stapes at the oval window causes disturbances in the perilymph, which causes deflection of the basilar membrane. The pillar cells attached to the basilar membrane move laterally in response to this deflection, in turn causing a lateral shearing of the stereocilia of the sensory hair cells of the organ of Corti against the tectorial membrane. Movement of the stereocilia is transduced into electrical impulses that travel via the cochlear nerve to the brain.

**Summary**

1. The ear is made up of three main parts: External, middle and internal ear.

2. Internal ear is composed of two compartments: The bony labyrinth, and membranous labyrinth, which lies within the bony labyrinth.

3. Bony labyrinth has three components: Three semicircular canals, the vestibule, and the cochlea.

4. The cochlea is snail-shell shaped and makes two and three-quarter turns around a central bony column known as the modiolus.

5. Spiral ganglion is embedded in the modiolus.

6. Membranous labyrinth is composed of two divisions: Vestibular labyrinth (saccule, utricle, and three semicircular ducts), and cochlear labyrinth (cochlear duct).

7. Cochlear duct contains hair cells in the spiral organ of Corti.

8. Movement of the stereocilia of hair cells is transduced into electrical impulses that travel via the cochlear nerve to the brain.

## Self Assessment

1. Perilymph is located in which of the following structures?
   a. Utricle
   b. Saccule
   c. Scala tympani
   d. Scala media

2. Which of the following is the function of vestibular membrane?
   a. Transmit sound to the oval window
   b. Maintain the gradient between the endolymph and perilymph
   c. Both of the above
   d. None of the above

3. Crista ampullaris is present in the:
   a. Semicircular duct
   b. Cochlear duct
   c. Utricle
   d. Saccule

4. Spiral ganglion contains which type of neurons?
   a. Unipolar
   b. Bipolar
   c. Multipolar
   d. None of the above

5. Organ of Corti is present in:
   a. Scala vestibuli
   b. Scala media
   c. Scala tympani
   d. Utricle

6. Organ of Corti is composed of:
   a. Rods and cones
   b. Hair cells and supporting cells
   c. Horizontal cells
   d. Amacrine cells

7. Membranous labyrinth is lined by which epithelium?
   a. Stratified cuboidal
   b. Simple columnar
   c. Simple squamous
   d. Pseudostratified

8. Modiolus is present in:
   a. Vestibule
   b. Semicircular canal
   c. Cochlea
   d. None of the above

9. Membranous labyrinth is present within the:
   a. Bony labyrinth
   b. Muscular labyrinth
   c. Vestibule
   d. Semicircular canals

10. How many semicircular ducts are present within the semicircular canals?
    a. 2                    b. 3
    c. 4                    d. 5

## Answers

1. c,     2. b,     3. a,     4. b,     5. b,     6. b,     7. c,     8. c,     9. a,
10. b

# Appendices

The following tables show the comparison between two or more structures:

**Table 1:** Light and electron microscope

| S. No. | Parameter | Light microscope | Electron microscope |
|--------|-----------|------------------|---------------------|
| 1 | Illumination | Light | Beam of electrons |
| 2 | Source | Low-voltage electric lamp or mirror | Heated tungsten filament |
| 3 | Focusing | Glass lenses | Electromagnets |
| 4 | Detection | Eye | Photographic plates (TEM) or CCD (SEM) |
| 5 | Magnification | 2,000X | 5,00,000X |
| 6 | Resolution | 0.2 μm | 0.2 nm (TEM) or 10 nm (SEM) |
| 7 | Staining | Colored dyes | Heavy metals |
| 8 | Cost | Less expensive | Very expensive |
| 9 | Size | Small and portable | Large and requires special rooms |
| 10 | Vacuum | Not required | Required (TEM) |

**Table 2:** Prokaryotic and eukaryotic cell

| S. No. | Parameter | Prokaryotic cell | Eukaryotic cell |
|--------|-----------|------------------|-----------------|
| 1 | Organisms | Bacteria | Humans, animals, fungi, plants |
| 2 | Size | ~1–10 μm | ~10–100 μm (nerve cells are meters long) |
| 3 | Nucleus | No real nucleus | Real nucleus with double membrane |
| 4 | DNA | Circular (usually) without proteins | Linear molecules (chromosomes) with histone proteins |
| 5 | RNA-/protein-synthesis | Coupled in cytoplasm | RNA-synthesis inside the nucleus, protein synthesis in cytoplasm |
| 6 | Ribosomes | 50S+30S | 60S+40S |
| 7 | Cytoskeleton | No cytoskeleton | Always has a cytoskeleton |
| 8 | Cell movement | Propelled by flagella | Cells are generally stationary except a few such as sperm cell |
| 9 | Mitochondria | Absent | Generally present |
| 10 | Chloroplasts | None | In algae and plants |

**Table 3:** Microtubules, intermediate filaments and microfilaments

| S. No. | Parameter | Microtubules | Intermediate filaments | Microfilaments |
|--------|-----------|--------------|------------------------|----------------|
| 1 | Diameter | 20–25 nm | 8–10 nm | 6–8 nm |
| 2 | Shape | Long, hollow, thin tubes | Long, straight or slightly bent filaments | Rod like |
| 3 | Location | Radiating from centrosomes and axonemes | Arranged throughout the cytoplasm, at desmosomes and inside the nuclear envelope | Concentrated beneath the cell membrane, and in cell extensions such as microvilli |
| 4 | Composition (types of protein) | α- and β-tubulin | Keratin, desmin, vimentin, laminin, glial fibrillary acidic protein and neurofilaments | G-actin and F-actin |
| 5 | Functions | Spindle formation, motion (ciliary and flagellar) and intracellular vesicular transport | Mechanical strength and support | Muscle contraction and motility in non-muscle cell |

**Table 4:** Mitosis and meiosis

| S. No. | Parameter | Mitosis | Meiosis |
|--------|-----------|---------|---------|
| 1 | Site | All cells, including sex cells up to certain stages | Only sex cells during reduction of chromosome number from 2n to n |
| 2 | Result of cell division of mother cell | One division forms two daughter cells | Two divisions form four meiotic products or haploid gametes |
| 3 | Mother cell | Either haploid or diploid | Always diploid |
| 4 | Number of chromosomes after division | Remains same | Remains one-half |
| 5 | S-phase | S-phase in which the amount of DNA is duplicated | Only in meiosis I |
| 6 | Pairing of homologous chromosomes | No pairing | Complete pairing of all homologous chromosomes |
| 7 | Crossing-over | Not occur | At least one crossing-over per homologous pair of chromosomes |
| 8 | Separation of centromeres | During anaphase | The centromeres do separate during anaphase II, but not during anaphase I |
| 9 | Genotype of the daughter cells | Same that of the mother cells | Differ from the mother cell |

**Table 5:** Serous and mucous acini

| S. No. | Parameter | Serous acini | Mucous acini |
|---|---|---|---|
| 1 | Size and shape | Smaller in size and rounded in shape | Larger in size and more variable in shape |
| 2 | Type of acini | Compound alveolar | Compound tubular or tubuloalveolar |
| 3 | Shape of lining cells | Cells are pyramidal in shape | Cells are truncated columnar in shape |
| 4 | Number of cells within an acinus | Cells are relatively more in number | Cells are relatively fewer in number |
| 5 | Cytoplasm | Cytoplasm depicts basal basophilia and apical eosinophilia | Cytoplasm is pale and vacuolated |
| 6 | Nuclei | Nuclei are rounded and centrally placed | Nuclei are flattened and peripherally placed |
| 7 | Lumen | Hardly visible | Mostly visible |
| 8 | Presence of demilune | Serous acini may be present as demilune on one aspect of some mucous acini | Mucous acini are not present as demilune |
| 9 | Staining | Darkly stained | Lightly stained |
| 10 | Biphasic staining | Present | Not present |
| 11 | Secretion | Secretes thin, watery saliva | Secretes thick, viscous saliva |

**Table 6:** Cilia and microvilli

| S. No. | Parameter | Cilia | Microvilli |
|---|---|---|---|
| 1 | Length | 5–10 µm (motile), 2–3 µm (non-motile) | 0.5–1.0 µm |
| 2 | Diameter | 0.2 µm | 0.08 µm |
| 3 | Shape | Cylindrical | Finger like |
| 4 | Motility | Motile and non-motile | Non-motile |
| 5 | Arrangement | Long and loosely arranged | Small and closely packed |
| 6 | Cytoskeleton | Rich in microtubules | Rich in microfilaments |
| 7 | Microscopic appearance | Cilia are seen even under light microscope | Seen under an electron microscope only |
| 8 | Functions | Transportation of secretion or cells or foreign particles (motile), sensors for mechanical and chemical signals (non-motile) | Absorption |
| 9 | Examples | Respiratory tract, oviducts, ventricle of brain (motile); epithelial cells of the rete testis, bile duct epithelium, retinal rods, and vestibular hair cells (non-motile) | Intestinal epithelium, gall bladder, and proximal convoluted tubule |

**Table 7:** Microvilli and stereocilia

| S. No. | Parameter | Microvilli | Stereocilia |
|--------|-----------|-----------|-------------|
| 1 | Length | Length is less | Unusually long microvilli |
| 2 | Villin | Present at the tip | Absent at the tip |
| 3 | Erzin | Absent | Erzin attaches the actin filaments to plasma membrane |
| 4 | $\alpha$-actinin | Absent | Actin bundles are attached to the cross bridges formed by $\alpha$-actinin |
| 5 | Microscopic appearance | Can be seen only with an electron microscope | Can be seen with a light microscope |

**Table 8:** Epithelium and supporting tissue

| S. No. | Parameter | Epithelium | Supporting tissue |
|--------|-----------|-----------|-------------------|
| 1 | Number of cells | A large number of cells are present | Number of cells are less |
| 2 | Matrix | Absent or negligible in amount | Present in large amount |
| 3 | Basement membrane | Cells rest on a basement membrane | The basement membrane is absent |
| 4 | Blood vessels | It is devoid of blood vessels (avascular) | It has many blood vessels (highly vascularized) |
| 5 | Exposure to outside environment | It is exposed to the outside environment (skin) | It is never exposed to the outside environment |
| 6 | Cell polarity | Most of the epithelial cells display functional and morphological polarity | Connective tissue cells do not show any polarity |
| 7 | Derivation | It is derived from all three germ layers, i.e. ectoderm, endoderm, and mesoderm | It is mainly derived from mesoderm |

**Table 9:** Collagen, elastic and reticular fibers

| S. No. | Parameter | Collagen fibers | Elastic fibers | Reticular fibers |
|--------|-----------|-----------------|----------------|------------------|
| 1 | Structure | Fibers are present in the form of wavy bundles; may be branched or anastomose with neighboring fibers. But individual fiber does not branch | Fibers are fine and branch to form a network | Fibers are very delicate and form fine networks |
| 2 | Fibrils | Fiber shows the presence of fibrils | Fibrils are not seen in fiber | A few fibrils may be seen |

(Contd.)

| S. No. | Parameter | Collagen fibers | Elastic fibers | Reticular fibers |
|---|---|---|---|---|
| | **Table 9:** Collagen, elastic and reticular fibers (*Contd.*) |
| 3 | Striations | Transverse striations are present | Not present | The striations are present |
| 4 | Appearance | Colorless, white fibers | Yellow fibers | Seen only with silver staining (argyrophilic fibers) |
| 5 | Physical properties | Fibers are flexible, yet have great tensile strength | Fibers have considerable elasticity, but a little tensile strength | Little elasticity and tensile strength |
| 6 | Stain: H and E<br>Orcein<br>Silver | Pink<br>–<br>– | –<br>Dark brown<br>– | –<br>–<br>Black |
| 7 | Distribution | Present in capsule, ligaments, tendons, and dermis | Present in aorta, lung, and ligamentum nuchae | Present in spleen, lymph node, and red bone marrow |

**Table 10:** White (unilocular) and brown (multilocular) adipose tissue

| S. No. | Parameter | White adipose tissue | Brown adipose tissue |
|---|---|---|---|
| 1 | Size of cells | Cells are larger in size | Cells are smaller in size |
| 2 | Nucleus | The nucleus is pushed to the periphery with the cytoplasm | The nucleus is centrally placed |
| 3 | Mitochondria | Contains less number of mitochondria | Contains numerous mitochondria |
| 4 | Lipid droplet | It contains a large single central lipid droplet | It contains a great number of lipid droplets of many sizes |
| 5 | Free ribosome | More in number | Few in number |
| 6 | Occurrence | Found in adults | Found in children |
| 7 | Function | Associated with energy production | Associated with heat production |

**Table 11:** Tendon and ligament

| S. No. | Parameter | Tendon | Ligament |
|---|---|---|---|
| 1 | Location | Attach skeletal muscle to bone | Connect bone to bone at the joints |
| 2 | Structure | Made up of bundles of collagen fibers | Along with collagen a few elastic fibers are also present |
| 3 | Amount of matrix | Less matrix per unit area | More matrix per unit area |
| 4 | Fibroblasts | Larger (20–25 μm) in size | Smaller (12–15 μm) in size |
| 5 | Level of organization | More organized | Less organized |
| 6 | Functions | Serve to move the bone or structure | Serve to hold the structure together and keep them stable |

**Table 12:** Hyaline cartilage, elastic cartilage and fibrocartilage

| S. No. | Parameter | Hyaline cartilage | Elastic cartilage | Fibrocartilage |
|---|---|---|---|---|
| 1 | Types of fibers | Type II collagen fibers | Elastic fibers with type II collagen fibers | Type I collagen fibers |
| 2 | Number of cells | Maximum number of cells | Moderate number of cells | Less number of cells |
| 3 | Major cells | Chondroblasts, chondrocytes | Chondroblasts, chondrocytes | Chondrocytes, fibroblasts |
| 4 | Chondrocytes | Mainly present in isogenous groups | Present singly, and in isogenous groups | Present singly, in pairs, and in isogenous groups |
| 5 | Perichondrium | Perichondrium present in most places except in articular cartilages and at the direct junction of cartilage with bone (costal cartilage, and epiphyseal plate) | Perichondrium present | Perichondrium absent |
| 6 | Matrix | Intensely metachromatic, contains proteoglycan aggrecan and calcify with aging | Intensely metachromatic, contains proteoglycan aggrecan and does not calcify with aging | Less metachromatic, contains proteoglycan versican and calcification occurs during repair of bone |
| 7 | Appearance | Bluish white color | Yellowish color | Glistening white |
| 8 | Locations | Trachea, bronchi, costal cartilages, thyroid cartilage, in the nasal septum, cartilage of larynx (cricoid and most of arytenoid), and articular ends of bones | Pinna of the ear, epiglottis, external acoustic meatus and auditory tube | At the sites, where tendons are inserted into the bone and in the intervertebral discs (annulus fibrosus), the pubic symphysis, glenoidal labrum, acetabular labrum, and the menisci of the knee joint |
| 9 | Functions | Reduces friction at joints, responsible for longitudinal growth of long bones and provide flexibility to rib | Maintains the shape of the organ and provides support to the organ, with elasticity | Provides strength and also capable of resisting compression and tearing forces |

**Table 13:** Cartilage and bone

| S. No. | Parameter | Cartilage | Bone |
|--------|-----------|-----------|------|
| 1 | Physical property | It is a firm but flexible tissue | It is a very hard tissue |
| 2 | Ground substance | No mineralization and highly hydrated (80%) | Mineralized and less hydrated (7%) |
| 3 | Fibers | Type I collagen fibers, type II collagen fibers, and elastic fibers | Type I collagen fibers |
| 4 | Lamellae | Collagen fibers are not organized to form lamellae | Collagen fibers are organized in lamellae |
| 5 | Vascularity | Avascular, nutrients received via diffusion | Highly vascular |
| 6 | Growth | Appositional, and interstitial | Appositional only |
| 7 | Nerves | Absent | Present |
| 8 | Communication between cells | No communication between cells | Cells communicate via gap junctions |

**Table 14:** Compact and spongy bone

| S. No. | Parameter | Compact bone | Spongy bone |
|--------|-----------|--------------|-------------|
| 1 | Density | Dense like ivory | Porous like sponge |
| 2 | Haversian system | Present | Absent |
| 3 | Bony trabeculae | Absent | Present |
| 4 | Weight | 75–80% of human skeleton | 20–25% of human skeleton |
| 5 | Arrangement of bony lamellae | Regular | Irregular |
| 6 | Marrow cavity | Single, central | Many, irregular |
| 7 | Bone marrow | Yellow | Red |
| 8 | Location in bone | Outer region | Inner region |

**Table 15:** Red, white and intermediate muscle fiber

| S. No. | Parameter | Red muscle fiber | White muscle fiber | Intermediate muscle fiber |
|--------|-----------|------------------|--------------------|--------------------------|
| 1 | Diameter | Smaller in diameter | Larger in diameter | Intermediate in diameter |
| 2 | Mitochondria | Numerous mitochondria are present | Only a few mitochondria are present | Numerous mitochondria are present |
| 3 | Myoglobin | Rich in myoglobin | Contains less myoglobin | Rich in myoglobin |
| 4 | Amount of glycogen | Low | Considerable | High |
| 5 | Speed of contraction | Slow contraction | Rapid contraction | Rapid contraction |
| 6 | Rate of fatigue | Slow | Fast | Intermediate |
| 7 | Generation of ATP | Aerobic glycolysis (oxidative phosphorylation of fatty acids) | Anaerobic glycolysis | Anaerobic glycolysis |
| 8 | Location | Muscles of the limbs, and back | Muscles of eyeball, and fingers | Muscles of leg |

**Table 16:** Skeletal, smooth and cardiac muscle fibers

| S. No. | Parameter | Skeletal muscle | Smooth muscle | Cardiac muscle |
|---|---|---|---|---|
| 1 | Shape | Long, cylindrical, and unbranched | Spindle shaped, and unbranched | Short, cylindrical, and show branching |
| 2 | Length | 1 mm to 30 cm | 20–500 µm | 85–100 µm |
| 3 | Diameter | 10–100 µm | 10–20 µm | 15 µm |
| 4 | Nuclei | Multinucleated, elongated, and peripherally located | Single, elongated, and centrally located | Single, oval, and centrally located |
| 5 | Intercalated disc | Absent | Absent | Present |
| 6 | T tubules | Present, at the junction of A- and I-band | Absent | Present, at Z-lines |
| 7 | Cell junctions | Absent | Gap junctions present | Through intercalated disc (fascia adherens, desmosomes, and gap junctions) |
| 8 | Striations | Cross striations are present | Striations absent | Less prominent cross striations are present |
| 9 | Control of contraction | Voluntary | Involuntary | Involuntary |
| 10 | Contraction | Quicker and faster | Slow and sustained | Rhythmic contraction |
| 11 | Location | Limbs, tongue | Walls of respiratory and digestive tracts | Heart |

**Table 17:** Elastic artery, muscular artery, arteriole and metarteriole

| S. No. | Parameter | Elastic artery | Muscular artery | Arteriole | Metarteriole |
|---|---|---|---|---|---|
| 1 | Subendothelial connective tissue layer | Thick | Thin | Very thin | Absent |
| 2 | Internal elastic lamina | Not clearly visible | Clearly visible | Absent except in largest arterioles | Absent |
| 3 | Concentric fenestrated elastic lamellae | 50 or more in number | Absent | Absent | Absent |
| 4 | Smooth muscle fibers | Present in between the elastic fibers | 10–40 layers of smooth muscle fibers | 1–5 layers of smooth muscle fibers | Incomplete rings of smooth muscle fibers |
| 5 | External elastic lamina | Not clearly visible | Clearly visible | Absent | Absent |
| 6 | Tunica adventitia | Thin | Thick | Very thin | Absent |
| 7 | Vasa vasorum | Present and prominent | Present and not prominent | Absent | Absent |

**Table18:** Continuous capillary, fenestrated capillary and sinusoidal capillary

| S. No. | Parameter | Continuous capillary | Fenestrated capillary | Sinusoidal capillary |
|---|---|---|---|---|
| 1 | Diameter | Small | Small | Large |
| 2 | Regularity of cross section | Regular | Regular | Irregular |
| 3 | Intercellular gaps | Absent | Absent | Present and variable |
| 4 | Fenestrations | Absent | Numerous | Variable |
| 5 | Basal lamina | Prominent and continuous | Prominent and continuous | Scanty or absent |
| 6 | Exchange between blood and tissues | Through cytoplasm of endothelial cells (transcytosis) | Through diffusion across diaphragm | Through pores without any barrier |
| 7 | Locations | Muscles, brain and connective tissue | Endocrine glands, pancreas and kidney | Liver, bone marrow and spleen |

**Table 19:** Arteries and veins

| S. No. | Parameter | Arteries | Veins |
|---|---|---|---|
| 1 | Lumen | Lumen is almost circular | Lumen is collapsed or irregular |
| 2 | Thickness of wall | Thicker | Thinner |
| 3 | Situation | Mostly deeply situated | Both superficially and deeply situated |
| 4 | Direction of blood | Away from heart except pulmonary trunk and pulmonary arteries | Towards the heart except pulmonary veins |
| 5 | Three coats | All arteries have well defined three coats | Small and medium-sized arteries have not well defined three coats |
| 6 | Tunica intima | Often corrugated or scalloped after death | Never scalloped |
| 7 | Endothelial lining | Well defined | Not so well defined |
| 8 | Internal elastic lamina | Prominent in some arteries | Never so prominent |
| 9 | Tunica media | Form 2/3 of the thickness of wall | Form 1/3 of the thickness of the wall |
| 10 | External elastic lamina | Distinct | Not well defined |
| 11 | Tunica adventitia | Form 1/3 of the thickness of wall | Form 2/3 of the thickness of wall |
| 12 | Extent of vasa vasorum | Supply extend up to outer 2/3 of tunica media | Supply extend up to tunica intima |
| 13 | Valves | None | Present in the veins of medium-sized caliber, especially those of extremities |
| 14 | Wall thickness to lumen size ratio | Except in large arteries, the wall is thicker than lumen | The wall is thinner than Lumen |
| 15 | Blood | Carries oxygenated blood | Carries deoxygenated blood |
| 16 | Flow of blood | Spurty flow of blood | Sluggish flow of blood |
| 17 | Blood pressure | Blood move with pressure | Blood move under very low pressure |

**Table 20:** Blood and lymph

| S. No. | Parameter | Blood | Lymph |
|---|---|---|---|
| 1 | Course | It is pumped throughout the body by the heart | It flows through the veins in a passive manner |
| 2 | Movement | It flows through the body in a circular motion | It moves in a single direction |
| 3 | Constituents | It contains liquid plasma, red blood cells, white blood cells and platelets | It is a whitish and clear liquid |
| 4 | Function | It transports oxygen throughout the body | It removes waste from the system |
| 5 | Seen with naked eyes | Blood can be seen if there is damage to the vessels | Lymph cannot be seen with the naked eyes |
| 6 | Purification | The kidneys purify the blood | Lymph is purified in the lymph nodes |

**Table 21:** Blood capillaries and lymphatic capillaries

| S. No. | Parameter | Blood capillaries | Lymphatic capillaries |
|---|---|---|---|
| 1 | Appearance | Reddish, so can be seen easily | Colorless, so difficult to see |
| 2 | Diameter | Small | Large |
| 3 | Basement membrane | Well developed | Poorly developed |
| 4 | Content | Blood | Lymph |
| 5 | Function | Add tissue fluid to intercellular spaces | Absorb tissue fluid from intercellular spaces |

**Table 22:** Lymph node, spleen, thymus and palatine tonsil

| S. No. | Parameter | Lymph node | Spleen | Thymus | Palatine tonsil |
|---|---|---|---|---|---|
| 1 | Outer covering | Capsule | Capsule | Capsule | Stratified squamous nonkeratinized epithelium |
| 2 | Trabeculae or Septa | Thin trabeculae present | Abundant thick trabeculae with blood vessels | Incomplete septa are present | Both are absent |
| 3 | Cortex and medulla | Present | Absent | Present | Absent |
| 4 | Lymphatic nodules | Present | Present | Absent | Present |
| 5 | White and red pulp | Absent | Present | Absent | Absent |
| 6 | Cords and sinuses | Present | Present | Absent | Absent |
| 7 | Lymphatic vessels | Afferent and efferent | A few efferent only | A few efferent only | Efferent only |
| 8 | Unique structures | Subcapsular sinus | Malpighian corpuscle | Hassall's corpuscle | Tonsillar crypts |

| S. No. | Parameter | Thin skin | Thick skin |
|--------|-----------|-----------|------------|
| | **Table 23:** Thin and thick skin | | |
| 1 | Epidermal layers | Stratum spinosum and corneum are thin. Stratum lucidum is absent | Stratum spinosum and corneum are thick. Stratum lucidum is present |
| 2 | Epidermal thickness | ~0.1 mm | 1 mm or more |
| 3 | Epidermal ridges | Absent | Present |
| 4 | Hairs | Present | Absent |
| 5 | Merocrine sweat glands | Few | Many |
| 6 | Sebaceous glands | Present | Absent |
| 7 | Sensory receptors | Less | More |
| 8 | Distribution | Whole body except palm and sole | Present only in palm and sole |

**Table 24:** Various parts of respiratory system

| S. No. Parameter | Vestibule | Nasal-fossa | Olfactory mucosa | Paranasal sinuses | Naso-pharynx | Larynx | Trachea and primary bronchi | Intra-pulmonary bronchus | Terminal bronchiole | Respiratory bronchiole | Alveoli |
|---|---|---|---|---|---|---|---|---|---|---|---|
| 1 Epithelium | Stratified squamous keratinized | Pseudostratified columnar ciliated | Pseudostratified columnar ciliated | Pseudostratified columnar ciliated (thinner) | Pseudostratified columnar ciliated | Pseudostratified columnar ciliated and stratified squamous non-keratinized | Pseudostratified columnar ciliated | Pseudostratified columnar ciliated | Simple cuboidal (with a few cilia), and more number of Clara cells | Simple cuboidal and Clara cells | Simple squamous |
| 2 Goblet cells | Absent | Present | Absent | Present | Present | Present | Present | Present | Absent | Absent | Absent |
| 3 Ciliated cells | Absent | Present | Absent | Present | Present | Present | Present | Present | Present | Absent | Absent |
| 4 Glands | Sebaceous and sweat glands | Sero-mucous glands | Bowman's glands | Sero-mucous glands | Mucous and serous glands | Mucous and sero-mucous glands | Mucous and sero-mucous glands | Mucous and sero-mucous glands | Absent | Absent | Absent |
| 5 Skeleton | Hyaline cartilage | Bone | Bone | Bone | Muscle | Hyaline and elastic cartilage | Hyaline cartilage (C-shaped) | Hyaline cartilage (irregular plates) | Absent | Absent | Absent |

**Table 25:** Filiform, fungiform, circumvallate and foliate papilla

| S. No. | Parameter | Filiform papilla | Fungiform papilla | Circumvallate papilla | Foliate papilla |
|---|---|---|---|---|---|
| 1 | Distribution | Anterior 2/3. These are most numerous papillae | Anterior 2/3 (among filiform). These are more numerous at tip | In front of and parallel to the sulcus terminalis | Posterolateral margin (rudimentary in men, but well developed in lagomorphs) |
| 2 | Shape | Conical (with keratinization on tip) | Like a mushroom | Dome shaped (surrounded by a circular sulcus) | Leaf shaped |
| 3 | Secondary connective tissue papillae | On all surfaces | On all surfaces | Only on its top surface | On all surfaces |
| 4 | Taste buds | Absent | Few on the free surface | On the sides | On the sides |
| 5 | Glandular association | Absent | Present (serous) | Present (serous— von Ebner's gland) | Present (serous) |

**Table 26:** Cardia, fundus and pylorus of stomach

| S. No. | Parameter | Cardia | Fundus | Pylorus |
|---|---|---|---|---|
| 1 | Gland | Very short gland ½ is body and ½ is duct | Tubular gland. Lower 3/4 is secretory and upper 1/4 is conducting | Coiled pyloric glands. Lower 1/3 is secretory and upper 2/3 is conducting |
| 2 | Cells of gland | Mucous cells and a few parietal cells | Undifferentiated, mucous neck, parietal, chief, and a few argentaffin cells | Mucous cells, and fewer parietal, and argentaffin cells |
| 3 | Muscularis externa | Inner oblique, middle circular, and outer longitudinal | Inner oblique, middle circular, and outer longitudinal | Circular muscle layer thickened to form pyloric sphincter |

**Table 27:** Pylorus and duodenum

| S. No. | Parameter | Pylorus | Duodenum |
|---|---|---|---|
| 1 | Lining epithelium | All the cells of surface epithelium look alike. It dips in to form deep pits | Cells of the surface epithelium do not look alike. It evaginates to form villi of varying heights. It also invaginates to form crypts |
| 2 | Columnar cells | Columnar cells do not exhibit striated (brush) border | Columnar cells exhibit striated border |
| 3 | Goblet cells | No goblet cells | Goblet cells present |
| 4 | Submucosa | Submucosa only contains connective tissue, nerve fibers, and fine blood vessels | Submucosa contains mucus secreting Brunner's glands |
| 5 | Muscularis externa | Thickened middle circular coat to form pyloric sphincter | Outer longitudinal, and inner circular layer of smooth muscle fibers are present |

**Table 28:** Duodenum, jejunum and ileum

| S. No. | Parameter | Duodenum | Jejunum | Ileum |
|---|---|---|---|---|
| 1 | Epithelium | Columnar epithelium with striated border and a few goblet cells are seen | Columnar epithelium with striated border and goblet cells are seen | Columnar epithelium with striated border and goblet cells are more |
| 2 | Villi | Broad, tall, and leaf-shaped villi | Villi have clubbed end | Villi are shorter and finger shaped |
| 3 | Lymphatic tissue in lamina propria | Scattered lymphocytes are present | Scattered lymphocytes, and large number of lymphatic follicles are present | Peyer's patches are present |
| 4 | Submucosa | Mucus secreting Brunner's glands are typical feature | Only connective tissue, blood vessels, and nerves | Peyer's patches extend in the submucosa |

**Table 29:** Small and large intestine

| S. No. | Parameter | Small intestine | Large intestine |
|---|---|---|---|
| 1 | Villi | Villi are present | Villi are absent |
| 2 | Crypts of Lieberkühn | Crypts of Lieberkühn are fewer and less deep | Crypts of Lieberkühn are deeper and more in number |
| 3 | Goblet cells | Goblet cells are less in number | Goblet cells are more in number |
| 4 | Taenia coli | Longitudinal coat of muscularis externa is uniformly thick | Longitudinal coat of muscularis externa is thickened to form three taenia coli |
| 5 | Sacculations | No sacculations | Taenia are shorter than the length of the large intestine, so sacculations appear |
| 6 | Appendices epiploicae | No appendices epiploicae | Peritoneal pouches filled with fat are present. These are called appendices epiploicae |

**Table 30:** Pancreas and parotid gland

| S. No. | Parameter | Pancreas | Parotid gland |
|---|---|---|---|
| 1 | Connective tissue | Relatively less, as septa are a few and thin | Relatively more due to numerous thick septa |
| 2 | Islets of Langerhans | Present and are a characteristic feature | Absent |
| 3 | Centroacinar cells | Present in between the cells and lumen of serous acini | Absent |
| 4 | Lobes and lobules | Only lobules are present | Both are present |

**Table 31:** Proximal convoluted tubule and distal convoluted tubule

| S. No. | Parameter | Proximal convoluted tubule | Distal convoluted tubule |
|---|---|---|---|
| 1 | Sections | More sections, as it is highly convoluted | Less sections, as it is less convoluted |
| 2 | Lining cells | Truncated broad base with brush border | Cuboidal with no brush border |
| 3 | Nucleus | Large, spherical, and centrally located | Small, spherical, and centrally located |
| 4 | Lumen | Hardly visible | Clearly visible |
| 5 | Cytoplasm | Strongly eosinophilic | Less eosinophilic |
| 6 | Cell outlines | Not distinct | Distinct |
| 7 | Diameter | 45–60 μm | 30–50 μm |

**Table 32:** Sperm and semen

| S. No. | Parameter | Sperm | Semen |
|---|---|---|---|
| 1 | Definition | Male reproductive cell | Seminal fluid that contains millions of sperms |
| 2 | Functions | Genetic bearer and haploid cell | Nourishment of sperm cells |
| 3 | Visibility | Not visible with eye (microscopic) | Easily visible fluid |

**Table 33:** Non-lactating mammary gland and lactating mammary gland

| S. No. | Parameter | Non-lactating mammary gland | Lactating mammary gland |
|---|---|---|---|
| 1 | Size of glandular alveoli | Small | Glandular alveoli are large |
| 2 | Lumen of glandular alveoli | Does not contain anything | Contain eosinophilic (milk) secretion |
| 3 | Duct system | Well developed | Not well developed |
| 4 | Lobules | Poorly defined | Clearly demarcated |
| 5 | Stroma | More | Less |

**Table 34:** Nervous and endocrine system

| S. No. | Parameter | Nervous system | Endocrine system |
|---|---|---|---|
| 1 | Mode of information transfer | Nerve impulse and neurotransmitter release at specific site | Hormone released into bloodstream |
| 2 | Receptor location in body | Internal and external | Internal |
| | **Effects:** | | |
| 3 | Location | Localized | Entire body |
| 4 | Targets | Nerve, gland, and muscle cells | All tissues |
| | **Time for:** | | |
| 5 | Onset | Immediate (milliseconds) | Gradual (seconds to hours) |
| 6 | Duration | Short-term (milliseconds to minutes) | Long-term (minute to days) |
| 7 | Recovery | Immediate (as soon as signal removed) | Slow (continues after signal removed) |

| S. No. | Parameter | Axon | Dendrite |
|---|---|---|---|
| | | **Table 35:** Axon and dendrite | |
| 1 | Number in a neuron | Only one axon | Usually multiple |
| 2 | Diameter | It has uniform diameter | Its thickness reduces with its division |
| 3 | Surface | Smooth | It bears many small spine-like projections |
| 4 | Nerve impulse | Travels away from the cell body | Travels towards the cell body |
| 5 | Nissl bodies | Absent | Present |
| 6 | Branches | Rarely branch, but ends by dividing into fine processes | Branch profusely |

| S. No. | Parameter | Dorsal ganglion | Autonomic ganglion |
|---|---|---|---|
| | | **Table 36:** Dorsal (spinal) and autonomic (sympathetic) ganglion | |
| 1 | Type of neurons | Pseudounipolar | Multipolar |
| 2 | Cell body | Large and rounded | Smaller and irregular |
| 3 | Nucleus | Central | Eccentric |
| 4 | Satellite cells | Forms a complete layer around each neuron | Forms an incomplete layer around each neuron |
| 5 | Nerve fibers | Thick and myelinated | Thin and unmyelinated |
| 6 | Arrangement of neurons | Present in groups | Scattered |
| 7 | Synapses | Absent | Present |
| 8 | Locations | Dorsal roots of spinal nerves, and in paths of V, VII, IX, and X cranial nerves | Along the sympathetic trunk |

| S. No. | Parameter | Protoplasmic astrocytes | Fibrous astrocytes | Oligodendrocytes | Microglia |
|---|---|---|---|---|---|
| | | **Table 37:** Protoplasmic astrocytes, fibrous astrocytes, oligodendrocytes and microglia | | | |
| 1 | Cell size | Large | Large | Medium | Small |
| 2 | Shape of nucleus | Oval (lightly stained) | Oval (lightly stained) | Small spherical (darkly stained) | Small elongated (darkest) |
| 3 | Cytoplasmic processes | Many short, thick processes | Many long, slender processes | A few delicate processes | Short, thin processes with spines |
| 4 | Occurrence (predominant in) | Grey matter | White matter | Grey and white matter | Grey matter |
| 5 | Functions | Help to establish the blood–brain barrier, and may contribute to its maintenance | Healing, and scar formation after injury in the central nervous system | Myelinaton | Phagocytosis |
| 6 | Embryological origin | Neuroectoderm | Neuroectoderm | Neuroectoderm | Bone marrow |

## APPENDIX II: QUICK REVIEW

### Simple Squamous Epithelium (Fig. 4.1A, B)

- Single layer of flattened (height of the cells is very less in comparison to width) cells.

- Cells are thin, so nucleus forms a bulging on the cell surface.

- These epithelial cells are present in lining of the heart (endocardium), blood and lymphatic vessels (endothelium), and lining of pleural, pericardial, and peritoneal cavities (mesothelium).

### Simple Cuboidal Epithelium (Fig. 4.3A, B)

- Single layer of cube-like (height, width and depth of the cells are approximately equal) cells.

- Nuclei are rounded and centrally placed.

- These epithelial cells are present in thyroid follicles (active), and covering of the ovary.

### Simple Columnar Epithelium (Fig. 4.4A, B)

- Single layer of column-like (height of the cells is more than the width) cells.

- Nuclei are oval and basally placed.

- These epithelial cells with cilia are present in uterine tubes and uterus, and without cilia are present in the digestive tract.

### Pseudostratified Columnar Epithelium (Fig. 4.5A, B)

- The cells vary in height, so the nuclei lie at different levels.

- It appears multilayered but actually made up of single layer of epithelial cells.

- These epithelial cells are present in most of the upper respiratory tract.

### Stratified Squamous Keratinized Epithelium (Fig. 4.6A, B)

- More than one layer of cells in which basal cells are cuboidal or columnar, intermediate cells polyhedral, and superficial cells are flat.

- Nuclei are oval in the basal cells, rounded in the intermediate cells, and superficial cells have no nuclei, as they are filled with tough keratin protein.

- This epithelium is present in the epidermis of the skin.

### Stratified Squamous Nonkeratinized Epithelium (Fig. 4.7A, B)

- More than one layer of cells in which basal cells are cuboidal or columnar, intermediate cells polyhedral, and superficial cells are flat.

- Nuclei are oval in the basal cells, rounded in the intermediate cells, and flattened in the superficial cells.
- This epithelium is present in lining of the mouth, esophagus, and vagina

## Transitional Epithelium (Urothelium) (Fig. 4.10A, B)

- More than one layer of cells in which basal cells are cuboidal or columnar, intermediate cells polyhedral, and superficial cells are dome shaped.
- Superficial cells are transitory when under no tension cells are dome (umbrella or pear) shaped and under tension superficial cells become flattened.
- This epithelium is present in the urinary tract from renal calyces to the urethra.

## Goblet Cells (Fig. 4.12A to C)

- Shape of goblet cells is like a glass or chalice.
- They are distended at their apex because of mucigen granules and narrow base contain nucleus.
- When stained with H and E, they look empty and with PAS + hematoxylin stain they look magenta in color.

## Loose Areolar Tissue (Fig. 5.6A to C)

- Thick wavy bundles of collagen fibers and straight, short branching elastic fibers are present.
- Large number of connective tissue cells (fibroblasts and mast cells) and a large amount of ground substance are present.
- This tissue is present in mesentry, adventitial layer of blood vessels, and in lamina propria of gastrointestinal tract.

## Tendon (Fig. 5.10A, B)

- Parallel arrangements of bundles of collagen fibers are present.
- Rows of flattened nuclei of fibroblast are present in between collagen bundles.
- Less amount of ground substance is present.

## Embryonic Connective Tissue (Fig. 5.5A, B)

- Stellate-shaped mesenchymal cells with oval nuclei are present.
- Delicate branching cytoplasmic extensions from cells form an interlocking network throughout.
- Faint background is due to the amorphous ground substance.

## White/Unilocular Adipose Tissue (Fig. 5.7A, B)

- Fat cells are polyhedral and look empty as the fat present in them gets dissolved during preparation of section.
- Cytoplasm is present at the periphery as a thin rim and flattened nuclei lie in the thickened part of this rim.
- This tissue is found subcutaneously throughout the body except over the eyelid, penis, and scrotum.

## Brown/Multilocular Adipose Tissue (Fig. 5.8A, B)

- Fat cells are polyhedral and nuclei are spherical and centrally placed.

- Multiple droplets filled with fat are present but look empty as the fat present in them gets dissolved during preparation of section.
- This tissue is present in the axilla, between the shoulder blades, in the inguinal region, and in the region of the neck.

### Reticular Tissue (Fig. 5.9A, B)

- Delicate network of reticular fibers along with spindle-shaped reticular cells are present.
- Reticular fibers are not visible with H and E stain, but can be seen easily stained black by impregnation of silver salts.
- This tissue is present in the liver, spleen, and lymph nodes.

### Hyaline Cartilage (Fig. 6.1A, B)

- Cartilage is formed by cells (chondrocytes), and matrix (basophilic and homogenous). It is surrounded from all sides by a connective tissue layer known as perichondrium.
- Chondrocytes which are located superficially are ovoid. Those located deeper are more spherical in shape and may occur in isogenous groups (cell nests).
- It is present in trachea, bronchi, costal cartilages, and thyroid cartilage.

### Elastic Cartilage (Fig. 6.4A, B)

- Cartilage is formed by cells (chondrocytes), and matrix (contain plenty of elastic fibers). It is surrounded from all sides by a connective tissue layer known as perichondrium.
- Chondrocytes are more abundant and bigger in size and are present singly, and in isogenous groups.
- It is present in pinna of the ear, epiglottis, external acoustic meatus and auditory tube.

### Fibrocartilage (Fig. 6.6A, B)

- Perichondrium is absent.
- It is made up of parallel running bundles of collagen fibers, and chondrocytes (lies between bundles).
- It is often present at the sites, where tendons are inserted into the bone. It is also present in the intervertebral discs (annulus fibrosus), the symphysis pubis, glenoidal labrum, acetabular labrum, and the menisci of the knee joint.

### Compact Bone (TS) (Figs 7.3A, B and 7.5A, B)

- Bone is covered by periosteum and haversian system is present.
- Three layers of lamellae are present: Circumferential, concentric, and interstitial. In between the lamellae osteocytes are present.
- This bone forms diaphysis of long bones. It also forms a thin layer on the external surface of short, flat and irregular bones in which the core is made up of spongy bone.

### Compact Bone (LS) (Fig. 7.6)

- Longitudinal running canals are haversian canals, while horizontally running canals are Volkmann's canals.
- Osteocytes are present.
- This bone forms diaphysis of long bones. It also forms a thin layer on the external surface of short, flat and irregular bones in which the core is made up of spongy bone.

**Spongy Bone** (Fig. 7.7A, B)

- Presence of bony trabeculae separated by marrow spaces containing bone marrow. Osteocytes are present in the trabecular matrix, while osteoblasts and osteoclasts lie on the surface of the trabeculae.
- Haversian system and lamellar arrangement is absent.
- This bone mainly forms epiphysis of long bones. All short, flat, and irregular bones consist of a core of spongy bone. A thin rim around the marrow cavity of the diaphysis of long bone consists of spongy bone.

**Bone Growth in Length** (Fig. 7.10A, B)

- Epiphyseal plate of cartilage is responsible for longitudinal growth of long bone.
- Epiphyseal plate shows various zones, i.e. resting, proliferative, hypertrophic, calcification, and ossification.
- Osteoblasts cover the remnants of calcified cartilage and form bone on it.

**Skeletal Muscle (LS)** (Fig. 8.1A, B)

- Muscle fibers are long, cylindrical, and unbranched.
- Prominent transverse striations showing alternative dark (A) and light (I) band.
- Multiple elongated nuclei lie at the periphery.

**Skeletal Muscle (TS)** (Fig. 8.3A, C)

- Fibers are irregular in outline with peripherally located nuclei.
- Individual muscle fibers are invested by endomysium and bundles of muscle fibers are surrounded by perimysium.
- Whole muscle is surrounded by epimysium.

**Smooth Muscle (LS)** (Fig. 8.9A, B)

- Muscle fibers are long, spindle shaped, and striations are absent.
- Nucleus is elongated and present in the widest part of the fiber.
- Fibers are arranged in such a way that near the central wide part of a fiber, thin tapering end of neighboring fibers are placed.

**Smooth Muscle (TS)** (Fig. 8.10A, B)

- Fibers are oval in outline.
- Nuclei are centrally placed.
- Nuclei are not visible in all muscle fibers; they are only visible if the plane of section passes through them.

**Cardiac Muscle (LS)** (Fig. 8.11A, C)

- Muscle fibers are long, cylindrical, and branched with a few striations.
- Nuclei are one or two, oval and centrally placed.
- Fibers are joined serially end to end by intercalated disc (step-like pattern).

**Cardiac Muscle (TS)** (Fig. 8.11B, D)

- Fibers are irregular in outline.

- Nuclei are centrally placed.
- Nuclei are not visible in all muscle fibers.

### Muscle Spindle (Fig. 8.6A, B)

- The nuclear chain fibers are present whose nuclei line up in a row.
- The nuclear bag fibers showing nuclei in the center.
- It is present in skeletal muscle and it is the sense organ for measuring the level of contraction.

### Heart (Fig. 10.2)

- It is lined by three layers. From inner to outer side these are: Endocardium, myocardium, and epicardium.
- Myocardium is the thickest middle layer of the heart and it is composed of cardiac muscle fibers.
- Endocardium and epicardium are made by simple squamous epithelium and a connective tissue layer.

### Elastic/Conducting Artery (Fig. 10.6A, B)

- Innermost layer (tunica intima) is made up of endothelium and subendothelial connective tissue layer.
- Middle layer (tunica media) is thickest and contains 50 or more (number increases with age) concentric elastic lamellae made up of elastin.
- Outermost layer (tunica adventitia) is relatively thin and contains abundant vasa vasorum.

### Muscular/Distributing Artery (Fig. 10.7A, B)

- Subendothelial connective tissue layer is thin or absent.
- Internal and external elastic laminas are well defined.
- Tunica media is the thickest and consists of 10–40 concentric layers of smooth muscle fibers.

### Arteriole (Fig. 10.8)

- Small artery whose luminal diameters usually equal the wall thickness.
- Tunica media is composed of 1–5 layers of smooth muscle fibers.
- Tunica adventitia is relatively thin.

### Large Veins (Fig. 10.11)

- Lumen is partially collapsed and even RBCs can be seen. Subendothelial layer is thick.
- Tunica media is thin and contains a few layers of smooth muscle fibers.
- Tunica adventitia is thick and contains vasa vasorum.

### Medium to Small Sized Veins (Fig. 10.12)

- Lumen is partially collapsed and even RBCs can be seen. Subendothelial layer is inconspicuous.
- Tunica media is thin and contains a few layers of smooth muscle fibers.
- Tunica adventitia forms the main bulk and contains vasa vasorum.

### Venule (Fig. 10.13)

- Tunica intima is made by endothelial cells.
- Tunica media is made up by 1–3 layers of smooth muscle fibers.
- Tunica adventitia is thick.

**Lymph Node** (Fig. 11.4A, B)

- Just beneath the capsule a subcapsular (marginal) sinus is present.
- Outer part is cortex with well developed lymphatic nodules.
- Inner part is medulla with medullary cords and sinuses.

**Palatine Tonsils** (Fig. 11.7A, B)

- Capsule is absent.
- Deep tonsillar crypts lined by stratified squamous nonkeratinized epithelium.
- Just beneath the epithelium lies aggregation of lymphatic nodules.

**Thymus** (Fig. 11.8A, B)

- Capsule with incomplete septa dividing it into many lobules.
- Lobules with darkly stained outer cortex and lightly stained inner medulla.
- Hassall's corpuscles are present in the medulla.

**Spleen** (Fig. 11.10A, B)

- It is enclosed by a well-developed capsule with trabeculae.
- White pulp contains lymphatic nodules with eccentric arteriole.
- Red pulp contains splenic cords and a large number of sinusoids.

**Thick Skin** (Fig. 12.4A, B)

- Thick epidermis is made by stratified squamous keratinized epithelium, in which stratum corneum is thick.
- Numerous sweat glands are present in the dermis.
- Hair follicles and sebaceous glands are absent.

**Thin Skin** (Fig. 12.3A, B)

- Thin epidermis is made by stratified squamous keratinized epithelium, in which stratum corneum and stratum spinosum are thin and stratum lucidum is absent.
- Hair follicles, sebaceous glands, and arrector pili muscle are present.
- Epidermal and dermal ridges are unmarked.

**Tactile Corpuscle of Meissner** (Fig. 12.1A, B)

- Encapsulated body with a pinecone-shaped structure.
- Their long axis is perpendicular to the skin's surface.
- These receptors are present in lips, external genitalia, and nipple.

**Lamellar Corpuscle** (Fig. 12.2A, B)

- Encapsulated body with a unique onion-shaped structure.
- Each corpuscle is having a central myelinated axon, which is surrounded by concentric lamellae of compact collagen fibers.
- These are present in hypodermis.

**Hair (TS)** (Fig. 12.7A, B)

- In the center (cortex) looks dark black in color due to the presence of pigment cells.

- The broad external dermal root sheath is separated from connective tissue by a glassy membrane.
- Internal root sheath contains eosinophilic keratohyaline granules.

### Hair (LS) (Fig. 12.8A, B)

- Central core (medulla) is formed by 2–3 layers of shrunken cornified cells and it is surrounded by layers of pigment cells (dark brown to black).
- At the base lie a bulbous expansion; the hair bulb, enclosing the hair papilla.
- Sebaceous glands associated with hair follicles are present.

### Sebaceous Gland or Oil Gland (Fig. 12.12A, B)

- Pear-shaped structure associated with upper parts of the hair follicles.
- Form by clusters of large vacuolated cells.
- These glands can be found everywhere on the body except for the palms and the soles.

### Merocrine or Eccrine Sweat Gland (Fig. 12.9A, B)

- Secretory portion of the gland lies deep in the dermis and lined by cuboidal or low columnar epithelium.
- Duct directly opens on the skin surface and lined by stratified cuboidal epithelium.
- These glands are found over the entire body.

### Apocrine Sweat Gland (Fig. 12.10A, B)

- Much larger than merocrine sweat glands.
- The glands are embedded in the subcutaneous tissue, and their duct empties the sweat into the upper part of the hair follicle.
- These are present in the axillary, pubic, and perianal regions.

### Olfactory Mucosa (Fig. 13.1A, B)

- It is lined by pseudostratified columnar epithelium with olfactory hair.
- In the lamina propria serous Bowman's glands are present.
- This mucosa is present in the roof of the nasal cavity, either side of the nasal septum and superior nasal concha.

### Epiglottis (Fig. 13.2A, B)

- It is the tongue-shaped superior portion of the larynx with elastic cartilage in the middle.
- Anterior or lingual surface, the apex and approximately upper half of the posterior surface is lined by stratified squamous nonkeratinized epithelium.
- The posterior surface (lower half) is lined by pseudostratified columnar ciliated epithelium with goblet cells.

### Trachea (Fig. 13.3A to C)

- It is a tubular structure with posterior flattening and lined by ciliated pseudostratified columnar epithelium with goblet cells.
- C-shaped hyaline cartilage ring is present.
- The open ends of cartilage are connected by fibroelastic ligament and a band of smooth muscle (trachealis muscle).

## Lung (Fig. 13.4A, B)

- Honey comb appearance of pulmonary alveoli and they are lined by simple squamous epithelium.
- Outer surface is covered by the serous membrane, called pleura composed of mesothelial cells.
- Sections of intrapulmonary bronchus, bronchioles, and respiratory bronchioles are present.

## Intrapulmonary Bronchus (Fig. 13.5)

- It is rounded in outline and do not show a posterior flattening.
- It is lined by ciliated pseudostratified columnar epithelium with a few goblet cells.
- Irregular plates of hyaline cartilage are present.

## Terminal and Respiratory Bronchiole (Fig. 13.6A, B)

- Terminal bronchiole is lined by ciliated cuboidal cells along with non-ciliated clara cells.
- Respiratory bronchiole is lined by ciliated cuboidal cells along with non-ciliated clara cells. Wall of these bronchioles are interrupted by thin-walled outpocketings, known as alveoli.
- Hyaline cartilage and goblet cells are absent.

## Alveoli (Fig. 13.7A, B)

- Honey comb appearance.
- Lined by simple squamous epithelium.
- Interalveolar septa contains a large number of capillaries.

## Lip (Fig. 14.1)

- The core of lip is composed of skeletal muscle (orbicularis oris).
- Its external surface is covered by thin skin and internally its surface is covered by mucous membrane.
- The submucosa contains many small mucous and mucoserous salivary (labial) glands.

## Tongue (Fig. 14.3A, B)

- Dorsal surface is covered by the stratified squamous epithelium with a number of small eminences (papillae).
- Core of the tongue consists of bundles of skeletal muscle fibers arranged in vertical, transverse and longitudinal planes.
- The ventral surface of the tongue is smooth and thin in comparison to the dorsal surface and lined by nonkeratinized stratified squamous epithelium.

## Filiform and Fungiform Papillae (Fig. 14.4A, B)

- Filiform papillae are conical papillae and keratinized on their tips.
- Fungiform papillae resemble a mushroom of the common edible variety and covered by stratified squamous nonkeratinized epithelium.
- Filiform papillae have no taste buds, while fungiform papillae have 1–5 taste buds associated with them on their free surface.

## Circumvallate Papillae (Fig. 14.5A, B)

- These papillae are dome shaped and lined by stratified squamous nonkeratinized epithelium.
- Numerous taste buds arranged around the sides of the papilla.

- These papillae are surrounded by a deep circular sulcus or trench or moat, which is flushed by the secretion of serous glands (von Ebner).

## Taste Buds (Fig. 14.6A, B)

- These are barrel-shaped bodies, which are embedded in the whole thickness of the epithelium.
- Each bud communicates with the exterior through the taste pores.
- These are composed of three types of cells: Supportive or sustentacular cells, taste or gustatory cells, and basal cells.

## Tooth (LS) (Fig. 14.7A, B)

- In the center pulp cavity is present.
- Pulp cavity is surrounded by dentin.
- Enamel covers the crown and cementum covers the root of the tongue.

## Developing Tooth (Bud Stage) (Fig. 14.8)

- Tooth buds looks like little knobs.
- Each tooth bud is lined by low columnar cells and in center lies polygonal cells.
- These buds are embedded in the connective tissue (ectomesenchyme).

## Developing Tooth (Cap Stage) (Fig. 14.9A, B)

- Enamel organ takes the shape of cap.
- Cells at the convexity of cap are cuboidal (outer enamel epithelium) and at the concavity are tall columnar (inner enamel epithelium).
- In the center lies network of star-shaped cells, called stellate reticulum.

## Developing Tooth (Bell Stage) (Fig. 14.10A, B)

- Enamel organ takes the shape of bell and now crown shape can be identified.
- In the center pulp cavity is present.
- Ameloblasts form the enamel, and odontoblasts form the dentin.

## Esophagus (Fig. 14.13A to D)

- Lined with stratified squamous nonkeratinized epithelium.
- Mucus secreting esophageal glands are present in the submucosa.
- Muscularis externa consists of inner circular and outer longitudinal layers.

## Gastro-esophageal Junction (Fig. 14.12A, B)

- Abrupt transition from stratified squamous nonkeratinized epithelium (esophagus) to simple columnar epithelium (stomach).
- Esophageal glands are present in the submucosa and esophageal cardiac glands (esophagus), and cardiac glands (stomach) are present in the lamina propria.
- Transition in muscularis mucosae from longitudinal layer (esophagus) to inner circular and outer longitudinal layers (stomach).

## Cardiac Part of Stomach (Fig. 14.15)

- Lined by simple columnar epithelium.
- The gastric pits are shallow.
- Cardiac glands are present in the lamina propria.

## Fundic Part of Stomach (Fig. 14.16A, B)

- The gastric pits are not deep, and they extend into the one-fourth of the thickness of the mucosa.
- Parietal cells with eosinophilic cytoplasm often bulge outwards (in lamina propria) creating a beaded appearance.
- Chief cells with basophilic cytoplasm at the base.

## Pyloric Part of Stomach (Fig. 14.18)

- The gastric pits are deep and occupy two-thirds of the thickness of the mucosa.
- Lined by simple columnar epithelium.
- Pyloric glands are present in the lamina propria.

## Duodeno-pyloric Junction (Fig. 14.19A, B)

- At the pyloric region, the middle circular layer thickened to form the pyloric sphincter.
- Pyloric glands are present in the pylorus and duodenum contains villi.
- Brunner's glands are present in the submucosa.

## Duodenum (Fig. 14.22A, B)

- Villi are broad, tall, and leaf-shaped and lined by simple columnar cells and a few goblet cells.
- Brunner's glands are present in the submucosa.
- Intestinal glands are present in the lamina propria.

## Jejunum (Fig. 14.23A, B)

- Villi are clubbed shaped and lined by simple columnar cells and a few goblet cells.
- Brunner's glands and Peyer's patches are absent.
- Solitary lymphatic nodules and intestinal glands are present in the lamina propria.

## Ileum (Fig. 14.24A, B)

- Villi are shorter and appear more fingers like.
- Villi are lined by simple columnar cells and goblet cells.
- Peyer's patches are present in the submucosa.

## Colon (Fig. 14.25A, B)

- Villi are absent.
- Lined by simple columnar cells with plenty of goblet cells.
- The inner circular layer of muscularis externa is thin and outer longitudinal layer is gathered into three bands, called taenia coli.

## Rectum (Fig. 14.26A, B)

- Villi are absent and crypts are deeper and a few in number.
- Abundant goblet cells are present.
- Taenia coli are absent.

## Recto-anal Junction (Fig. 14.27A, B)

- Abrupt transition from simple columnar epithelium (rectum) to stratified squamous nonkeratinized epithelium (anus).

- Muscularis mucosae is absent.
- Submucosa of anal canal contains prominent venous sinuses.

### Appendix (Fig. 14.28A, B)

- The lumen is small and usually of irregular outline, often contains cellular debris. Whole lumen can be seen in the section.
- The lamina propria is occupied by many large and small lymphoid nodules that may extend in the submucosa.
- The muscularis mucosa is incomplete and muscularis externa is thin but contains usual two layers.

### Parotid Gland (Fig. 14.29A, B)

- Serous acini with small lumen are present.
- Septa divide the gland into lobes and lobules.
- A large number of ducts is present.

### Submandibular Gland (Fig. 14.30A, B)

- Many serous and a few mucous acini are present.
- At some places serous demilunes are also present.
- A few ducts are present.

### Sublingual Gland (Fig. 14.31A, B)

- Mucous acini with large lumen are present.
- At some places serous demilunes are also present.
- Very few ducts are present.

### Liver (Fig. 14.32A to D)

- Polygonal hepatic lobules with central vein in the center.
- Hepatic cords formed by hepatocytes are present and in between the cords sinusoids are present.
- At the angles lie portal triads (branches of the hepatic artery, portal vein (venule) and interlobular bile duct).

### Gall Bladder (Fig. 14.36A, B)

- Abundant mucosal folds lined by simple columnar epithelium with brush border are present.
- Muscularis externa is composed of randomly arranged smooth muscle fibers with interlacing collagen and elastic fibers.
- The muscularis mucosae and submucosa are absent.

### Pancreas (Fig. 14.37A, B)

- Numerous darkly stained serous acini are present.
- In between the serous acini lightly stained islets are present.
- Centroacinar cells are present in the serous acini.

### Kidney (Fig. 15.2A, B)

- Covered by a dense collagenous capsule.
- Outer part is cortex, which contains renal corpuscles, PCT and DCT.
- Inner part is medulla, which contains Henle's loop, and collecting ducts.

## Kidney—Cortex (Fig. 15.4A, B)

- Glomeruli surrounded by double walled Bowman's capsule are present.
- PCT is lined by low columnar epithelium with brush border.
- DCT is lined by simple cuboidal epithelium without any brush border.

## Kidney-Medulla (Fig. 15.7)

- Collecting tubules (simple cuboidal epithelium) and collecting ducts (simple columnar epithelium) are present.
- Thin (simple squamous epithelium) and thick (simple cuboidal epithelium) segments of loop of Henle are present.
- Vasa recta lined by endothelium are present.

## Ureter (Fig. 15.9)

- Mucosa has several longitudinal folds, giving the lumen a stellate shape in the cross-section.
- The lining of the mucosa is transitional epithelium.
- Inner longitudinal and outer circular layers of smooth muscle fibers are present.

## Urinary Bladder (Fig. 15.10A, B)

- The lining epithelium is transitional.
- The mucous membrane is thrown into numerous folds (rugae).
- Three smooth muscle tunics, i.e. transverse, oblique, and longitudinal, interweave in the muscularis externa and are difficult to distinguish.

## Male Urethra (Fig. 15.11A, B)

- It consists of 3 parts: Prostatic, membranous, and spongy. Prostatic part is lined by transitional epithelium but changes to a pseudostratified columnar or stratified columnar in rest of the urethra.
- Lamina propria contains mucous glands (Littre's gland).
- The muscle coat consists of outer circular and inner longitudinal layers of smooth muscle fibers and well defined only in the membranous and prostatic parts.

## Female Urethra (Fig. 15.12)

- The lining epithelium is mainly stratified columnar or pseudostratified.
- Lamina propria contains mucous glands (Littre's gland).
- The muscle coat consists of an outer circular and inner longitudinal layers of smooth muscle.

## Testis (Fig. 16.3A, B)

- Numerous seminiferous tubules are present.
- Interstitial cells of Leydig are present in between the seminiferous tubules.
- Spermatogenic cells in various stages of development are present in the tubules.

## Seminiferous Tubules (Fig. 16.2A, B)

- Spermatogenic cells in various stages of development are present in the tubules.
- Sertoli cells are present whose nuclei are oriented perpendicular to wall of the tubule.
- Interstitial cells of Leydig are present in between the seminiferous tubules.

**Straight Tubule and Rete Testis** (Fig. 16.4A, B)

- Straight tubule is lined by simple columnar epithelium.
- Rete testis is lined by single layer of cuboidal to columnar cells.
- Cells of straight tubule resemble Sertoli cells.

**Efferent Ductules** (Fig. 16.9A, B)

- Lined by ciliated tall columnar cells and cuboidal cells.
- The lumen of ductule is irregular due to the difference in the height of the cells.
- One or two layers of smooth muscle fibers surround each ductule.

**Epididymis** (Fig. 16.10A to C)

- Ducts are lined by pseudostratified columnar epithelium.
- Sperms are present in the lumen.
- Thin layer of smooth muscle fibers surrounds the lobules.

**Vas Deferens** (Fig. 16.11)

- Lumen is irregular as the mucosa forms low longitudinal folds.
- Lined by pseudostratified columnar epithelium with long stereocilia.
- The muscle layer consists of thin inner and outer longitudinal layers along with thick middle circular layer of smooth muscle.

**Seminal Vesicle** (Fig. 16.12A to C)

- The mucosa shows thin, branching and anastomosing folds.
- Lined by pseudostratified columnar epithelium
- The muscle layer consists of inner circular and outer longitudinal layers of smooth muscle.

**Prostate** (Fig. 16.13 B)

- Prostatic acini lined by cuboidal or columnar epithelium is present.
- In the lumen of the secretory alveoli prostatic concretions (corpora amylacea) are present.
- Fibromuscular stroma is present surrounding the acini.

**Bulbourethral Glands** (Fig. 16.14)

- Covered by capsule from which septa arises and divide each gland into several lobules.
- Glands are lined by simple columnar epithelium.
- Excretory ducts lined by simple cuboidal epithelium are present.

**Penis** (Fig. 16.15)

- Two corpora cavernosa are present.
- One corpus spongiosum containing spongy urethra is present.
- Penis is surrounded by epidermis, dermis, and dartos muscle. Three corpora are surrounded by thick tunica albuginea.

**Ovary** (Fig. 17.1)

- It is covered by a single layer of cuboidal epithelium (germinal epithelium).

- Outer cortex contains various stages of development, i.e. primordial, primary, secondary, and mature Graafian follicle.
- Inner medulla contains typical fibroblasts, strands of smooth muscle, and many elastic fibers.

### Primordial and Primary Follicle (Fig. 17.2)

- Primordial follicles are present in large numbers in the cortex and contain primay oocyte surrounded by single layer of flattened follicular cells.
- Primary follicles contain primary oocyte surrounded by zona pellucida.
- Connective tissue stroma is present in between the follicles.

### Secondary Follicle (Fig. 17.3A, B)

- Small intercellular spaces are present in between the granulosa cells.
- Primary oocyte lies eccentric in postition.
- The primary oocyte is surrounded by a small group of granulosa cells (cumulus oophorus) that project out from the wall into the fluid-filled antrum.

### Graafian Follicle (Fig. 17.4A, B)

- It is largest in size.
- Secondary oocyte lies eccentric in postition.
- The oocyte is now floating freely in the follicular antrum.

### Corpus Luteum (Fig. 17.5A, B)

- Small deeply stained theca lutein cells are present at the periphery.
- Large lightly stained granulosa lutein cells are present in the center.
- Numerous capillaries are present in between the lutein cells.

### Fallopian Tube (Oviduct or Uterine Tube) (Fig. 17.6A, B)

- Mucosa is highly branched and folded.
- Lined by a simple columnar epithelium; some of the cells are ciliated.
- Muscularis externa has poorly defined inner circular and outer longitudinal smooth muscle layers.

### Isthmus of Fallopian Tube (Fig. 17.7A, B)

- Mucosa is highly branched and folded.
- Lined by a simple columnar epithelium; some of the cells are ciliated.
- Muscularis externa has poorly defined inner circular and outer longitudinal smooth muscle layers.

### Uterus—Proliferative Phase (Fig. 17.8A, B)

- Endometrium lined by simple columnar epithelium.
- Lamina propria contains simple tubular uterine glands.
- Thick myometrium with numerous blood vessels are present.

### Uterus—Secretory Phase (Fig. 17.9A, B)

- Thick endometrium (due to secretion of glands) lined by simple columnar epithelium.
- Lamina propria contains serrated glands and spiral arteries.
- Thick myometrium with numerous blood vessels are present.

## Uterus—Menstrual Phase (Fig. 17.10A, B)

- Epithelium is broken with blood in the lumen.
- Superficial two-thirds part of endometrium is shed off.
- Thick myometrium with numerous blood vessels are present.

## Uterus—Menopause Phase (Fig. 17.11A, B)

- Endometrium regresses and consists of only basal layer.
- The uterine glands also regress.
- Thick myometrium with numerous blood vessels are present.

## Cervix (Fig. 17.12A, B)

- Lined by simple columnar epithelium with cilia.
- Mucosa contains mucous cervical glands.
- The mucosa rests upon myometrium which is mainly composed of dense collagenous connective tissue containing many elastic fibers and only a few smooth muscle fibers.

## Cervico-vaginal Junction (Fig. 17.13A, B)

- Transition from simple columnar epithelium (cervix) to stratified squamous nonkeratinized epithelium (vagina).
- Mucosa of cervix contains mucous cervical glands.
- The surface cells in the vagina continuously desquamate.

## Vagina (Fig. 17.14)

- Lined by stratified squamous nonkeratinized epithelium.
- The surface cells in the vagina continuously desquamate.
- Muscularis externa is composed of interlacing bundles of smooth muscle fibers. On the inner side, the fibers are mainly circularly arranged and thin, while on the outer side, fibers are longitudinally arranged and thick.

## Early Placenta (Fig. 17.15A, B)

- Numerous villi are present.
- Villi are lined by cytotrophoblast and syncytiotrophoblast.
- Maternal red blood cells lie in between the villi.

## Late Placenta (Fig. 17.16A, B)

- Villi are mainly lined by syncytiotrophoblast.
- Maternal red blood cells lie in between the villi.
- Core of the villi contains fetal blood vessels, mesenchyme, and macrophage.

## Umbilical Cord (Fig. 17.18A, B)

- One umbilical vein and two umbilical arteries are present.
- It is filled with gelatinous embryonic connective tissue, known as Wharton's jelly.
- It is lined by flattened amniotic epithelial cells.

## Mammary (Non-lactating) Gland (Fig. 17.19A to C)

- More connective tissue and less glandular tissue.
- Alveoli are poorly defined.
- Plenty of fat cells are present and lobules are ill defined.

## Mammary (Lactating) Gland (Fig. 17.20A to C)

- More glandular tissue and less connective tissue.
- Compactly packed alveoli are having distended lumen containing milk.
- The alveoli are lined by cuboidal or columnar epithelium.

## Pituitary Gland (Fig. 18.4A, B)

- Pars distalis contain acidophils, basophils, and chromophobes.
- Pars intermedia contain colloid filled cysts that are lined by cuboidal epithelium.
- Pars nervosa contain nerve fibers, and pituicytes.

## Thyroid Gland (Fig. 18.8A, B, C, D)

- Thyroid follicle lined by cuboidal epithelial cells.
- Eosinophilic colloid is present in the follicles.
- Parafollicular cells are present either in between follicular epithelium and basement membrane or in the scanty connective tissue.

## Parathyroid Gland (Fig. 18.9A, B)

- Plenty of small rounded chief cells whose cytoplasm is weakly acidophilic.
- Less number of polyhedral oxyphil cells whose cytoplasm is strongly acidophilic.
- A considerable number of fat cells are also present.

## Suprarenal Gland (Fig. 18.10A, B)

- Outermost capsule with trabeculae.
- Outer layer is cortex which shows zona glomerulosa (cells are present in curved column), zona fasciculata (radially arranged cords of spongiocytes), and zona reticularis (anastomosing cell cords).
- Inner layer is medulla which contains small clusters of chromaffin cells.

## Cerebrum (Fig. 19.1)

- Grey matter is located on the surface as cerebral cortex and white matter is present in the more central regions.
- The cortex is having six layers, i.e. molecular layer, outer granular layer, outer pyramidal layer, inner granular layer, inner pyramidal layer, and fusiform cell layer.
- Inner pyramidal layer consists of cell bodies of large pyramidal cells (giant pyramidal cells of Betz).

## Cerebellum (Fig. 19.3A to D)

- Grey matter is located on the surface as cerebellar cortex and white matter is present in the center as medulla.
- Grey matter contains outer light staining molecular layer, single layer of Purkinje cells, and inner darkly stained granular layer.
- Medulla is lightly stained.

## Spinal Cord (Fig. 19.4A to E)

- Outer white matter contains processes of neurons.
- Inner grey matter is H-shaped and contains cell bodies of neurons.
- Central canal is present in the grey commissure.

## Dorsal Root Ganglia (Fig. 19.5)

- Groups of rounded pseudounipolar neurons of varying sizes are present.
- Satellite cells are well defined and nucleus is centrally placed in neurons.
- Groups of neurons are separated by bundles of myelinated nerve fibers.

## Autonomic Ganglia (Fig. 19.6)

- Scattered multipolar neurons are present.
- Satellite cells are poorly defined and nucleus is eccentrically placed in neurons.
- In between neurons lie unmyelinated nerve fibers.

## Peripheral Nerve—H and E Stain (Fig. 19.7A)

- Each bundle of nerve fibers are surrounded by a dense connective tissue sheath called the perineurium.
- Axons of nerve fibers are darkly stained and present in the center.
- Empty space encircling the axon is unstained myelin sheath.

## Peripheral Nerve—Osmic Acid Stain (Fig. 19.7B)

- Black circles are the myelin sheaths of nerve fibers.
- Empty space in the circle of myelin sheath is the axon of nerve fibers.
- Each bundle of nerve fibers are surrounded by a dense connective tissue sheath called the perineurium.

## Neuron (Fig. 19.9)

- Showing cell bodies with multiple processes.
- Cytoplasm of neurons is rich in basophilic Nissl bodies.
- Nissl bodies are absent in axon hillock and axon.

## The Cornea (Fig. 20.2A, B)

- The anterior surface is lined by a stratified squamous nonkeratinized epithelium.
- The posterior surface is lined by an endothelium.
- Stroma is the thickest layer and consists of 200– 250 layers of regularly organized collagen fibers.

## Sclera and Choroid (Fig. 20.3A, B)

- Sclera consists of bundles of type I collagen fibers alternating with networks of elastic fibers.
- Connective tissue cells and pigment cells (melanocytes) are numerous in choroid and the melanocytes give the choroid its dark color.
- Small blood vessels are especially frequent in the innermost part (choriocapillary layer) of the choroid.

## Ciliary Body (Fig. 20.4A, B)

- It is an inward extension of the choroid at the level of lens.
- Ciliary processes extend from its anterior two-thirds towards the lens.
- It contains a considerable amount of dark staining melanin pigment.

## Iris (Fig. 20.5A to D)

- Anterior surface is rough and irregular and formed by incomplete layer of fibroblasts and melanocytes.
- Connective tissue stroma is highly vascularized.
- Posterior surface contains highly pigmented cells.

## Retina (Fig. 20.6A, B)

- Outermost layer is of single layer of cuboidal pigmented cells containing melanin granules.
- Inside this lies layer of rods and cones.
- Six more layers are present, i.e. outer nuclear layer, outer plexiform layer, inner nuclear layer, inner plexiform layer, ganglion cell layer, and nerve fiber layer.

## Lens (Fig. 20.8A, B)

- Lens capsule is transparent and homogenous.
- Just beneath the capsule on anterior surface lies simple cuboidal epithelium.
- Nucleated lens fibers are present.

## Eyelids (Fig. 20.9)

- Outer surface is covered by skin, whereas inner surface is covered by palpebral conjunctiva (stratified columnar epithelium).
- Orbicularis occuli muscle lies in the core.
- The margin of the eyelids contains eyelashes arranged in rows of three or four, but they are without arrector pili muscles.

## Lacrimal Gland (Fig. 20.10)

- Lumen is distended.
- Serous acini are lined by column-shaped cells.
- Well-developed myoepithelial cells surround the acini.

## Spiral Ganglion (Fig. 21.3A, B)

- It is a spiral-shaped mass of nerve cell bodies lying in a canal of the modiolus.
- Ganglion cells have the typical appearance of dorsal root ganglion cells.
- Afferent nerve fibers entering from organ of Corti and efferent passing to the center of modiolus can be seen.

## Macula Sacculi (Fig. 21.4A, B)

- It is composed of two types of neuroepithelial cells called type I and type II hair cells, and some supporting cells.
- It is covered by a thick gelatinous glycoprotein layer, known as the otolithic membrane.
- Otolithic membrane contains small crystals of calcium carbonate, known as otoliths (earstones or earsand or otoconia).

## Ampullary Crest (Fig. 21.5A, B)

- It is covered by sensory epithelium containing neuroepithelial hair cells and supporting cells.
- It is covered by a thicker glycoprotein layer and this layer has a conical form called cupula.
- Otoliths are absent.

## Cochlea (Fig. 21.2A, B)

- It can be identified by its snail-shell like shape.
- Modiolus forms the center of the cochlea.
- Each turn contains three compartments: Scala vestibuli above, scala tympani below and scala media in the middle.

## The Spiral Organ of Corti (Fig. 21.6)

- It contains scala vestibuli above, scala tympani below, and scala media in the middle.
- It is a complex epithelial layer and lies on the floor of the scala media.
- It is formed by: Hair (neuroepithelial) cells, phalangeal cells, and pillar cells.

# Index